EARLY ORTHODONTIC TREATMENT

Contributors

Leonard S. Fishman, DDS
Clinical Associate Professor
Division of Orthodontics
Department of Dentistry
Eastman Dental Center
University of Rochester

Mark A. Moss, DDS, PhD
Assistant Professor
Departments of Dentistry and Community
   and Preventive Medicine
Eastman Dental Center
University of Rochester

Scott Stein, DDS
Clinical Instructor
Division of Orthodontics
Department of Dentistry
Eastman Dental Center
University of Rochester

Ross H. Tallents, DDS
Professor, Department of Dentistry
Program Director, Temporomandibular Joint
   Disorders
Divisions of Orthodontics and Prosthodontics
Eastman Dental Center
University of Rochester

EARLY ORTHODONTIC TREATMENT

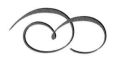

J. Daniel Subtelny, DDS, MS
Program Director and Professor
Division of Orthodontics
Department of Dentistry
Eastman Dental Center
University of Rochester

Quintessence Publishing Co, Inc
Chicago, Berlin, London, Tokyo, Paris, Barcelona, São Paulo, Moscow, Prague, and Warsaw

Library of Congress Cataloging-in-Publication Data

Subtelny, J. Daniel.
    Early orthodontic treatment / by J. Daniel Subtelny.
        p. ; cm.
    Includes bibliographical references and index.
    ISBN 0-86715-372-5
    1. Malocclusion in children. 2. Malocclusion—Treatment. 3. Children—Dental care. 4.
Orthodontics, Corrective. I. Title.
    [DNLM: 1. Malocclusion—therapy—Adolescence. 2. Malocclusion—therapy—Child. 3.
Mandible—abnormalities—Adolescence. 4. Mandible—abnormalities—Child. 5.
Maxilla—abnormalities—Adolescence. 6. Maxilla—abnormalities—Child. 7. Orthodontics,
Corrective—methods—Adolescence. 8. Orthodontics, Corrective—methods—Child. WU
440 S941e 2000]
RK523 .S826 2000
617.6'43'0083—dc21

99-047276

© 2000 Quintessence Publishing Co, Inc

Quintessence Publishing Co, Inc
551 Kimberly Drive
Carol Stream, Illinois 60188

Editor/Production: Arinne Dickson
Design: Michael Shanahan

Printed in the USA

Contents

Preface

An old adage states, "hindsight is better than foresight." Applying this adage to orthodontic treatment, we can say that hindsight should serve as a foundation upon which to develop better foresight. This is particularly true in treating patients at early age levels, where the orthodontist, using knowledge developed through experience, careful observation, and earlier documentation (hindsight), must foretell the result of treatment (foresight).

I am a long-time advocate of early orthodontic treatment, probably related in part to my interest in craniofacial growth and dysmorphology. In my 40+ years in private practice and education, I have had considerable experience with long-term treatment of early orthodontic cases. Much information needs to be added to our pool of knowledge regarding early orthodontics; despite its importance, this area still is not, and in truth may never be, fully comprehended. Certainly, long-term observations of early orthodontic treatment are lacking, consistent with the fact that such treatment has not been routinely pursued. However, the need has recently become more pronounced. The desirability of initiating orthodontic treatment at an early age is becoming more generally accepted as a means of gaining the greatest possible control over form and function and changes with time. It seems logical to assume that, to at-tain the greatest possible alteration in form incident to achieving the greatest possible adaptation in function, certain problems should be treated early to take advantage of the most craniofacial growth.

Many of our difficult orthodontic problems reside in maldeveloped and/or malrelated skeletal structures, or result from unfavorable functional adaptations that lead to adverse postural relationships. The dentition is what we see, and so we move teeth in an attempt to remove the "mal" and achieve an acceptable occlusion; however, we must consider that the causative mechanisms in the "mal" may lie elsewhere. Dental alignment may give a clue as to the cause and complexity of the problem; but the fact is that as the jaws go the teeth go, and where the jaws grow the teeth must also go.

An increasing number of severe malocclusions are skeletal (jaw) and/or "mal-growing" jaw malocclusions that manifest themselves as dental malrelationships. These become increasingly difficult to treat the longer the "mal-growth" continues; sometimes the desired outcome cannot be achieved. If these problems could be recognized and treated early, then it might be possible to minimize or even eliminate the consequences of undesirable craniofacial growth. In view of this possibility, this book presents several skeletal-related problems that might develop into overtly malrelated dentitions, as well as the more characteristic dentoalveolar malocclusions. Whenever possible, long-term treatments, along with appropriate diagnoses and treatment plans that permit at least partial correction of those malocclusions, will be presented.

In this book, the basic approach to early orthodontic treatment is not centered around technical procedures and the fabrication of appliances. Following a philosophy that "biology supersedes technology," the central focus of this book is jaws and jaw growth. The human head has two distinct and disjoined jaws, the maxilla and the mandible. One is stabilized, the other is capable of motion but is functionally related in occlusion. The dentition positioned within these two jaws brings into being either an acceptable occlusion or a malocclusion. The size, shape, and position of the two jaws will ultimately be the deciding factor in determining the presence or absence of a skeletal malocclusion.

Conceptually, jaw-related malocclusions and their treatment have not been discussed as fully as have the corrective procedures for the more recognizable and definitive dentoalveolar malocclusions. It is my contention that knowledge and orthodontic activity in this area will continue to increase. In the meantime, we must benefit from our lessons of the past and apply such knowledge toward the future.

The contributors of two chapters are gratefully acknowledged. Dr Leonard Fishman presents a unique approach to evaluating growth in the craniofacial complex and applying it to everyday use in private practice, education, and research. In another chapter Drs Scott Stein, Ross Tallents, and Mark Moss discuss some of the less understood disorders of the temporomandibular joint, an area much in need of new information to incorporate into our teaching and treatment. I have benefited tremendously from discussions with these and other colleagues at Eastman.

Good students are instrumental in making good teachers better thinkers, which in turn makes them better clinicians. Unquestionably, over the years, the students have left their imprint on many of the concepts and thought processes expressed throughout this book. Information from some of their research projects has been included. They too are gratefully acknowledged.

Each patient is a new lesson and a new teacher. Good patients teach us to practice what we teach and teach what we practice. Each patient has been valuable; some are prominent in this book. They are all gratefully acknowledged.

It is my hope that many young patients will reap benefits from the patients and concepts found in this book.

Part I

Maxillary Jaw Malocclusions

Chapter 1

Maxillary Skeletal Retrusion Malocclusions

Background to the Problem: Late vs Early Treatment

First to be considered is the complex problem of skeletal maxillary retrusion. Years ago a diagnosis of maxillary skeletal deficiency was in the formative stage, and mechanisms to treat it were less well formulated. Maxillary retrusion—a Class III dental malocclusion, but a nonskeletal mandibular prognathism—was an orthodontist's dilemma. Surgical mandibular retropositioning was frequently an unsatisfactory solution since it only served to create two retropositioned jaws and many times required extraction in both jaws to achieve a satisfactory occlusion. Eventually, surgical advancement of the maxillary complex became a potential resolution, but facially this procedure was frequently unable to compensate for retropositioned zygomas or small noses. Additionally, it might necessitate the undesirable extraction of maxillary teeth to achieve alignment in smaller maxillae. Early treatment was almost nonexistent and orthodontists awaited completion of growth to pursue orthognathic surgical correction. This can be exemplified by presenting the treatment of two brothers with similar jaw problems—skeletal maxillary retrusion, but with an approximate 12-year disparity in ages. It could be called "A Tale of Two Brothers"—a "Dickens" of a contrast.

Late treatment: Patient L.H.

The older brother (L.H.) was treated first. Based on a diagnosis of mandibular prognathism resulting in a Class III molar relation in a 16-year-old patient, the treatment plan called for a mandibular resection and surgical retropositioning. Utilizing contemporary cephalometric analyses[1-5] centering around the dentition and denture bases, the clinician failed to diagnose certain aspects of skeletal relations. Retrospectively, the initial lateral cephalogram clearly demonstrates maxillary skeletal retrusion (not diagnosed!); the level of the palatal plane was clearly above the anterior tubercle of the atlas, indicating vertical maxillary insufficiency (not diagnosed!) (Fig 1-1). Inadequate lower anterior facial height incident to the vertical insufficiency (resulting in mandibular overclosure, a prognathic chin, and forward positioning of the mandibular molar) was missed in the diagnostic process, as well as disparate posterior borders of the mandibular rami, suggesting skeletal or positional asymmetry. Also missed was an entry in the clinical notes that there was an excessive freeway space of 7 to 10 mm and that the lower face lacked adequate vertical dimension when the teeth were in occlusion—a clear case of overclosure into a Class III dental malocclusion.

Concomitant with the retruded position of point A, the fact that the maxillary second and

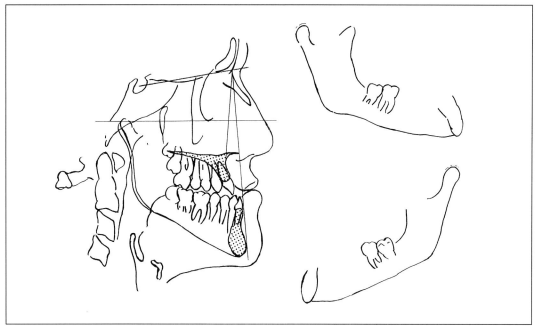

Fig 1-1 Patient L.H. Tracings of lateral cephalometric radiograph and oblique radiographs, taken prior to initiation of treatment (age 16 years) (1966).

third molars had not erupted whereas the mandibular second molars had (again an indication of maxillary deficiency) was likewise missed. The problem in this case from the beginning was inadequacy in diagnosis; the skeletal maxillary retrusion was concealed by the chin position and a Class III molar relationship.

Treatment was initiated with a maxillary palatal developer to attempt crossbite correction and a chin cup to be worn at night. At that time it was believed that the chin cup could retard further mandibular growth,[6] which we presently conceptualize not to be the case; chin-cup wear seems to result more in vertical mandibular repositioning.[7] Full-banded appliance therapy was subsequently undertaken in preparation for surgery. Following this, a mandibular sagittal split was successfully performed (Figs 1-2a and 1-2b). Now the asymmetric mandible was asymmetrically retropositioned to compensate for a smaller-than-normal maxilla. A positive overjet and a more acceptable anteroposterior dental occlusion were achieved, but unexpectedly the lower anterior facial height increased as the mandibular plane steepened (Fig 1-2c). With time, the mandibular dentition—seemingly due to continued mandibular growth—was observed to become positioned more anteriorly, approaching a negative overjet. This necessitated extraction of a mandibular incisor to reduce mandibular arch length (Fig 1-3). At this point the patient experienced a speech problem: a slurring of words and a tendency to lisp. We now surmise that the speech problem was caused by an intrusion on tongue space, influencing tongue function.

After approximately 2 years, treatment was completed, and the patient was retained (Fig 1-4) and dismissed (1973) (Fig 1-5). New records were obtained 20 years later (1992), revealing that the maxillary retrusive facial profile was still evident (Fig 1-6). The overjet was gone. The patient was observed to subconsciously retroposition his mandible in attempt to achieve an overjet, but did little more than effect an edge-to-edge occlusion. The mandibular incisor extraction site currently exhibits a depression in the crestal gingiva, a loss of alveolar crestal bone, an unsightly space, and possibly a periodontal problem. The buccal occlusion is not fully acceptable due to lack of adequate interdigitation, and a Class III tendency still exists in the canine region; the buccal crossbite remains.

Fig 1-2 Patient L.H. *(a)* Tracings of lateral cephalometric radiograph and oblique radiographs taken 1 month following a mandibular sagittal split (1969). *(b)* Tracings of lateral radiographs and superimposition before and after surgery. *(c)* Eight months after surgery.

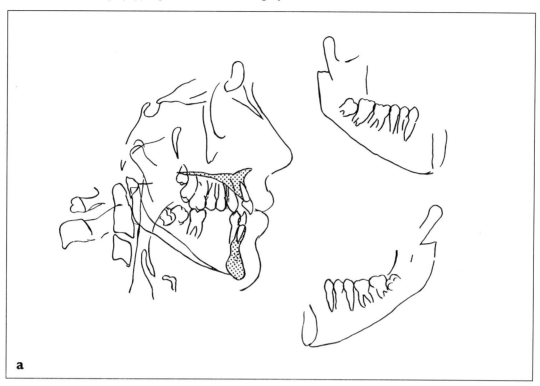

a

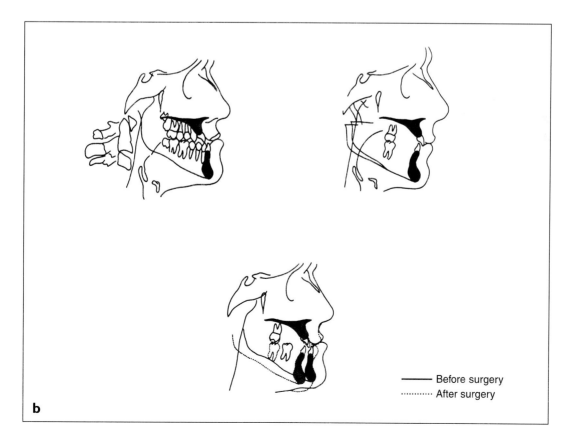

——— Before surgery
·········· After surgery

b

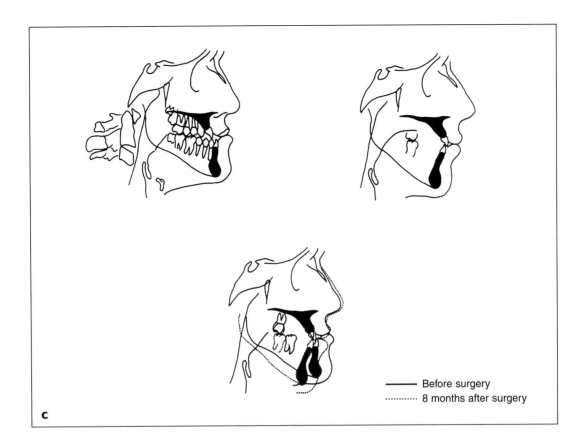

Before surgery
8 months after surgery

c

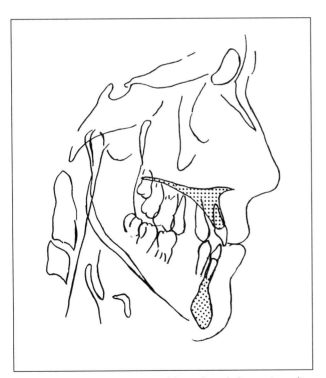

Fig 1-3 Patient L.H. Tracing of lateral cephalometric radiograph following one mandibular incisor extraction and recreation of an anterior dental overjet (1970).

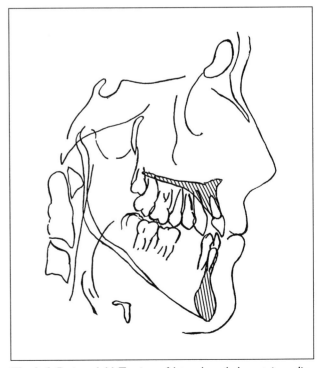

Fig 1-4 Patient L.H. Tracing of lateral cephalometric radiograph at retention (1971).

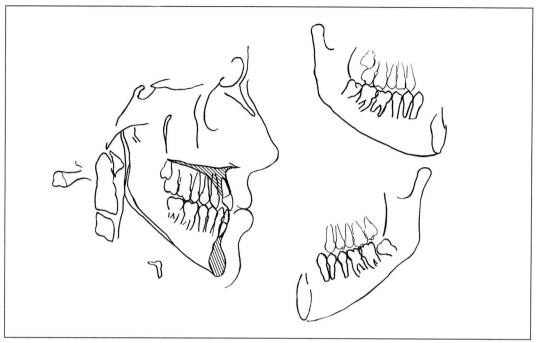

Fig 1-5 Patient L.H. Tracings of lateral cephalometric and right and left oblique radiographs taken at time of dismissal (1973).

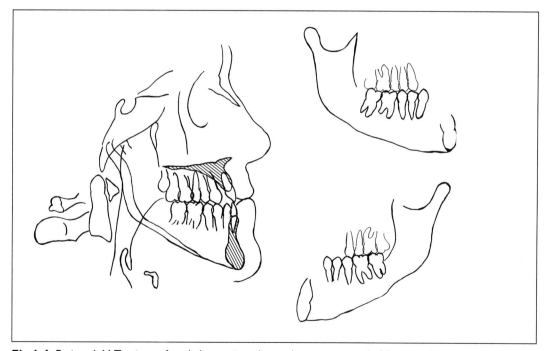

Fig 1-6 Patient L.H. Tracings of cephalometric radiographs approximately 20 years after dismissal from orthodontic care (1992).

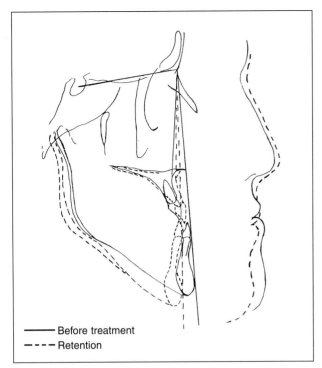

Fig 1-7 Patient L.H. Superimposition of lateral cephalometric radiographs, denoting changes in dentofacial skeletal relationships and soft tissue profile relationships before treatment and at retention, a period after mandibular surgical setback.

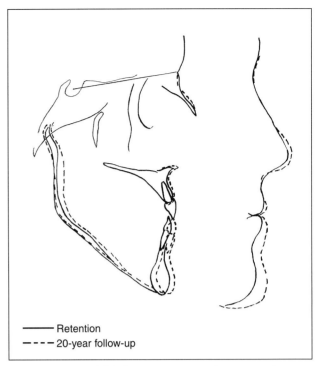

Fig 1-8 Patient L.H. Superimposition of tracings, denoting changes in skeletal profile relationships from retention to follow-up, approximately 20 years later.

The basic problem in this case was that a patient having skeletal maxillary retrusion was treated for skeletal mandibular prognathism because of a Class III molar occlusion. At that time, maxillary surgical advancement and orthopedic therapy were not usual orthodontic procedures—Class III occlusions were usually corrected by surgical mandibular retropositioning. A related factor was the retropositioning of the mandibular occlusion, causing an increase in lower anterior facial height; this made it more tenuous to achieve an adequate overbite to help maintain the anteroposterior occlusal correction. Of benefit was a reduction in the prognathic soft tissue profile (Figs 1-7 and 1-8). But treatment was directed toward the dentition and, unfortunately, the wrong jaw!

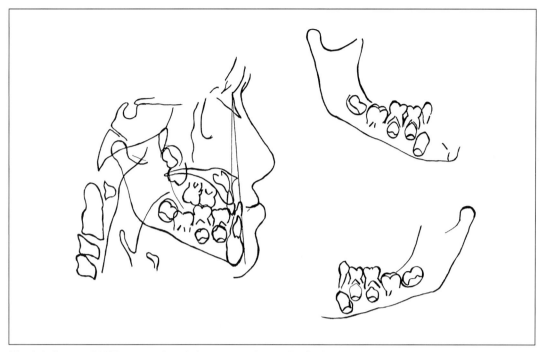

Fig 1-9 Patient P.H. Tracings of cephalometric radiographs (lateral and obliques) taken prior to treatment, age 6 years 11 months. Mandibular prognathism and vertical overclosure are evident.

Early treatment: Patient P.H.

In 1972, when it came time to treat the younger brother (P.H.), the parents were cognizant of the ramifications of growth. The patient was brought in at age 7, exhibiting mandibular overclosure, a Class III malocclusion, and an anterior crossbite of the deciduous dentition. The parents expressly desired that, if possible, surgery be avoided.

Initial records revealed mandibular overclosure (through a 9- to 10-mm freeway space), resulting in a severe anterior crossbite. A prognathic, concave facial pattern with a diagnosable skeletal maxillary retrusion was noted (Fig 1-9), along with a profile sorely in need of increased vertical dimension. It was decided to initiate early orthodontic treatment; a high-pull chin cup was placed to position the chin down and back to permit eruption of the posterior teeth into the excessive freeway space. The chin cup was *not* used to counteract mandibular growth, because our studies indicate that it causes a downward repositioning of the mandible and it is possible to maintain that position via molar eruption. A mandibular bite plane was used to anteriorly position the maxillary incisors, especially during eruption of the permanent teeth.

Considerable improvement was noted, so a maxillary lingual arch with anteriorly placed hooks was constructed after first permanent molar eruption. Vertical hooks were placed on the chin cup, and, with elastics to the lingual arch hooks, the chin cup was used as a reverse headgear. With improvement, the maxillary arch was retained with a bite plate, the patient was placed in a resting phase, and a decision was made to extract the mandibular deciduous canines.

After incisor eruption and during eruption of other permanent teeth, several periods of treatment were undertaken (Fig 1-10). By this time, the possibility of developing point A by advancing the anterior dentition with labial root torque had become known[8] (Fig 1-11). Additionally, the possibility of face-mask therapy to encourage development of the nasomaxillary complex[9,10] was under investigation and clinical evaluation. Both were introduced as part of the younger brother's orthodontic therapy.

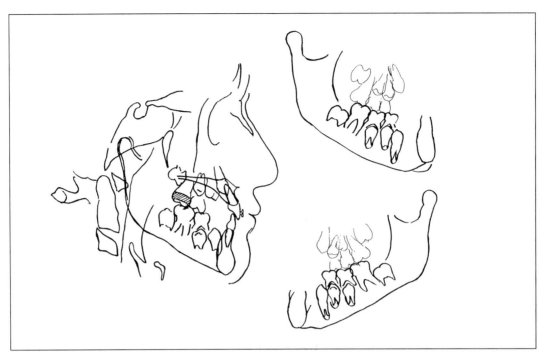

Fig 1-10 Patient P.H. Tracings of radiographs after several periods of early orthodontic treatment and subsequent to the eruption of permanent incisors.

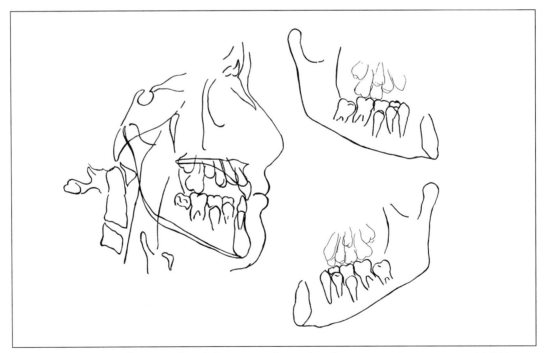

Fig 1-11 Patient P.H. Tracings of cephalometric radiographs when some advancement and labial root torque of the maxillary incisors had been achieved.

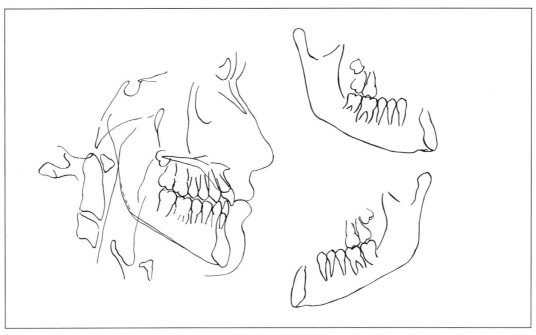

Fig 1-12 Patient P.H. Cephalometric tracings indicating attainment of satisfactory skeletal and soft tissue profile relationships and an acceptable anteroposterior occlusion.

After full permanent-dentition eruption and alignment, maxillary incisor labial root torque was maintained, and several on-and-off periods of face-mask therapy were initiated. Despite continuing mandibular growth, molar eruption causing mandibular vertical repositioning maintained acceptable anteroposterior interocclusal relationships. Reinitiation of face-mask therapy to compensate for mandibular growth was undertaken several times over the many intermittent periods of treatment. At various times, extraction of mandibular premolars or a mandibular incisor was considered but never undertaken. Subsequently, retention with face-mask inclusion was placed.

The result was highly gratifying (Fig 1-12). An acceptable facial profile was achieved. Orthognathic surgery was obviated, making parents and patient happy. The occlusion was acceptable both anteroposteriorly and vertically. One problem in occlusion became obvious—a posterior crossbite but, because it did not cause any mandibular malpositioning or displacement that would impair function, it was not considered clinically significant. Further, it was not feasibly

treatable at the later age. The crossbite was the result of not compensating for inadequate nasomaxillary width by failing to orthopedically open the midpalatal suture. This would have achieved the width needed to accommodate continued mandibular growth. With this growth, a wider part of the mandibular dental arch had been positioned more anteriorly, resulting in a posterior dental crossbite. However, despite the crossbite, a highly acceptable result was evident 10 years out of retention (Figs 1-13 to 1-15).

In comparing the brothers (1992), one sees that the older one still finds it necessary to retrude his mandible to achieve occlusion. He is more retruded in facial appearance, particularly in the nasomaxillary region, still more "chinny." His occlusion seems stable, but not as well articulated as the younger boy's—not a fully satisfying result (Fig 1-16). It might be argued that today a surgical maxillary advancement might have given the older brother a better result. This is questionable, since it would have required a reduced maxillary dentoalveolar complex incident to extraction which, by itself, is not desirable in a skeletal maxillary retrusion.

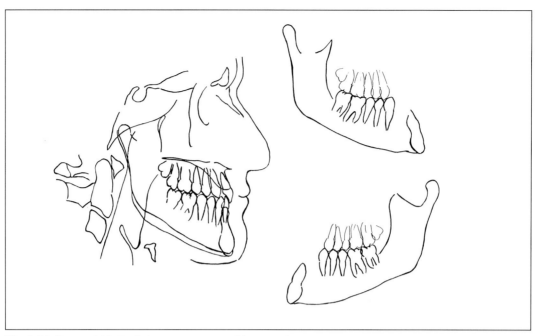

Fig 1-13 Patient P.H. Cephalometric tracings 10 years after removal of retention and dismissal.

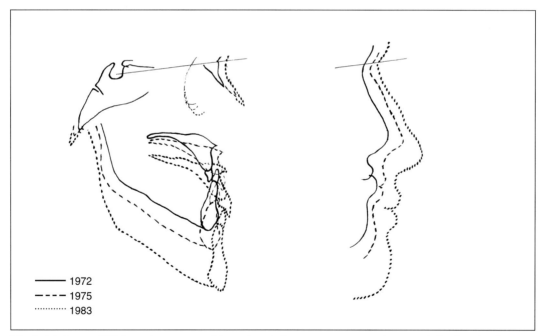

——— 1972
---- 1975
············ 1983

Fig 1-14 Patient P.H. Superimposition of lateral cephalometric tracings indicating skeletal and soft tissue profile changes incident to growth and orthodontic therapy from initiation of treatment until completion. Some maxillary development and vertical growth of the mandible is evident.

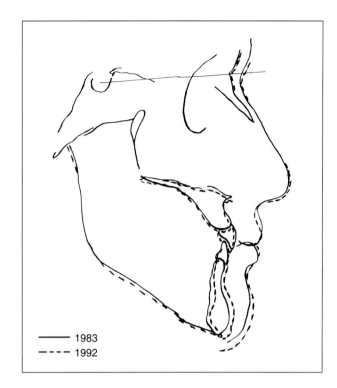

Fig 1-15 Patient P.H. Superimposition of cephalometric radiographs taken at the time of dismissal in 1983 and 9 years later. Residual mandibular development has resulted in a more forward position of the chin as well as some soft tissue change and adaptation in the profile.

——— 1983
- - - - 1992

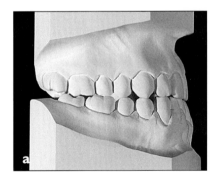

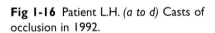

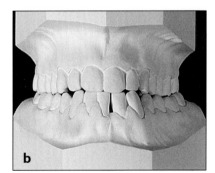

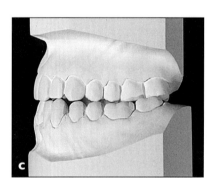

Fig 1-16 Patient L.H. *(a to d)* Casts of occlusion in 1992.

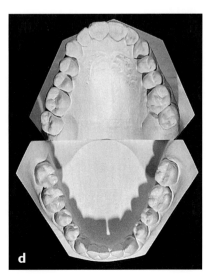

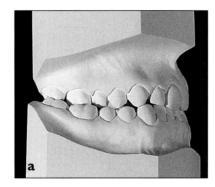 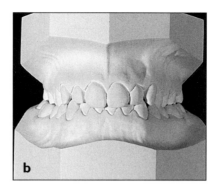 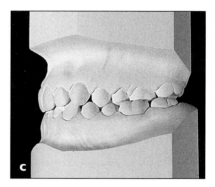

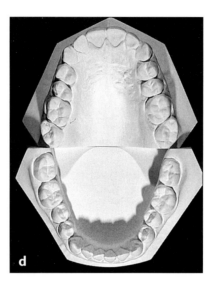

Fig 1-17 Patient P.H. *(a to d)* Casts of occlusion in 1992.

The younger brother exhibited a significantly more satisfying result with a better occlusion (Fig 1-17), better facial appearance, better function in that there is no mandibular repositioning, and a decidedly more esthetic occlusion. There were some negative aspects of the younger boy's treatment: a longer treatment time, several periods of treatment over the years, and, of course, a posterior crossbite. However, despite these detriments, a more acceptable result was achieved, with a potentially greater benefit to the form and function of the occlusion.

Development of Point A and the Nasomaxillary Complex

Diagnosis of maxillary insufficiency: Clues

To date, little consideration has been given to the potential of stimulating maxillary development in patients exhibiting midfacial retrusion incident to inadequate forward growth of the maxillary skeletal complex. Reference is made to patients having insufficient facial convexity at early ages. Many times evaluation reveals a real

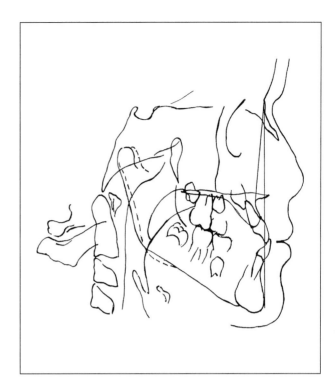

Fig 1-18 Cephalometric tracing of a maxillary retrusion patient at an early age.

maxillary insufficiency with a retrusive relationship of point A to the forehead, along with anterior crossbites of varying degrees. In many of these patients the maxillary incisors, although in crossbite, are not retroclined, but may actually exhibit considerable proclination. In other patients they approximate an edge-to-edge incisal relationship (Fig 1-18).

In orthodontic diagnosis, the lateral cephalometric radiograph is valuable in providing a method of objectively evaluating skeletal components of the face and of appraising the skeletal profile. From the cephalometric radiograph one can obtain an immediate indication of the relative sizes of the skeletal jaws, as well as the relative position of these parts to each other, to the cranial base, and to the bony facial profile. Without question, facial appearance is dependent not only on mandibular position but also on the anteroposterior relationship of the maxilla to the cranium and the mandible. Within limits, a retruded maxilla may still present a semblance of facial balance. It should be emphasized that in some instances we may be dealing with the relationships of the skeletal

components of the jaws, while in other instances we are relating the two denture bases to each other, as well as to the profile. We must determine whether the skeletal jaws are too far forward or too far back, or some combination of each. This, of course, has obvious clinical implications insofar as diagnosis and treatment planning are concerned.

In evaluating jaw relationships, orthodontists have thus far paid attention almost exclusively to anteroposterior relationships of the molars. They tend to think exclusively in terms of Class I, II, or III molar relationships and frequently forget that there are other dimensions that contribute to facial form, specifically, the anteroposterior relationships of the jaws. Certain analyses may be of assistance in evaluating anteroposterior maxillary dimensions if used judiciously.

Normal maxillary growth has been described as paralleling the forward growth of nasion. Brodie,[11] Lande,[12] and Ricketts[13] have shown that angle SNA changes very little with growth. University of Michigan standards of facial growth also reveal little change in SNA from ages 6 to 16. Using the SNA angle to evaluate the anteroposterior position of the maxilla should be done with a degree of caution. SN, an anterior cranial base plane, can vary considerably in angulation and thereby misrepresent the exact location of the most anterior point of the maxilla. As such, it does not truly represent the relationship of the maxilla to the forehead. It seems that the nasion–point A plane (NA) relative to the Frankfort horizontal plane (FH) (as propounded by Lande[12]) might be more representative of the anteroposterior position of the forepart of the maxilla. Lande's study of 34 persons aged 4 to 17 demonstrated very little anteroposterior maxillary change.[12]

Preparation for face-mask therapy

A relatively high rate of success has recently been achieved by the use of appliances similar to that advocated by Delaire[9] and Verdon and Salagnac[10] for the correction of maxillary skeletal insufficiency. In particular, the Delaire face mask—an extraoral orthopedic appliance—has been specifically designed to stimulate forward maxillary development. Clinically, both in private practice and in the orthodontic department of the Eastman Dental Center, recent results have encouraged continued use and evaluation and have led to the development of adjunctive treatment procedures. Foremost, it was found advantageous, prior to face-mask use, to increase maxillary incisor labial root torque and concomitantly develop point A.[8] Advancement of the maxillary denture base (the junction of alveolar and basal bone—specifically point A) is contingent on advancing the incisor apices without going through the labial plate of bone. This movement cannot be accomplished by simply placing labial root torque in the arch wire because the crown may move lingually rather than the root labially. As a consequence, we found it necessary to tie forward, causing a slight forward movement of the incisal edge, while the strong labial root torque caused the apex to move anteriorly to a greater extent; this effectively uprighted the incisor without permitting lingual movement of the incisal edge (Fig 1-19).

Achieving labial root torque provided many treatment advantages. First, advancing the incisors and point A frequently created sufficient additional space for the placement of teeth in an otherwise inadequate arch, for example, partially blocked-out canines (Fig 1-20), premolars, even lingually locked maxillary lateral incisors. This, of course, is highly desirable in cases of skeletal maxillary retrusion. Point A is back and, if sufficient arch length cannot be achieved, then extractions may be necessary to achieve alignment, which can only serve to further retroposition point A and possibly incur a negative overjet. Arch length becomes evident with progressive tying forward to the first or second deciduous molars or other anteriorly located teeth.

In our clinical treatment, the desirability of first attaining maxillary incisor labial root torque did not become evident until we noticed that attempts to advance maxillary incisors in maxillary retrusive cases resulted in gingival stripping, recession, or clefts. It was also thought that a Tweed "toehold" had been achieved in the maxillary bone prior to face-mask use, thereby having a greater influence on the bone itself. At present, except in the deciduous dentition, anterior labial root torque is consistently established before undertaking maxillary skeletal advancement.

Face-mask therapy in the treatment of maxillary retrusion: Timing

Incisor labial root torque with advancement promotes observable development of point A[14]; subsequent face-mask therapy is then initiated to orthopedically achieve anterior maxillary development. As the face mask rests against the forehead and chin, heavy elastics (of about 1 to 1.5 lb per side, as suggested by Verdon and Salagnac[10]) attached to hooks distal to the maxillary incisors produce a downward and forward force on the maxillary complex (Fig 1-21). The hooks are placed distal to the laterals since, in previous clinical trials when elastics were placed posteriorly, it was found that an eruptive force was placed on the posterior teeth and undesired tendencies toward an anterior open bite ensued. Elastic forces placed more anteriorly cause more of a downward (as well as forward) force on the anterior of the maxillary arch—the antithesis of producing open bites.

Fig 1-19 *(a)* Placement of anterior labial root torque and ligature ties to initiate forward movement of incisors, causing forward movement of apices. *(b)* Stronger influence on forward movement of apex by tightening the ligature tie forward with pliers.

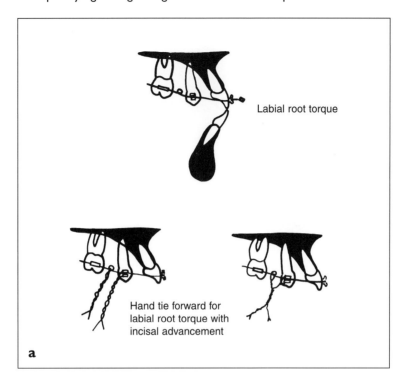

Labial root torque

Hand tie forward for labial root torque with incisal advancement

a

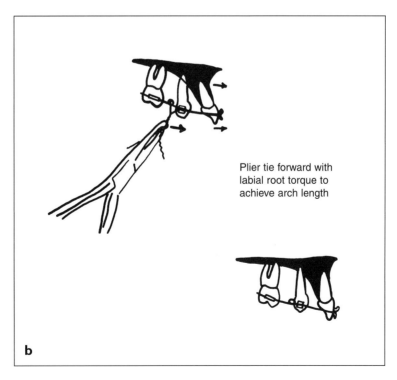

Plier tie forward with labial root torque to achieve arch length

b

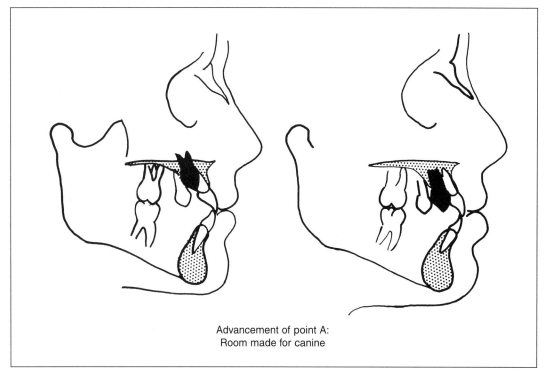

Advancement of point A:
Room made for canine

Fig 1-20 Cephalometric tracings indicating space made for permanent canine by advancing maxillary incisors with labial root torque and increasing arch length.

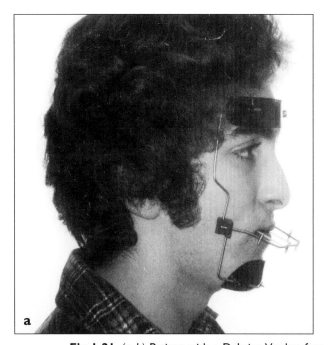 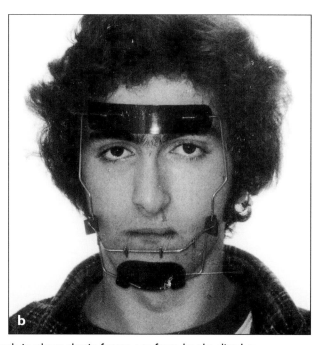

Fig 1-21 *(a, b)* Patient with a DeLaire-Verdon face mask in place; elastic forces are from hooks distal to the lateral incisors. (From Bardach J and Morris HL. *Multidisciplinary Management of Cleft Lip and Palate,*1990. Reprinted with permission from Saunders.)

Several investigations,[15–20] undertaken in the Eastman Dental Center orthodontic department to evaluate the effect of face-mask therapy on the maxillary skeletal complex and mandibular position, determined that both the maxillary dental arch and its skeletal complex can be advanced by this means, depending on the stage of maturation. The younger patients, those who had not reached their peak of pubertal growth, exhibited the greatest amount of anteroposterior skeletal maxillary development and interarch correction. The youngest age group especially (approximately 5 to 7 years old and in the deciduous or early mixed dentition) showed a substantial increase in the distance from the pterygomaxillary fissure to point A with face-mask use. A concomitant increase in the SNA, NA-FH, and basion-nasion–point A angles indicated a significant change in the forward positioning of skeletal point A. Although this could reflect the forward positioning of the erupting permanent incisors, it should be noted that, after face-mask therapy, they seemed to erupt into a more advantageous position anterior to the mandibular incisors.

A study was undertaken at the Eastman Dental Center to determine the optimal time for initiation of face-mask therapy.[18] Rather than evaluating changes relative to chronologic age, which introduces a large variable in timing, changes were analyzed relative to stages of maturation, as developed by Fishman.[21–23] Fishman has shown the fallibility in using chronologic age as a determinant, demonstrating that chronologically young patients can be average, accelerated, or delayed in their maturational levels. Accordingly, he developed a longitudinal series of 11 skeletal maturity indicators (SMIs), using hand-wrist films, to identify an individual's maturational stage and correlate it with rates of craniofacial growth. The progression of SMIs represents increasing percentage amounts of completed craniofacial growth, thus creating a basis for determining the amount of growth completed as well as the amount remaining. Glauser[18] determined that the optimal time for initiation of face-mask therapy was during the prepubertal growth spurt, SMI stages 0 to 3, followed by the time of peak growth velocity, stages 4 to 7. The greatest skeletal correction in

the forward positioning of point A was during the SMI period 0 to 3, obviously the period (prepubertal growth spurt) when face-mask treatment should be started to achieve maximum skeletal advancement of point A.

The subjects in the transitional stage of dental development, approximately 9 to 10 years of age, demonstrated the most dramatic changes in maxillary skeletal development. In these cases, the linear measurement from the pterygomaxillary fissure to point A increased substantially; in addition, SNA, NA-FH, and basion-nasion–point A angles increased much more than would be expected incident to normal growth when compared with the University of Michigan growth studies. Evaluation of this age group had led to the recommendation that face-mask therapy be initiated at least by the beginning of the adolescent growth spurt, for at this stage greater changes in development of the maxillary region might be anticipated. Although skeletal maxillary development by face-mask use was observed in individuals past the peak of pubertal growth, this seemed to be more slowly achieved and of a lesser amount. At later ages—late adolescent and early adulthood, as previously reported—face-mask therapy was helpful, but little enhancement of maxillary development could be anticipated and changes seemed to be limited to dentoalveolar arch advancement. Maxillary incisor labial root torque was maintained throughout treatment because it was felt that the anterior dentition could reinforce the face-mask therapy by maintaining forward pressure in the region of point A and thereby encourage anterior maxillary development, as well as forward arch movement.

Outcomes of early face-mask treatment

Once again, mandibular position was found to be a strong factor in the correction of maxillary retrusion[7]: cephalometric records clearly indicate that some of the correction occurs incident to a change in the posture of the growing mandible. Under the influence of the chin-cup aspect of the face mask, a greater-than-normal increase in the mandibular plane angle and in lower anterior facial height was generally noted, correlated to a degree with the length of time

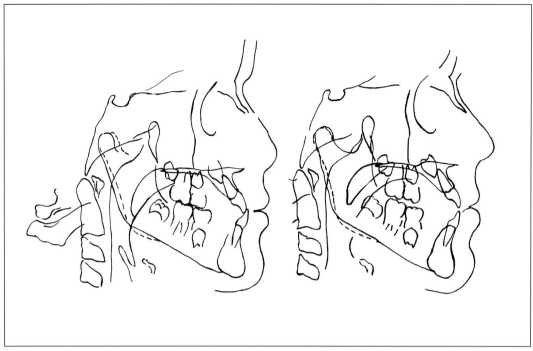

Fig 1-22 Patient R.S. Cephalometric tracings of a young individual with maxillary retrusion taken in occlusion *(left)* and rest *(right)* prior to orthodontic treatment.

of face-mask use. Concomitant with the increment in lower facial height, a substantial increase in the angle of convexity was noted. Some of the more dramatic changes were noted during the transitional dentition stage, also at later ages, and to some extent when growth was essentially completed.

Much of the increment in lower facial height was the result of molar eruption, with the maxillary molars erupting more frequently than the mandibular molars, and with twice the increment. This finding explains the occasional development of an anterior open bite, especially when the face mask was used too long in an effort to achieve overcorrection of the maxillary dental retrusion. At the present time, anteroposterior overcorrection is no longer sought if a vertical discrepancy is developing; so overbite is watched carefully. Although some variation was noted, the face mask tended to posture the chin in a more downward (thus, less forward) direction with continued facial growth, while achieving midface advancement. The overall effect was helpful in creating a notable improvement

in facial appearance that overcame the maxillary retrusive configuration (Figs 1-22 to 1-27).

The correction of considerable midface retrusion may not be achievable by face-mask therapy alone, yet may not be severe enough to contemplate the adjunct of surgical repositioning. Of course, in severe cases, orthodontic correction may be beyond the realm of possibility, making orthognathic surgery a necessity. In borderline cases with further growth expected, however, additional orthodontic procedures should be considered. Whereas extraction in the maxillary arch is not recommended, first premolars in the mandibular arch have frequently been removed to reduce arch dimensions and to retroposition the anteriors. If the first premolars are erupting (or have erupted), and the overjet achieved through face-mask correction still seems inadequate and considerable mandibular growth is anticipated, then this orthodontic procedure should be considered. In summary, extractions may be undertaken in the mandibular arch, but are not considered in the maxillary arch if they can be avoided (Figs 1-28 to 1-32).

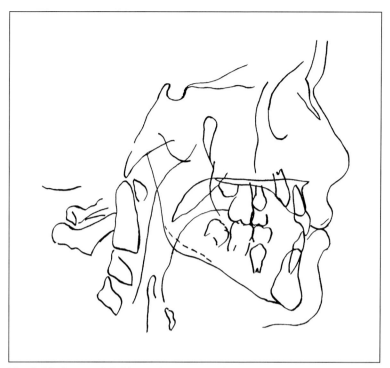

Fig 1-23 Patient R.S. Head plate tracing following establishment of labial root torque and face-mask therapy to correct skeletal malrelationships incident to the retruded position of point A.

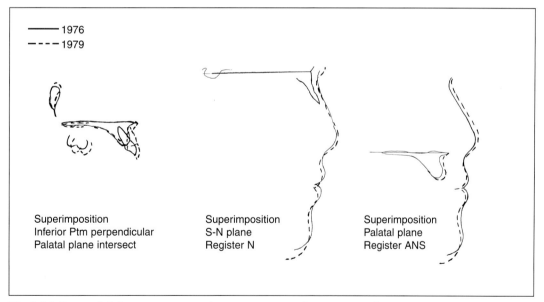

—— 1976
- - - 1979

Superimposition
Inferior Ptm perpendicular
Palatal plane intersect

Superimposition
S-N plane
Register N

Superimposition
Palatal plane
Register ANS

Fig 1-24 Patient R.S. Superimposition of tracings at start of treatment and initial retention, indicating maxillary dental, skeletal, and soft tissue profile changes.

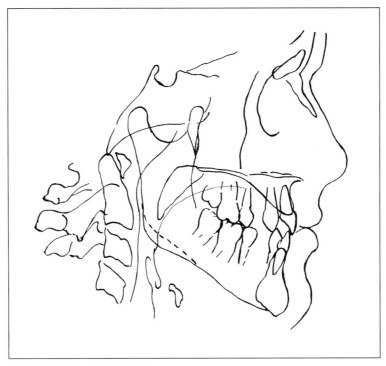

Fig 1-25 Patient R.S. Tracing obtained after a second period of orthodontic treatment and retention.

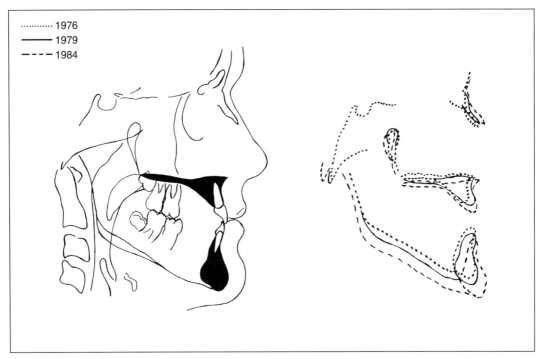

Fig 1-26 Tracing of R.S. taken after a period of removal from retention and at time of dismissal. Superimpositions indicate changes in skeletal relationships from initiation of treatment and time of dismissal.

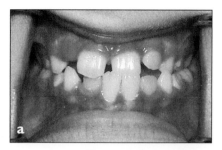
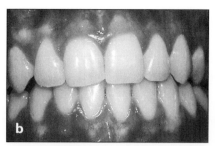
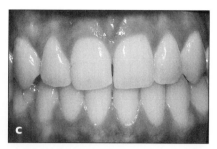

Fig 1-27 Patient R.S. *(a)* Intraoral photograph at start. *(b)* Intraoral photograph at retention. *(c)* Photograph of occlusion at dismissal.

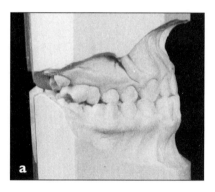
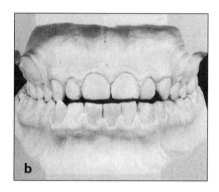
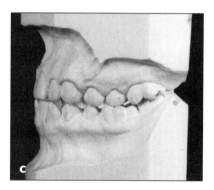

Fig 1-28 Patient K.D. *(a to d)* Casts and cephalometric radiograph of a young male teenager with maxillary skeletal Class III retrusion, proclined maxillary anteriors (note root canal), a midline discrepancy, and crossbite. It would have been desirable to start this patient at an earlier age, but facial growth was still projected.

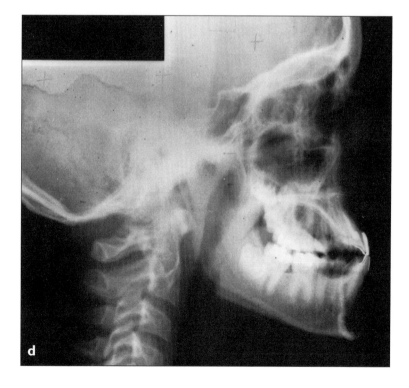

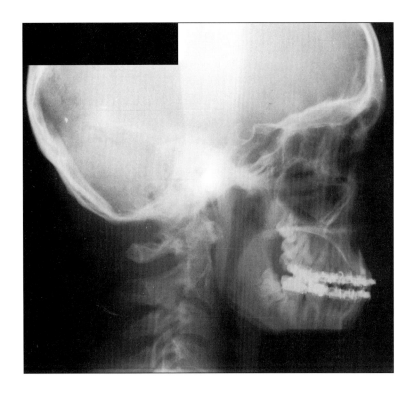

Fig 1-29 Patient K.D. Cephalometric centric radiograph taken a short time before retention. Note labial root torque (root canal) and bone dimly visible labially and apically to the incisor apex.

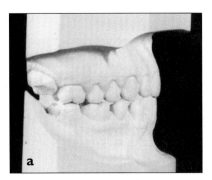
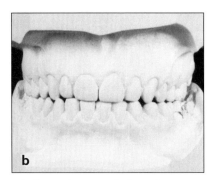
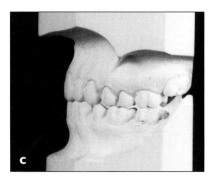

Fig 1-30 Patient K.D. *(a to c)* Casts after completion of treatment. The mandibular left first premolar and right second premolar were extracted to achieve midline correction. No extractions were undertaken in the maxillary arch.

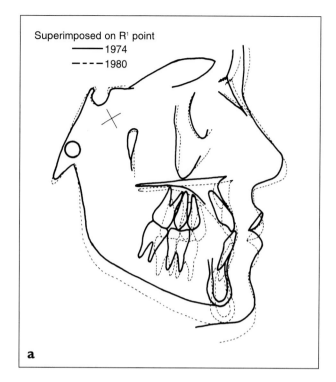

Superimposed on R¹ point
——— 1974
---- 1980

a

Fig 1-31 Patient K.D. *(a to c)* Superimpositions of lateral radiograph tracings revealing development of point A and downward positioning of mandibular symphysis, with change in skeletal and soft tissue profile relationships, as well as dental changes.

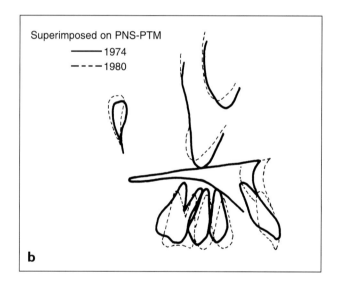

Superimposed on PNS-PTM
——— 1974
---- 1980

b

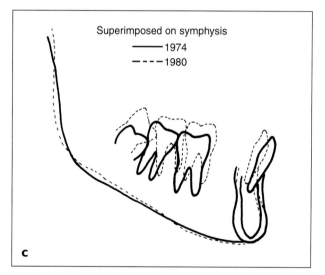

Superimposed on symphysis
——— 1974
---- 1980

c

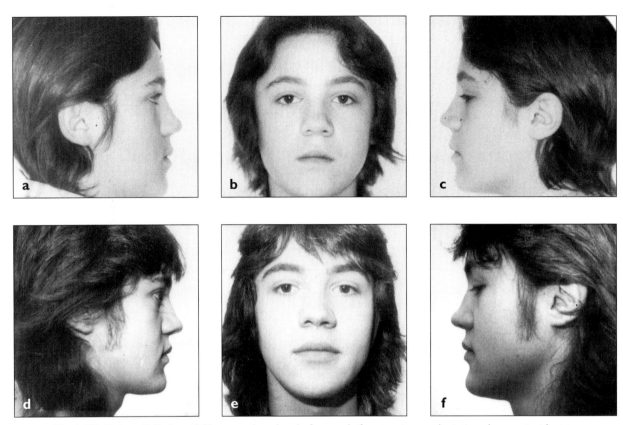

Fig 1-32 Patient K.D. *(a to f)* Photographs taken before and after treatment, depicting changes incident to growth and orthodontic-orthopedic correction.

This observation becomes more pertinent when we consider recent findings where, in many youngsters who had undergone face-mask therapy and were still growing, nasion seemed to develop forward, but the nasomaxillary complex remained virtually static and facial convexity decreased. After maxillary development has been achieved, the forward development of point A seems to be retained; however, the maxillary complex may not continue to express forward growth. Thus it may be necessary to once again institute face-mask therapy to further stimulate forward development of point A (Figs 1-33 and 1-34).

Not only can there be an anteroposterior problem with continued mandibular growth, but a problem in maxillary arch width can also de-velop, resulting in a posterior crossbite. This problem, if recognized early enough, can be prevented by conjunctive use of a maxillary palatal developer, whereby an attempt is made to increase maxillary width by orthopedically opening the midpalatal suture and inducing new bone development in that area. In some young patients with maxillary retrusion and deficient maxillary width, face-mask therapy has recently been instituted in conjunction with palatal developers having the downward and forward elastic force applied from the face mask directly to attachments on the expander (Fig 1-35). Recent studies[24] indicate that the midpalatal suture can be patent well into the adolescent stage of development.

Fig 1-33 Patient R. *(a)* Tracings of lateral cephalograms before *(left)* and after *(right)* correction of maxillary retrusion and anterior crossbite. *(b to e)* Occlusal and profile photographs at the start of orthodontic treatment.

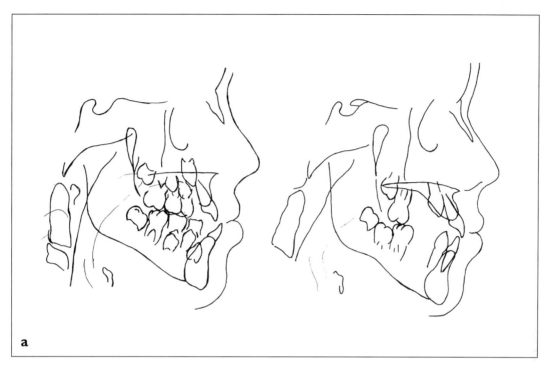

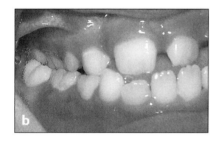
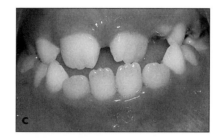
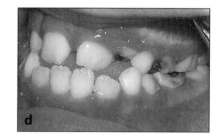

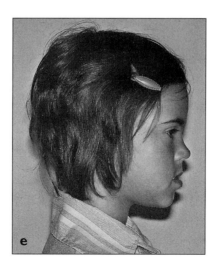

Fig 1-34 Patient R. *(a to e)* Occlusal and profile photographs after maxillary orthopedic advancement and mandibular first premolar extractions. Tracings indicate that, with continued mandibular growth, a loss of overjet, and an edge-to-edge incisor relationship is becoming evident. There is a need for additional advancement of point A and further orthodontic-orthopedic correction.

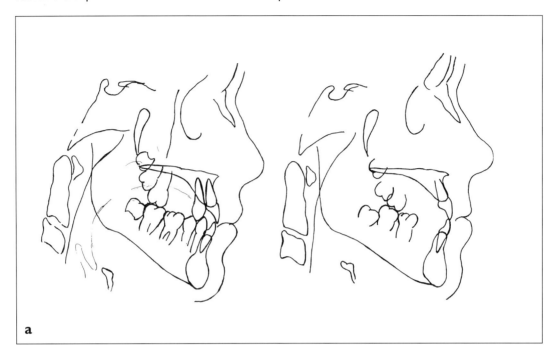

a

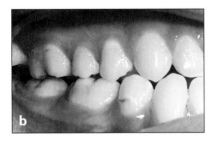

b

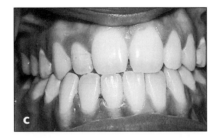

c

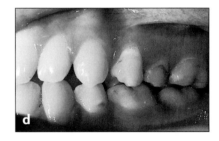

d

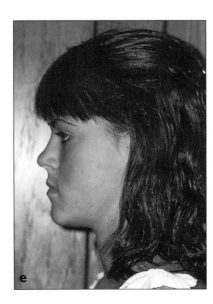

e

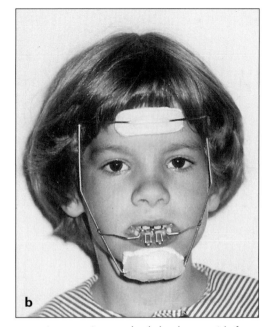

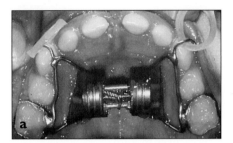

Fig 1-35 (a, b) A young patient with maxillary retrusion wearing a palatal developer with face-mask hooks to attain increment in both maxillary width and anteroposterior length.

The face mask has also been found to be useful in more conventional orthodontic procedures and as an anchorage adjunct. For example, in closing maxillary spaces, either due to congenitally missing teeth or extractions (and significant efforts must be made to prevent retropositioning of the maxillary anteriors), the face mask can help maintain a forward position of the anterior dentition while more posterior teeth are brought mesially to close spaces. Further, the face mask has been used to reduce (or even preclude) relapse after maxillary surgical advancement (Fig 1-36). A gradual repositioning of the maxilla has been noted in some cases after it has been surgically advanced, and it has been possible to orthodontically regain this loss by instituting face-mask therapy to create a forward-positioning force on the surgically treated maxilla (Fig 1-37).

Theoretically, the face mask creates a tension force that is conducive to bone "build up" and counteracts the pressures of the surrounding musculature and compressive forces of the healing fibrous tissue and the forming cicatricious tissue. The face mask has even worked advantageously, to a limited degree, in bringing a mandibular arch forward in cases where (1) mandibular anteriors have been positioned too far lingually during orthodontic tooth movement, (2) the mandibular dental arch has been positioned excessively distally, or (3) it is obviously undesirable to further retract the maxillary dentition. Correction of this overjet can be achieved by causing mandibular arch advancement with face-mask therapy. At any rate, face-mask use is not necessarily restricted to the development of point A.

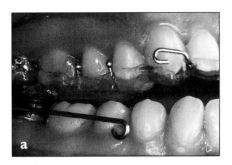
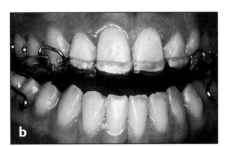
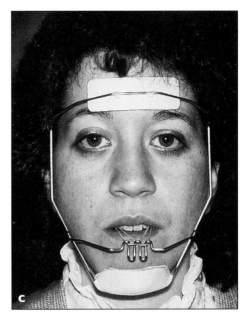

Fig 1-36 *(a to c)* An orthognathic surgery patient, subsequent to a maxillary advancement, wearing a removable appliance with face mask hooks and a nighttime face mask to regain and/or maintain a forward positioning of the maxilla.

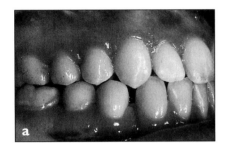
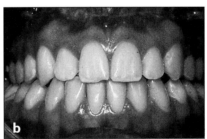
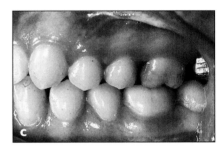

Fig 1-37 *(a to c)* Occlusal relationships of the patient in Fig 1-36 incident to regaining the forward position of the maxillary arch.

To summarize, skeletal development of the maxillary complex is strongly recommended during the transitional stage of dental development when the orthodontist can take advantage of considerable potential growth. This is specifically recommended for cases of skeletal maxillary retrusion, which must be differentiated from skeletal mandibular prognathism. In both instances, the patient may exhibit a developing or frank anterior crossbite, but for different reasons. In the skeletal maxillary retrusive patient, forward development of point A via face-mask therapy is recommended. In mandibular skeletal prognathism, if minimal, an attempt to redirect mandibular growth, possibly via a chin cup, is suggested. In both instances, mandibular repositioning and eruption of molars to maintain the vertical positioning of the chin are important aspects in the correction of the anteroposterior skeletal malrelationship.

References

1. Downs WB. Variations in facial relationships: Their significance in treatment and prognosis. Am J Orthod 1948;34:812.
2. Tweed CH. The Frankfort–mandibular incisor angle in orthodontic diagnosis, treatment planning and prognosis. Angle Orthod 1954;24:3.
3. Riedel RA. An analysis of dentofacial relationship. Am J Orthod 1957;43:103.
4. Ricketts RM. Cephalometric synthesis. Am J Orthod 1960;46:647.
5. Steiner CC. Cephalometrics for you and me. Am J Orthod 1953;39:729.
6. Graber LW. Chincap therapy for mandibular prognathism. Am J Orthod 1977;72(1):23–41.
7. Bowman CJ. Chincap and Reverse Headgear Therapy [senior research]. Rochester, NY: Eastman Dental Center, 1975.
8. Subtelny JD. Oral respiration: Facial maldevelopment and corrective dentofacial orthopedics. Angle Orthod 1980;50:147–164.
9. Delaire J. La croissance maxilaire: Deductions therapeutiques. Trans Eur Orthod Soc 1971;81–102.
10. Verdon P, Salagnac JM. Traitments originauz de quelques cas complexes: Utilisation successive des forces extra-orales (masque orthopédique de Delaire et plaque de Stephenson) et des forces légères (technique de Mollin). L'Orthodontic Francaise. 1977; 47(tome 2):802–811.
11. Brodie AG. Behavior of normal and abnormal facial growth patterns. Am J Orthod Oral Surg 1941;27:633.
12. Lande M. Growth behavior of the human bony facial profile as revealed by serial cephalometric roentgenology. Angle Orthod 1952;22:78–90.
13. Ricketts RM. The influence of orthodontic treatment on facial growth and development. Angle Orthod 1960;30:103–133.
14. Goldin B. Labial root torque: Effect on the maxilla and incisor root apex. Am J Orthod Dentofac Orthop 1989;95:208–219.
15. Fenn C. The Clinical and Cephalometric Results of Face Mask Therapy in the Dentofacial Region [senior research]. Rochester, NY: Eastman Dental Center, 1979.
16. Simonsen R. The Effects of Facemask Therapy [senior research]. Rochester, NY: Eastman Dental Center, 1982.
17. Galletto L. Cephalometric Evaluation of Dentofacial Changes Incident to Facemask Therapy [senior research]. Rochester, NY: Eastman Dental Center, 1988.
18. Glauser J. Timing of Facemask Therapy Based on Skeletal Maturation [senior research]. Rochester, NY: Eastman Dental Center, 1995.
19. Dingus B. An Evaluation of Skeletal and Dental Changes as a Result of Maxillary Protraction Therapy from Post Retention Records [senior research]. Rochester, NY: Eastman Dental Center, 1996.
20. Long S. The Soft Tissue Response Associated with Tie-Forward Mechanics and Protraction Facemask Therapy [senior research]. Rochester, NY: Eastman Dental Center, 1997.
21. Fishman LS. Chronological versus skeletal age: An evaluation of craniofacial growth. Angle Orthod 1979; 48:181–189.
22. Fishman LS. Radiographic evaluation of skeletal maturation: A clinically oriented study based on hand-wrist films. Angle Orthod 1982;52:88–112.
23. Fishman LS. Maturational patterns and prediction during adolescence. Angle Orthod 1987;57:178–193.
24. Revelo B, Fishman LS. Maturational evaluation of ossification of the midpalatal suture. Am J Orthod Dentofac Orthop 1994;105:288–292.

Chapter 2

Maxillary Skeletal Protrusion Malocclusions

The antithesis of maxillary skeletal retrusion and the accompanying malocclusion is, of course, the Class II dental malocclusion. It is a malocclusion that is not only prevalent but also one that the orthodontist feels relatively comfortable in treating. However, the Class II, division 1 malocclusion is varied enough to be the manifestation of a skeletal maxillary prognathism, a skeletal mandibular retrognathism (or a variable of both), or solely a dentoalveolar malocclusion; it therefore requires careful evaluation to determine the necessary treatment procedures (Fig 2-1).

The Class II Dilemma: Skeletal or Dentoalveolar?

Dentoalveolar Class II (early transitional dentition): Treatment procedures

When the Class II malocclusion is solely dentoalveolar in nature, it is an affirmation of the fact that the anteroposterior positions of the supporting skeletal jaws—the maxilla and the mandible—are in an acceptable relationship to each other. A dentoalveolar Class II is relegated to the dentition and to the anteroposterior position of the alveolar bone encompassing the roots of the teeth. It is the dentition and/or the denture bases—points A and B—that are dis-parate. Either the maxillary dentoalveolar complex (point A) is too far forward, the mandibular dentoalveolar complex (point B) is too far back, or there is some combination thereof. Angles SNA, SNB, and ANB are strictly ascribed to denture-base positions since point B is not indicative of the skeletal chin (pogonion) position.

Early treatment of Class II dentoalveolar malocclusions is really a lesson in diagnosis and growth. In these cases, orthodontic efforts may be the restraining of forward development of the maxillary dentition and its alveolar process with continued craniofacial growth (expressed by holding back point A) while concurrently permitting either forward mandibular dentoalveolar positioning or encouraging additional mandibular dentoalveolar development concomitant to mandibular growth. In other words, when treating early, we may attempt to either hold back point A in anticipation of the mandible "catching up," or we may try to supersede that forward mandibular growth with an even greater forward positioning of the mandibular dentition and point B.

Various treatment mechanisms can be used to correct Class II molar relationships, but these mechanisms usually also increase lower facial height. In some cases this could be advantageous; in other cases, not. In Class II cases needing increment in lower facial height, maxillary headgears can not only rotate and retract maxillary molars, but will also erupt them, increasing

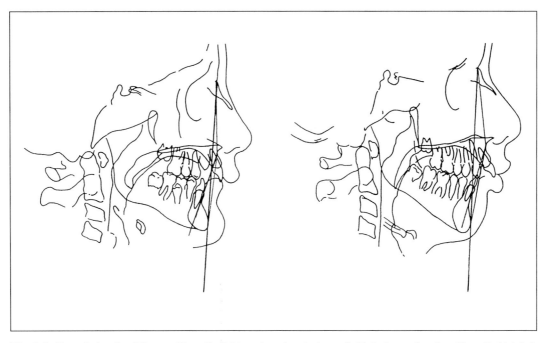

Fig 2-1 Two skeletally different Class II, division I malocclusions. *(left)* A dentoalveolar Class II. *(right)* A skeletal maxillary protrusion (Class II).

posterior dentoalveolar height as well as lower facial height. Again, the early transitional dentition period seems to offer the optimal time for positive results using headgear. Kopecky[1] showed that the greatest skeletal correction with headgear therapy was achieved during periods of peak growth velocity (skeletal maturity indicator [SMI] 4 to 7). At times, maxillary molar eruption must be augmented by mandibular molar eruption when considerable decrease of overbite and mandibular overclosure is desired. Achieving mandibular molar eruption may be more difficult in the presence of an excessive curve of Spee or a "two-step" plane of occlusion with depressed mandibular buccal segments. Lip bumpers can be used effectively to achieve mandibular molar eruption as well as attain added arch length, especially in patients having tight lower lip musculature. Using the lip bumper (Fig 2-2) as an intermediary, muscle forces of the lower lip can effect a distal (uprighting) movement of the mandibular molars, a forward movement of the mandibular incisors, or a combination of both—thus gaining additional arch length.[2] At early age levels, the lip bumper can be augmented with a maxillary bite plate to

take advantage of the natural eruptive process of the mandibular molars. The resulting increment of the mandibular posterior dentoalveolar height can reposition the chin downward, causing an increase in lower facial height, helping to reduce the overbite. However, this could also increase the overjet by positioning the symphysis slightly downward and backward which, of course, is counter to the direction of Class II treatment. Therefore, careful and educated judgment must be used; effects must be kept under scrutiny to preclude an increase in the posterior dentoalveolar height that would make Class II correction more difficult. In some cases the lip bumper can be used to remove the influence of the lower lip from the lingual of the maxillary incisors, aiding in lingual repositioning of these teeth and resulting in a more rapid reduction of overjet. Many times excellent results are achieved in early, or first phase, orthodontic treatment. However, the question arises: Are the treatment results stable over the long term, or do problems reveal themselves in succeeding years? Several cases with long-term records are presented to attempt an answer.

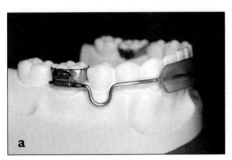

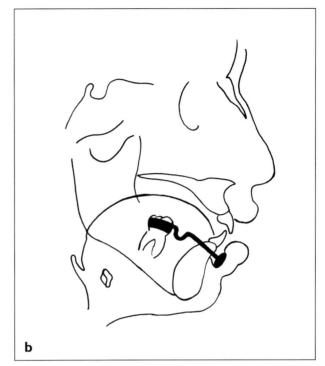

Fig 2-2 Patient A.D. *(a, b)* Mandibular lip bumper on a cast, and tracing of a lateral radiograph indicating lip bumper positioning.

Dentoalveolar Class II correction and long-term stability: Case presentations

Patient A.D. This patient presents a dentoalveolar Class II malocclusion with the maxilla and the chin in good relationship to nasion (Fig 2-3). Notably, the A-B relationship is disparate. Point A was determined to be in an acceptable relationship, but point B, the junction of the mandibular dentoalveolar process and the basal bone of the chin, was back. The mandibular dentition was retropositioned with retroclined mandibular incisors, insufficient eruption of maxillary molars (as determined by their root tips being above the palatal plane), and infraeruption of mandibular molars. The mandible moved into an overclosed position to achieve full occlusal contact (overclosure).

Treatment requirements: Mandibular incisor inclination needs to be improved by proclining these teeth, which also will reduce overjet. The mandibular dentoalveolar process needs to come forward, probably with continued mandibular growth, bringing point B forward and correcting the A-B disparity. At the same time, it was hoped that holding back the maxillary dentoalveolar process would also contribute to the correction of the overjet. Needed, as well, was increased mandibular posterior dentoalveolar height to preclude mandibular overclosure. In addition, increased mandibular arch length for placement of the mandibular dentition was an obvious requirement.

Outcome: An excellent outcome that achieved all the treatment requirements was evident at the time of retention. The headgear permitted a holding back of point A and the maxillary dentoalveolar process. The bite plate and conjunctive use of the lip bumper permitted the necessary eruption of the mandibular molars, as well as an increase in mandibular arch length

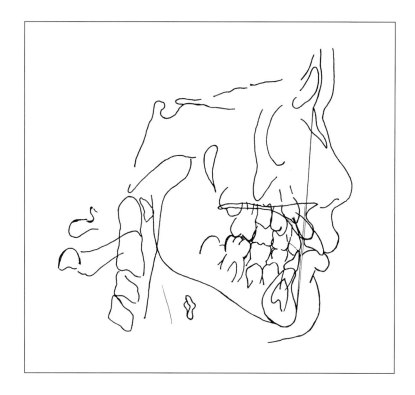

Fig 2-3 Cephalometric tracing of A.D., showing a dentoalveolar Class II malocclusion at the start of orthodontic treatment.

and a proclination of the mandibular incisors (Fig 2-4). Full orthodontic appliances permitted more precise adjustment of the occlusion while the desired downward and forward mandibular growth carried the dentoalveolar process into a good interocclusal relationship horizontally and vertically, with adequate opening of the bite as well (Figs 2-5a to 2-5l). Postretention evaluation (Fig 2-6) revealed that, relative to nasion, point A had come forward with continued craniofacial growth, (Fig 2-7) but the occlusion was maintained with continued forward mandibular growth; proportional vertical relationships were maintained with adequate molar eruption.

Over 20 years postretention, the occlusion was more than satisfactory, both functionally and esthetically, with a high degree of stability—all in all, a highly acceptable result (Fig 2-8). Advantageous mandibular growth—the right amount and the right direction—was obviously beneficial. Proper control and correction of dentoalveolar relationships allowed for correction of the Class II malocclusion. Early treatment followed by a secondary period of full appliance therapy for occlusal refinement served to achieve a very acceptable, long-term occlusion.

Figs 2-4 Patient A.D. *(a, b)* Mandibular casts (1961 and 1964, respectively) and *(c)* lateral cephalometric tracing (1964) depicting lip bumper effectiveness and changes in molar relationships. *(d)* Mandibular super-impositions indicate molar uprighting *(top)* and incisor proclination *(bottom)*.

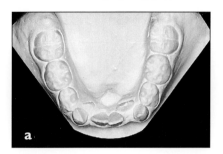
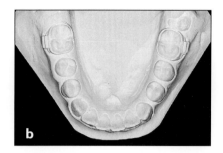

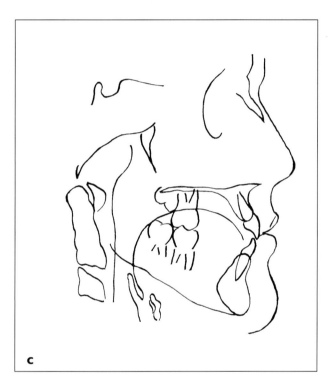
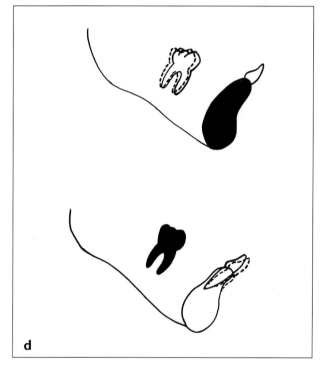

Fig 2-5 Patient A.D. *(a to f)* Lateral tracing and casts obtained in 1966, when full appliance therapy was initiated.

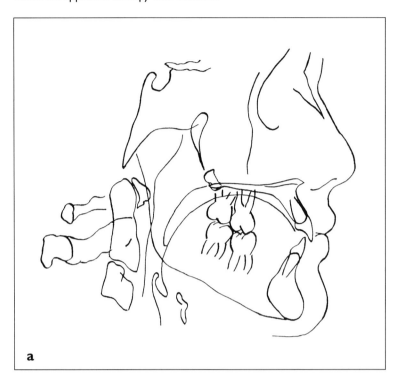

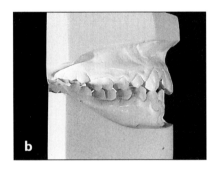

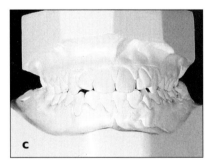

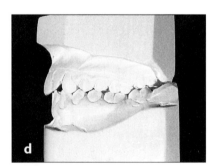

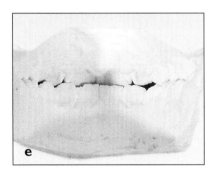

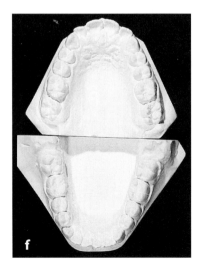

Fig 2-5 Patient A.D. *(g to l)* Lateral tracing and casts obtained in 1969, when retention was removed. Headgear bands were maintained throughout retention.

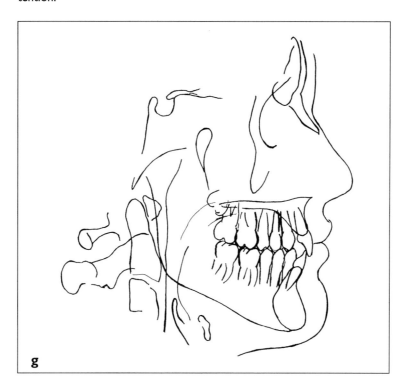

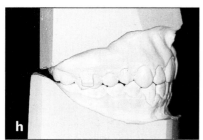
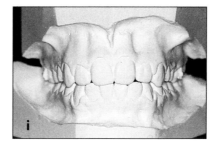
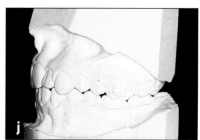

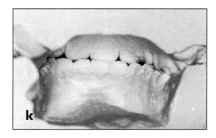
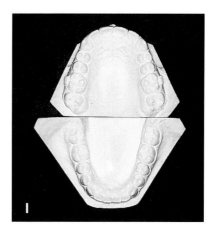

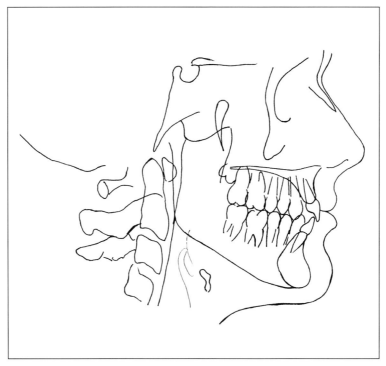

Fig 2-6 Patient A.D. Lateral cephalometric tracing obtained in 1972, 3 years after removal of retention.

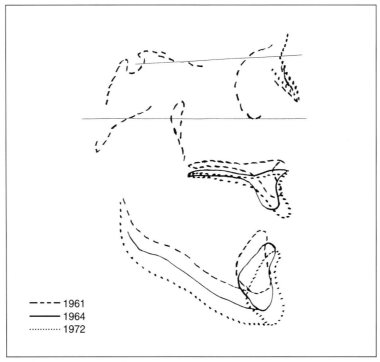

- - - - 1961
———— 1964
·············· 1972

Fig 2-7 Patient A.D. Superimpositions registering on nasion, revealing changes in position of point A and changing skeletal jaw relationships with continued growth.

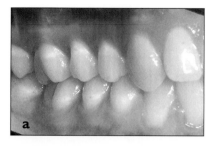
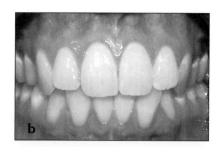
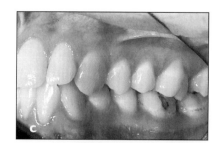
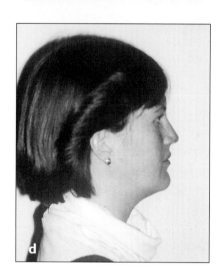

Fig 2-8 Patient A.D. *(a to d)* Intraoral photographs of the occlusion and profile photograph indicate a high degree of stability of the orthodontic result.

Patient S.B. The second patient to be presented, again, had a dentoalveolar Class II, division 1 malocclusion with a discernible mentalis habit. Cephalometric analysis indicated that the well-formed mandible was related nicely to the cranial base, as evidenced by a good facial angle; a chin button was duly noted. Point B, however, was back, indicating that the mandibular dentoalveolar process was positioned posteriorly on its basal bone, possibly incident to the mentalis habit (Fig 2-9). The maxilla was found to be in a very acceptable position (as indicated by SNA and Na-FH angles) and was found to be acceptably related to the total profile, considering the angle of convexity. A large ANB angle was evident, resulting primarily from a posteriorly positioned mandibular dentoalveolar process—not the skeletal chin per se. The mandibular incisors, when related to the A-pogonion plane, were placed bodily posteriorly as well as tipped lingually. This upright condition was seen again when the mandibular incisors were related to the mandibular plane. The relatively high AB–facial plane reading indicated that there was a disharmony between denture bases when related in the anteroposterior direction.

The information gathered indicated that the two jaws were in harmony when related to the cranial base, in that the maxilla and the chin were well related to each other. Again, the primary problem was that point B was positioned posteriorly on the mandible. The maxillary denture base was in an acceptable position, but the mandibular denture base was retropositioned. Of major concern was the movement necessary to correct the malrelationship of the dentition. In the analysis, point A was determined to be slightly forward, so it seemed logical to use headgear and growth to hold back point A. In the mandible, it seemed an obvious case for a lip bumper to counteract the influence of the mentalis habit and to permit the mandibular dentoalveolar process to be positioned forward,

Fig 2-9 Patient S.B. *(a to g)* Cephalometric tracing, facial photographs, and dental casts, exhibiting a dentoalveolar Class II with point B back, at start of treatment.

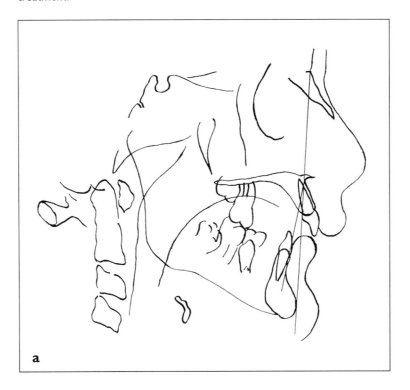

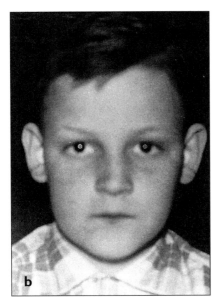

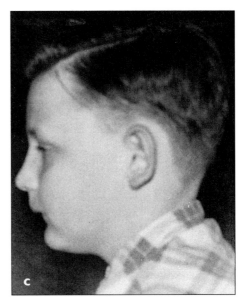

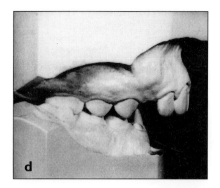

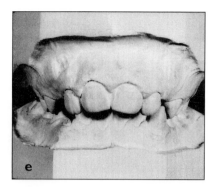

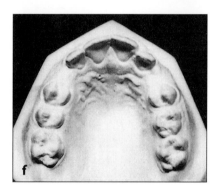

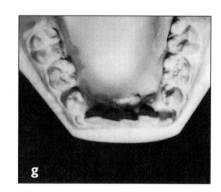

improving the position of point B and reducing overjet. Again, sufficient mandibular growth would be necessary to carry the mandibular denture forward to achieve occlusal correction.

Cephalometric appraisal at the time of retention showed the skeletal pattern to be essentially unchanged, although there was slight improvement in ANB and the AB–facial plane reading (Fig 2-10). The maxillary incisor, which initially showed good angular readings, still had good angulation but had been positioned posteriorly into a more harmonious relationship with the mandibular incisor. This tooth was found to be slightly procumbent, but its crown was well-related to the A-pogonion plane. The mandibular incisor root was still well-positioned between the cortical plates of the mandibular symphysis, indicating that good alveolar response in the area had been achieved.

Records taken 14 months after appliance removal (Fig 2-11) indicated that the teeth had settled into a very acceptable Class I relation-ship on both sides. The case appeared to be holding well, with no crowding, rotations, or slipped contacts. Analysis revealed that the anticipated mandibular growth had occurred, but not as much anteroposteriorly as had been hoped for. Registering on nasion or sella using the SN plane, we determined that a proportionately greater downward than forward positioning of the chin had occurred (Fig 2-12), which might have been anticipated in light of the mandibular configuration and the bending of the lower border of the mandible anterior to gonion. Some eruption of both maxillary and mandibular molars under appliance therapy added further to the increased vertical positioning of the chin. Obviously the cervical appliance was instrumental in restricting the forward movement of point A. Although limited, forward growth of the mandible, as well as the forward development of point B under lip bumper and appliance therapy, was sufficient to correct the Class II problem. Growth retardation of the max-

Fig 2-10 Patient S.B. *(a to h)* Lateral cephalometric tracing, facial photographs, and dental casts taken at time of retention.

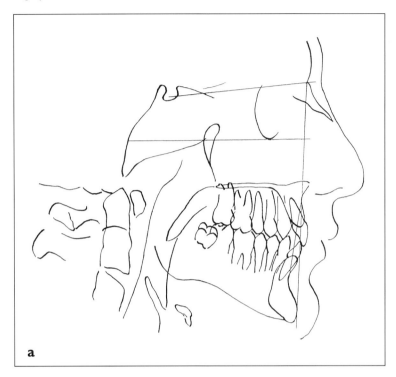

a

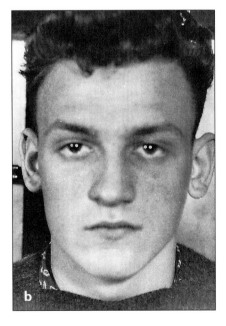

b

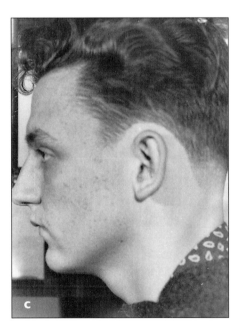

c

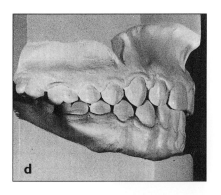
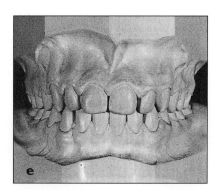
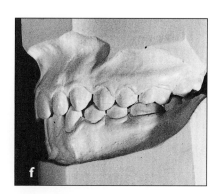

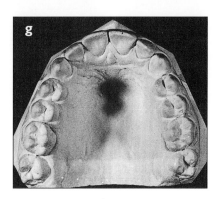
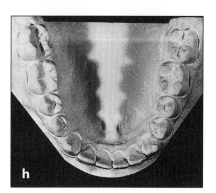

Fig 2-11 Patient S.B. *(a to g)* Lateral cephalometric tracing, facial photographs, and dental casts taken 14 months after orthodontic appliance removal.

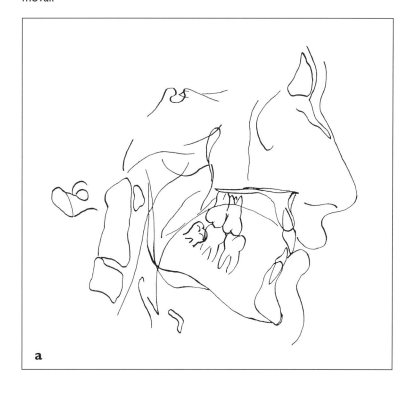

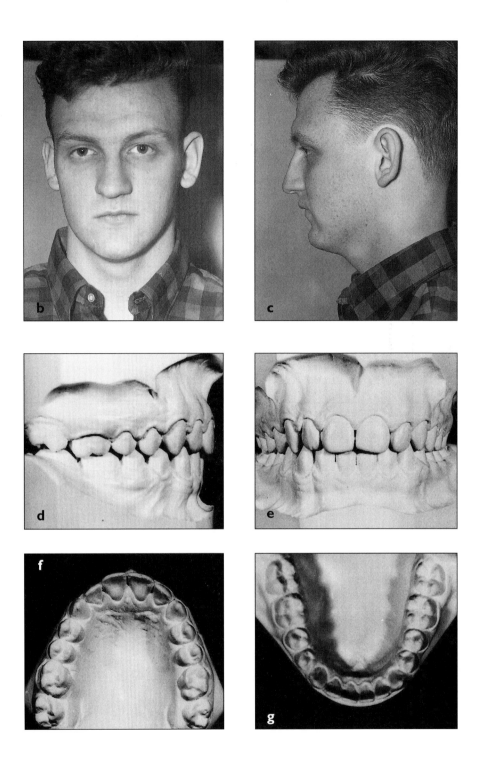

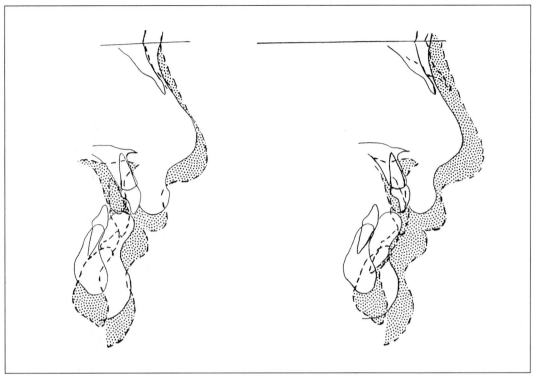

Fig 2-12 Patient S.B. Superimpositions of profile structures indicating the direction of chin positioning with progressive growth and orthodontic treatment.

illa was specific and adequately directed; in fact, point A was held back a little more than necessary. Tooth movement, coordinated with mandibular growth, was just sufficient to achieve the desired dentoalveolar correction.

Many years later, the Class II correction was highly stable and alignment of the arches was good (Fig 2-13). The small increase in overbite and overjet, apparently related to the limited and less-than-anticipated mandibular growth, was still within acceptable limits. Mandibular growth and changes incident to treatment had caused the chin to progress a little more downward than forward. It was fortunate that, with the retropositioning of point A during treatment, there was just enough forward mandibular growth to achieve good occlusal correction. Furthermore, additional maxillary growth during the 20-year postretention period, was limited, so that point A remained retropositioned relative to the cranium. There was proportionate forward growth of the mandible; though mini-

mal, it was sufficient to maintain good occlusal relationships. Although the bite closed a little with time, (and was a factor in the overbite increase), it helped bring the chin into a slightly more forward position.

All in all, the result was fortunate (Fig 2-14), but revealed that at times forward mandibular growth may not be sufficient to correct a Class II malocclusion without other alternatives. It also emphasizes that, in the correction of a Class II malocclusion, cognizance must be taken of the vertical direction of chin growth with treatment: the greater the amount of vertical versus anteroposterior positioning of the chin, the greater the potential for increase in overjet and the more difficult will be correction of the Class II malocclusion. The treatment result also points out that sometimes point A must be over-retracted to compensate for inadequate forward mandibular growth, with due consideration being given, of course, to the limitations imposed by the facial profile.

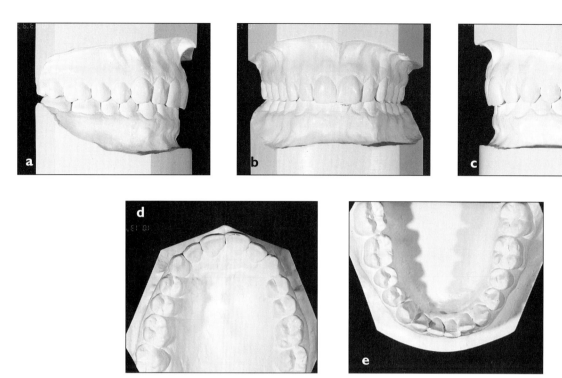

Fig 2-13 *(a to e)* Dental casts of S.B.'s occlusion nearly 20 years later.

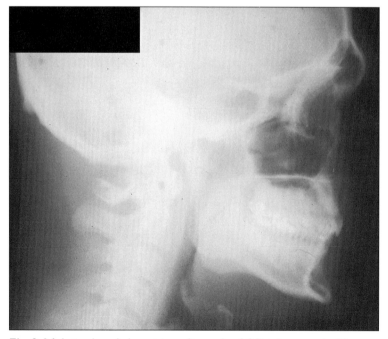

Fig 2-14 Lateral cephalometric radiograph of S.B. taken nearly 20 years later.

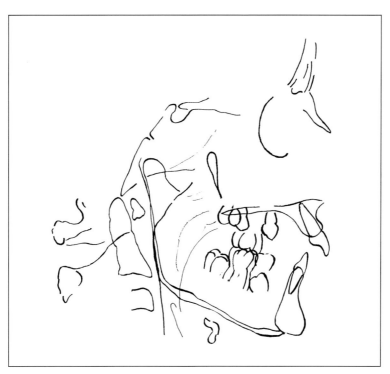

Fig 2-15 Lateral cephalometric tracing of E.D. at initiation of orthodontic treatment.

Patient E.D. An analysis of the casts revealed a Class II, division 1 malocclusion with 11 mm of overjet, ovoid arch form, and good arch symmetry. The cephalometric analysis (Fig 2-15) disclosed a mesognathic mandible, as shown by a facial angle of 86 degrees and a slightly prognathic maxilla (NA-FH, 90 degrees; SNA, 82 degrees) when related to the cranial base. The angle of convexity (+9 degrees) substantiated the prognathic relationship of the maxilla. The anteroposterior relationship of the denture bases, (AB–facial plane, 12 degrees) was not favorable. The mandibular plane, as well as the configuration of the mandible, indicated that growth had previously proceeded in a more forward than downward direction and, if this direction of growth were to continue, the anteroposterior relationship of the denture bases could

be rendered more favorable. This indicated that the patient must be treated without extraction, with the possibility of retracting the maxillary dentoalveolar process and discouraging forward growth of the maxilla. To correct the severe AB discrepancy, it was decided to minimally reposition point A and the maxillary dentoalveolar process; meanwhile, the mandibular denture base would be carried forward with growth, with the realization that the prominent chin could be an esthetic problem. Cervical traction to the maxillary molars established Class I molar relationships bilaterally incident to holding back forward development of point A.

By the time of retention, a mesognathic profile with slight midfacial soft tissue convexity was achieved (Fig 2-16). The profile appeared to be

Fig 2-16 Patient E.D. *(a, b)* Facial photographs at time of retention. *(c to f)* Dental casts depicting occlusal relationships at retention.

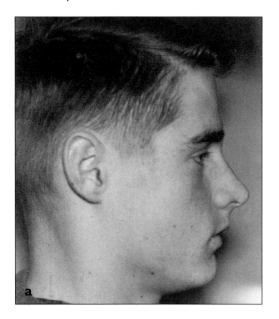
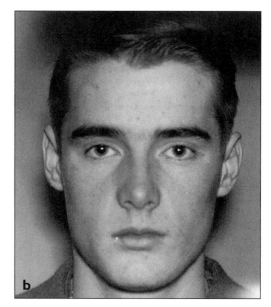

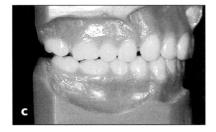
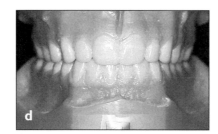
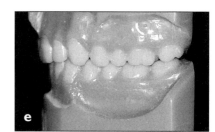

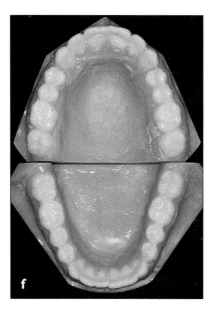

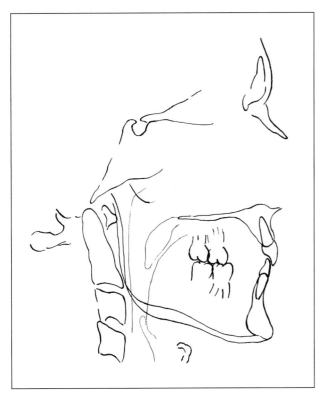

Fig 2-17 Patient E.D. Tracing of lateral cephalometric radiograph at time of retention.

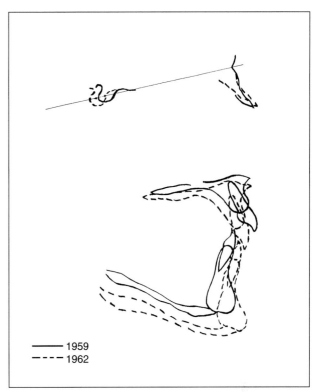

——— 1959
----- 1962

Fig 2-18 Superimposition of tracings of E.D. on the SN plane, registering on N, indicating the changed relationship of points A and B with growth and treatment.

esthetically pleasing and the occlusion corrected. Cephalometric appraisal indicated that the mandible had grown forward (manifested by a 2-degree increase in the facial angle [88 degrees]), and the maxilla had become less prognathic (as reflected by a 2-degree decrease in SNA [80 degrees]). Therapy had been successful in retropositioning point A. Concomitantly, a great change in the anteroposterior relationship of maxilla to mandible was noted by a decrease in the angle of convexity from +9 degrees to +1.5 degrees. The relationship of the denture bases (Fig 2-17), denoted by the AB–facial plane angle, showed a dramatic and highly desirable

change, partially incident to point B coming forward due to forward mandibular growth and appliance therapy (Fig 2-18). At the time of dismissal (Fig 2-19), a mesognathic mandible was found to be well related anteroposteriorly to the maxilla as well as to the cranial base, and the anteroposterior relationship of the denture bases remained relatively good. The interincisal angle had increased due to uprighting of the maxillary incisors, which had become more retruded relative to the AP plane.

Twenty years after dismissal, a successful occlusal result was still evident (Fig 2-20). However, strong forward growth of the mandible (with its

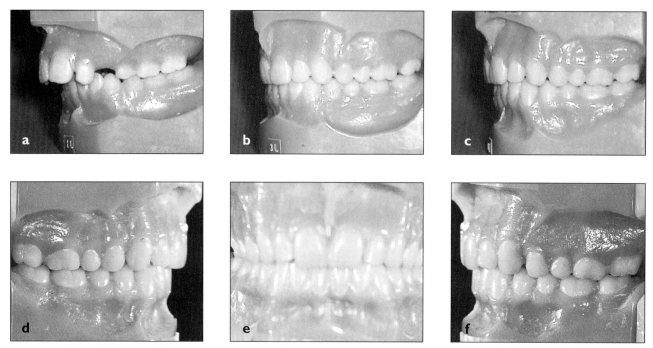

Fig 2-19 Patient E.D. *(a to c)* Lateral view of dental casts indicating changes in occlusion from the time of initiation of treatment to the time of dismissal. *(d to f)* Casts depicting occlusal relationships at the time of dismissal.

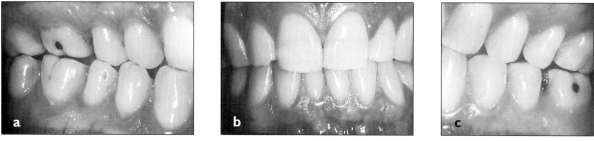

Fig 2-20 Patient E.D. *(a to c)* Intraoral photographs of the occlusion 20 years after orthodontic correction.

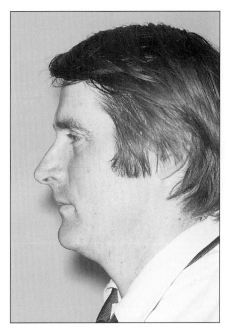

Fig 2-21 Patient E.D. Profile facial photo revealing concavity of soft tissue subsequent to growth of the nose and mandible.

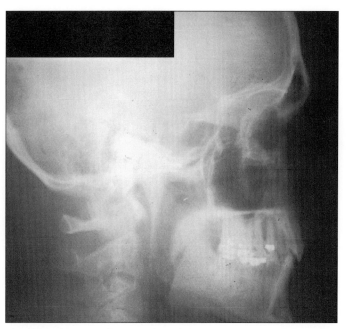

Fig 2-22 Patient E.D. Lateral cephalometric radiograph revealing underlying skeletal relationships.

chin button) and considerable growth of the nose had left their mark. These had caused the lips to be positioned farther back relative to the nose and chin than was desirable. This lip position had created a concave facial profile, despite the fact that no extractions had been undertaken (Fig 2-21). The lower face appeared to need more vertical dimension in the concavity between the nose and the chin (Fig 2-22). In the last analysis, with the anticipation of considerable horizontal mandibular growth, it might have been more expedient *(1)* to move point A back to a lesser degree, *(2)* to advance point B to a greater degree, and *(3)* to increase the posterior dentoalveolar heights, which, in turn, would have increased the vertical dimension of the posterior occlusion and achieved a more favorable configuration of the lips.

Indications were that a young male, whose mandibular configuration suggested greater proportional forward growth, might develop excessive facial concavity as a long-term result. Attempts should have been made to develop the mandibular dentoalveolar process more anteriorly in conjunction with greater increment of posterior dentoalveolar height. Facial appearance might have been enhanced, as well as the occlusion, which itself needed improvement.

Twenty years later, a deep bite was evident and consistent with the need for more lower facial height; in essence, there wasn't a sufficient increase in the mandibular plane angle. It is now judged that more Class II elastic therapy should have been instituted to accomplish this and to raise posterior buccal segments.

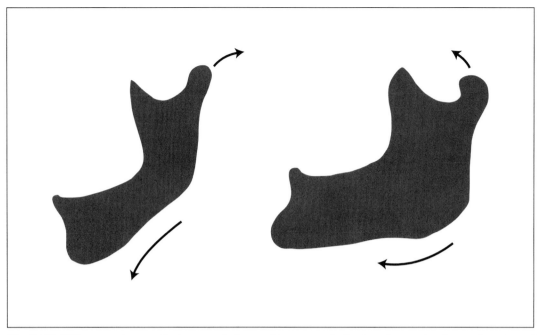

Fig 2-23 Differences in mandibular morphology, with arrows indicating the predominant direction of growth, vertical or horizontal, usually consistent with condylar morphology and spatial relationship of the ramus.

Growth and Class II correction

To a great extent, excellence and stability in early Class II treatment is contingent on the amount and direction of mandibular growth, both of which must rely on an educated guess. A distinct advantage in initiating early Class II treatment is the opportunity of seeing the apparent direction of mandibular growth; one can foresee the probability—or improbability—of the "help" of growth in the correction. One can hazard a guess, based on the shape of the mandible, whether the direction of growth will be favorable or not. Clues gleaned from radiographs (obliques) indicate that the morphology of the mandible (Fig 2-23) may minimize the guesswork on direction, leaving the amount of mandibular growth as the major remaining undetermined factor. Reasonable determinations of the potential amounts of residual mandibular growth may be forthcoming in future applications of skeletal maturity indicators,[3] but at present still reside in the realm of an educated guess. These educated guesses were reasonably good in the previously discussed cases.

Realistically, however, patients will be encountered where neither the amount nor the direction of mandibular growth will fulfill the needs for adequate correction. If point A cannot be held back sufficiently for Class II correction because of inadequate forward mandibular growth or because the chin may be positioning away from point A more vertically than horizontally, then decisions must be made to achieve adequate correction. For example, it may be decided that the extraction of maxillary first premolars may permit the degree of desired point A retraction to sufficiently improve the interrelationship of points A and B.

It should again be emphasized that initiation of treatment at early age levels (during the transitional dentition) affords the opportunity to observe and evaluate growth and positional changes so decisions can be more informed. In early treatment, the element of urgency in decision making does not exist; there is no immediate need to rush into extraction. Time is an ally to the orthodontist because maxillary permanent canines are usually the last teeth to erupt into the maxillary arch, exclusive of the second and third molars. During the course of early Class II treatment, it may become evident that the underlying problem is skeletal—either in the maxilla or the mandible—so a decision can be made whether the extraction of maxillary premolars can sufficiently compensate for the discordant anteroposterior positions of points A and B.

Case presentation: S.O.

This patient was started at an early age, when it became apparent that there would not be sufficient forward mandibular growth to compensate for an anteroposterior discrepancy in the relationship of points A and B. Initial cephalometric records indicated that the anteroposterior position of the mandible and the degree of convexity were very acceptable for this age; the maxilla and, of course, point A, were slightly forward of an ideal anteroposterior relationship with the cranium, indicating a slight skeletal maxillary protrusion (Fig 2-24). Upon evaluation of progress headplates taken after a period of early treatment, it was noted that there was insignificant forward mandibular growth and that the chin was positioning more downward and backward rather than forward relative to nasion. Initially, early treatment was directed toward holding back and/or retracting point A. This was accomplished. Headgear therapy had moved point A back slightly, but there was no possibility of further distalizing the maxillary first molars and it became obvious that the amount and direction of mandibular growth could not reduce the undesirable overjet. The occlusion was still a full Class II, with the first molars already tipped distally. The crowns of the developing maxillary second molars were situated directly at the root tips of the first molars; the developing third molars were high and close to the second molars (Fig 2-25).

Time to institute second phase of Class II treatment

It became apparent that a second phase of treatment was called for. Now the decision had to be made: Will the mandible grow sufficiently to preclude the need for extractions, or can the mandibular arch be advanced with Class II mechanics (surgical mandibular advancements were not undertaken at that time) to achieve satisfactory correction? In this case neither was deemed feasible, so it was decided to extract maxillary first premolars to retroposition point A and reduce the undesirable overjet. Subsequent to the extractions, the maxillary canines, then the incisors, were retracted to achieve a reduction of the overjet. An acceptable occlusion was achieved, albeit the molars were in a Class II relationship (Fig 2-26). Superimposition of progressive headplates on the S-N plane registering on nasion revealed that point A had been retracted dramatically relative to nasion. It was sorely needed, since the chin, relative to nasion, was observed to progress downward and somewhat posteriorly (Fig 2-27). The direction of mandibular growth insofar as profile and occlusion were concerned was definitively unfavorable and precluded any correction of overjet without maxillary extractions. In addition, later headplates revealed dramatically that antegonial notching (more on the left side than on the right) was developing—a clear indication of some mandibular growth disturbance (Fig 2-28).

This patient exhibited some degree of maxillary prognathism exacerbated by a mandible that developed in an unfavorable direction. Fifteen years later the occlusion is holding well, but the skeletal relationships have not improved with remaining growth (Fig 2-29), indicating that the course of treatment was the correct one. Even if surgery had been performed, it doesn't seem that a better result would have been achieved. The case also leads to the realization that all Class II malocclusions are not dentoalveolar in origin but may be related to maxillary skeletal prognathism, mandibular retrognathism, or a combination thereof.

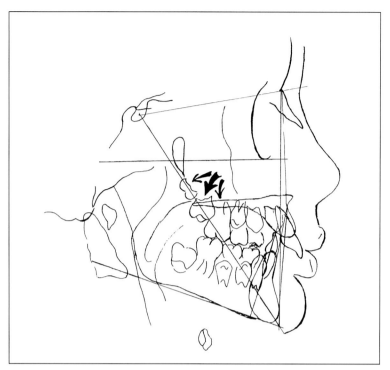

Fig 2-24 Tracing of cephalometric radiograph (S.O.) before treatment. Note the skeletal relationships of the jaws and relationship of the maxillary molars.

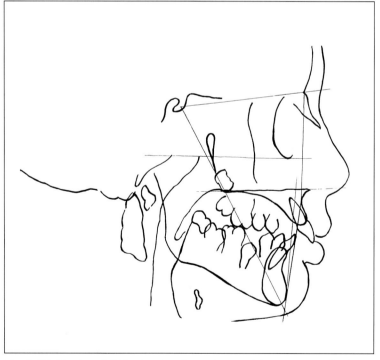

Fig 2-25 Tracing of S.O. after headgear therapy. Note continued relative positions of maxillary molars.

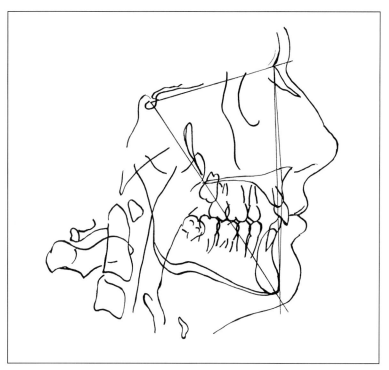

Fig 2-26 Patient S.O. Headplate tracing following removal of maxillary first premolars and retropositioning of incisors and point A to reduce anterior overjet.

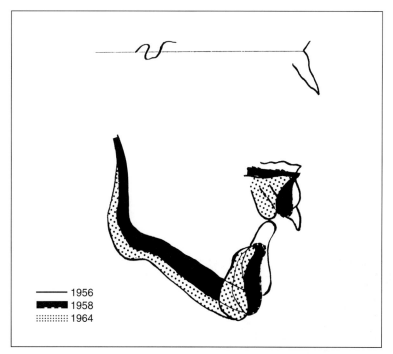

——— 1956
▬▬▬ 1958
::::::::: 1964

Fig 2-27 Patient S.O. Superimposed headplate tracings (registering on nasion) indicating skeletal profile changes incident to growth and orthodontic treatment.

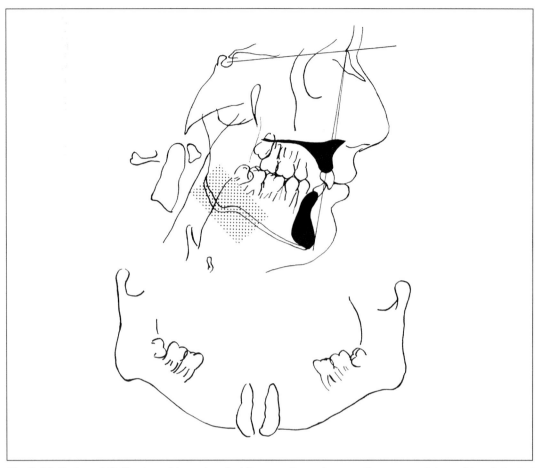

Fig 2-28 Patient S.O. Tracing of lateral and oblique radiographs revealing antegonial notching (stippled area).

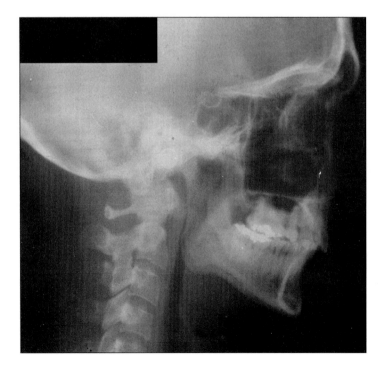

Fig 2-29 Patient S.O. Lateral cephalometric radiograph 15 years after removal of retention revealing continuance of mandibular skeletal discrepancies.

Class II Skeletal Problems: More than Dentoalveolar

Maxillary skeletal prognathism

Seemingly in a predominance of patients, the Class II malocclusion is caused by an exceptionally forward position of the maxilla, positioning the full maxillary dentition too far forward in the craniofacial profile[4]—maxillary skeletal prognathism. True maxillary prognathism, properly diagnosed, presents comparatively less challenge in treatment today than in years past. Forward positioning of the maxilla can readily be evaluated relative to the anterior cranial base by determining the anteroposterior relationship of point A to the forehead or, more specifically, nasion. A markedly excessive SNA angle can be indicative of this condition, likewise an excessive angular relationship between NA and Frankfort horizontal. At early maturational levels (during the transitional dentition), it is acknowledged that an acceptable face should have some degree of convexity; however, if the maxillary complex is excessively forward in relation to the anterior cranial base and the chin is in an acceptable relation to the forehead, then a true maxillary skeletal prognathism may exist. It represents a skeletal problem—an AB problem—in that point A is more forward of the mandibular landmark point B (as well as the skeletal chin) than is acceptable in relation to the rest of the skeletal facial profile. In those instances where true maxillary prognathism has been determined to exist, it has generally been our practice, after a period of early treatment, to extract first premolars in the maxillary arch to reposition point A by incisal retraction. At the same time, mandibular extractions have generally been avoided to prevent increment in overjet by not repositioning mandibular incisors. Throughout treatment, one should recognize that overeruption of the molars must be prevented to minimize repositioning the mandible and thereby increasing overjet and mandibular retrusion. As a consequence, Indiana and/or Nance holding arches have been placed not only to enhance anchorage, but equally to prevent maxillary molar eruption; likewise, where indicated, mandibular lingual arches have been

placed for the same reason. On occasion, a conjunctive bite block has been used. These cases, because of their relative prevalence, have gradually come under good orthodontic control with acceptable results.

Case presentation: W.C.

The following is an excellent example of treatment and long-term results in a case of maxillary prognathism. The distinguishing features of this Class II dental malocclusion were found in its skeletal relationships: the chin was in an acceptable position relative to the forehead, but the maxilla was protruded (Fig 2-30). The chin was slightly posterior relative to the forehead, with a facial angle of 85 degrees. The maxillary skeletal base was positioned excessively anterior to the forehead, with an NA-FH angle of 93 degrees (norm, 88 degrees) resulting in a convex skeletal profile (angle of convexity, +13 degrees). The two denture bases were poorly related to each other and to the profile, with an AB–facial plane angle of –11.5 degrees and an ANB angle of +8 degrees. Thus, the full maxillary dental arch was forward of a well-placed mandible with a well-formed mandibular dental arch. It was obviously desirable to retract point A to an acceptable relationship with the skeletal chin. Extraction of the maxillary first premolars would be an expedient way to retroposition point A, allowing for the greatest reduction in profile convexity and removing the overjet. To our mind, leaving the molars in a Class II relationship is perfectly acceptable; in these cases we have not found it necessary to finish in a Class I molar relationship to insure long-term stability and good functioning occlusion.

Initially headgear therapy was undertaken to restrict remaining maxillary horizontal growth, distalize the maxillary molars, and attempt to gain a more acceptable molar occlusion, as well as reduce the overjet. After 18 months of elastics and headgear wear, a Class I molar relationship had not been achieved, so a decision was made to extract maxillary first premolars. A lip bumper was placed to serve as anchorage for Class II elastics prior to fully bonding the mandibular arch. Following the extractions and retraction of the maxillary anteriors, a substan-

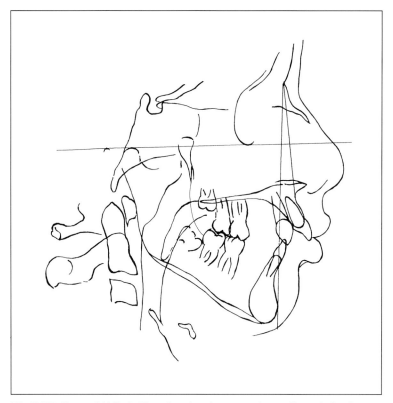

Fig 2-30 Patient W.C. A Class II malocclusion with maxillary skeletal prognathism.

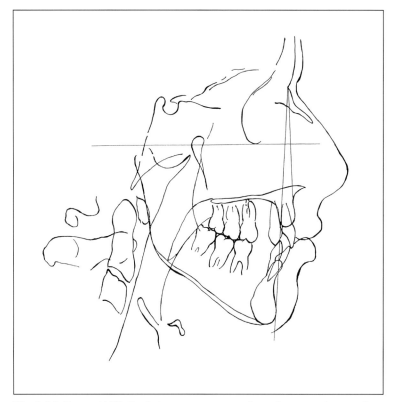

Fig 2-31 Patient W.C. Cephalometric tracing taken after completion of active orthodontic treatment.

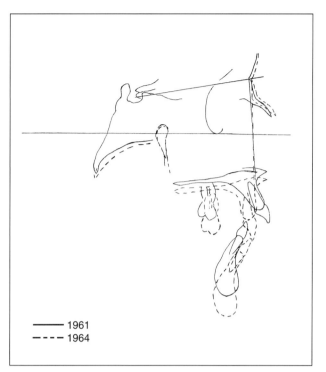

Fig 2-32 Patient W.C. Superimposition of 1964 tracing on 1961 tracing indicates a more posterior relationship of point A (1964), decreasing profile convexity.

1961
1964

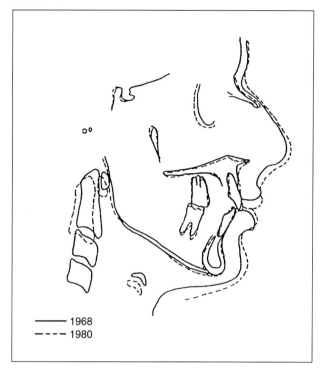

Fig 2-33 Patient W.C. Superimposition of 1968 and 1980 tracings indicating long-term changes in skeletal and soft tissue profiles.

1968
1980

tially improved facial profile was noted. Facial convexity was noticeably reduced (Fig 2-31). Class II molar and a Class I canine relationships were achieved incident to the removal of the maxillary first premolars. During active treatment, horizontal maxillary growth was largely held back. The NA-FH angle decreased (from 92 to 90 degrees) because of forward growth of nasion (Fig 2-32). Evaluation 2 years after retention showed continued facial growth. The maxilla grew forward, but so did the mandible. As a result, the angle of convexity remained essentially unchanged.

The patient returned to participate in an orthodontic and periodontic study conducted at the Eastman Dental Center 14 years after retention had been discontinued. Superimposition of lateral cephalometric tracings demonstrated a slight increase in vertical growth but no additional forward mandibular growth. The maxilla had grown slightly forward as well as vertically. As a result, the angle of convexity had increased from 8.5 to 10 degrees. Because of some in-

crease in soft tissue thickness over pogonion, this larger skeletal convexity was masked clinically (Fig 2-33). Moreover, after many years, the orthodontic correction had remained stable and acceptable in appearance as well as function (Fig 2-34). Some small changes were noted in the mandibular anteriors: the right central and lateral incisors had slipped contact and were rotated as well as out of their retained positions. A small space had appeared distal to the maxillary right lateral incisor, but this was due to a tooth-size discrepancy of a narrower-than-usual lateral incisor. The overbite was quite acceptable, and the overjet correction had largely maintained itself.

Class II Malocclusions and Mandibular Premolar Extractions

Extraction of teeth in Class II malocclusions, even in instances of crowding or potential arch length deficiencies, cannot be undertaken

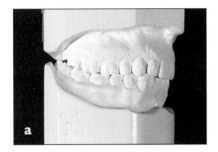
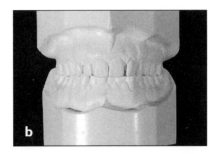
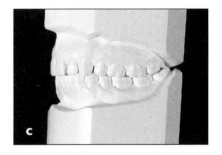
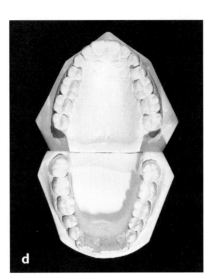

Fig 2-34 Patient W.C. Casts obtained 14 years after dismissal.

lightly, particularly in deep overbite cases. Much thought and extreme caution must be exercised because extraction of mandibular premolars creates the potential for maintaining or increasing the overjet since some retropositioning of the mandibular incisors can occur. If these teeth are maintained in position or brought forward to decrease overjet, then mandibular molars may need to be advanced considerably to achieve a Class I relationship. In the following example, extractions should not have been undertaken or, at most, should have been restricted to the maxillary arch; unfortunately, first premolars were taken out in the mandibular arch as well as the maxillary.

Patient L.S. A young female patient was first seen at the age of 11. She presented a retrognathic profile with minimal facial convexity. The perioral musculature appeared severely strained over the incisors when her lips were brought together (Fig 2-35). The lower lip touched

Ricketts' esthetic (E-) plane, while the upper lip lay 1 mm behind this plane. A maxillary second premolar was congenitally missing; the remaining second premolars were impacted. The initial casts showed Class II canines, considerable overjet, and excessive overbite. The cephalometric evaluation (Fig 2-36) indicated a retrognathic mandible (facial angle, 81 degrees) associated with a retrognathic maxilla (NA-FH, 82 degrees) when related to the cranial base. That the facial convexity was minimal was shown by the facial plane (NP) passing only 1.5 mm behind point A and by an angle of convexity of +3 degrees. Notably, there was considerable proclination and spacing of the maxillary anteriors (Fig 2-37) as well as an apparent arch length discrepancy in the mandibular arch, with blocked-out premolars. The maxillary first molars were markedly rotated mesiolingually and asymmetric anteroposteriorly. There was a deep bite, with the mandibular premolars and molars well

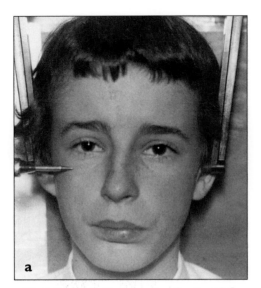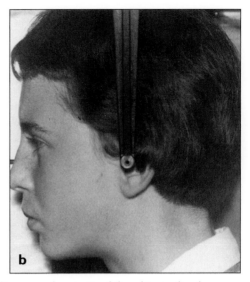

Fig 2-35 *(a, b)* Photographs of patient L.S., revealing muscular strain while achieving lip closure.

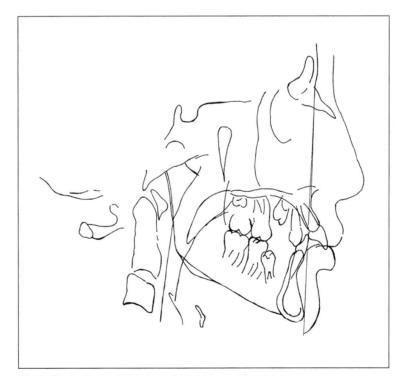

Fig 2-36 Patient L.S. Tracing of initial lateral headplate.

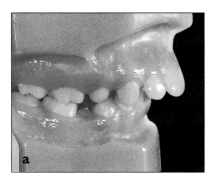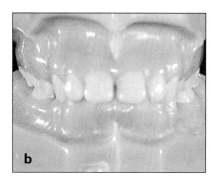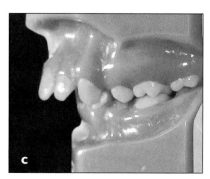

Fig 2-37 *(a to c)* Casts of L.S. at start of treatment.

below the level of the incisors and canines. The exceptionally large mandibular right second molar and the fullness and unattractive configuration of the lips (expressing considerable tension), prompted a decision to extract all four first premolars. The maxillary incisors were retracted, reducing lip tension and overjet and achieving dental alignment and a Class I molar relationship (Fig 2-38).

Maxillomandibular relationships and the potential growth of the mandible, as well as the deep bite due to overclosure, were not fully considered when the decision was made to extract the four premolars. The patient really had a skeletal maxillary retrusion with an NA-FH of 83 degrees and an SNA of 78 degrees. The mandible was likewise somewhat retrognathic, with a facial angle of 81 degrees, despite the presence of a chin button and an overclosed mandible. The mandibular denture base was back with an AB–facial plane angle of –11 degrees. The large overjet was due to a retropositioned mandibular dentoalveolar process (point B) positioned on a retrognathic mandible relative to a retruded maxilla. Ideally there should have been no extractions in this case, and an attempt should have been made to bring the mandibular dentoalveolar process forward to reduce the overjet; arch length increment should have been undertaken to place and align the mandibular

dentition. At best, only maxillary premolars should have been extracted to reduce the overjet, since correction of the overclosure would have brought the chin and point B to a slightly more retruded position by bringing the chin down and back. In this case, the latter would have been a more feasible approach since one maxillary premolar was congenitally missing. Because both jaws were being retruded in an overjet case, extraction in the mandibular arch to achieve a Class I molar relationship only increased the potential for maintaining the overjet and complicated the treatment process.

After treatment, an improvement in facial appearance was immediately obvious (Fig 2-39). Esthetics improved partly due to the patient's holding her head more erect. As a result, her profile appeared to be more mesognathic than initially indicated. The perioral musculature appeared unstrained when the lips were held in repose. The upper lip lay 6 mm, and the lower lip 5 mm, behind the E-plane. An acceptable, bilateral Class I molar occlusion was achieved, with improvement in overjet, overbite, and appearance.

Superimposition of headplate tracings (Fig 2-40) indicated that much of the improvement was incident to further retraction of point A which, at the time of retention, had moved posteriorly 1.5 mm. SNA had decreased 1 degree,

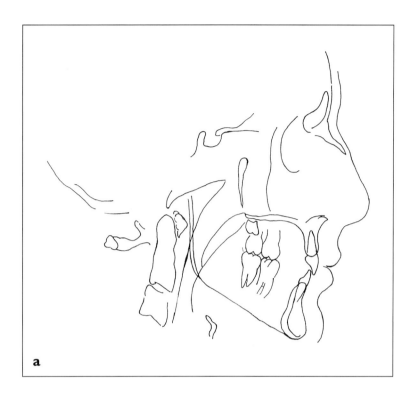

Fig 2-38 Patient L.S. *(a to d)* Cephalogram tracing and dental relationships after treatment.

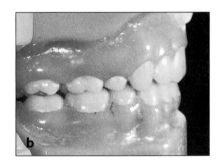 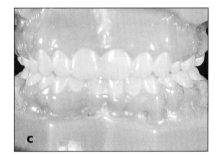 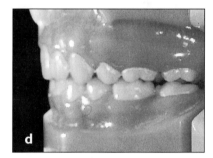

the angle of convexity 1.5 degrees, and AB–facial plane angle 3 degrees. Improving the occlusion to a Class I was primarily achieved by forward movement of the mandibular molars. Depression of mandibular incisors was noted, but there was no evidence of protraction, proclination, or retroclination of these teeth. One year out of retention, the patient still showed excellent results (Fig 2-41).

Twenty years later, the dentition was still observed to be very well aligned, and the Class I molar relation had held very well (Fig 2-42). However, major problems were noted. The bite had deepened significantly, and there was a no-

ticeable increase in overjet. With time and growth, the chin button had become more pronounced. Notably, a return of the deep overbite, an increased overjet, and mandibular anterior malalignment were evident. Overclosure, with some return of depressed mandibular buccal segments and a concomitant reduction in lower facial height was also noted. On the cephalometric headplate, some mandibular asymmetry was noted, and the occlusion exhibited a slight midline discrepancy (Fig 2-43).

Hindsight is better than foresight: there probably should not have been mandibular extractions. This patient had a retrognathic

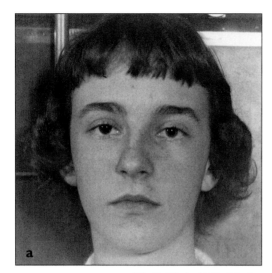 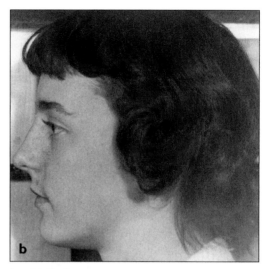

Fig 2-39 *(a, b)* Facial photographs of L.S. after treatment.

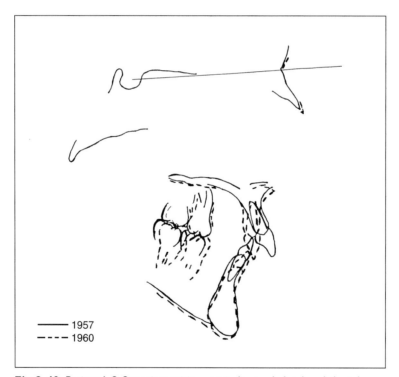

—— 1957
- - - - 1960

Fig 2-40 Patient L.S. Superimpositions to indicate skeletal and dental profile changes incident to treatment.

Fig 2-41 Patient L.S. *(a to l)* Views of occlusion before treatment, at retention, and 1 year after retention removal.

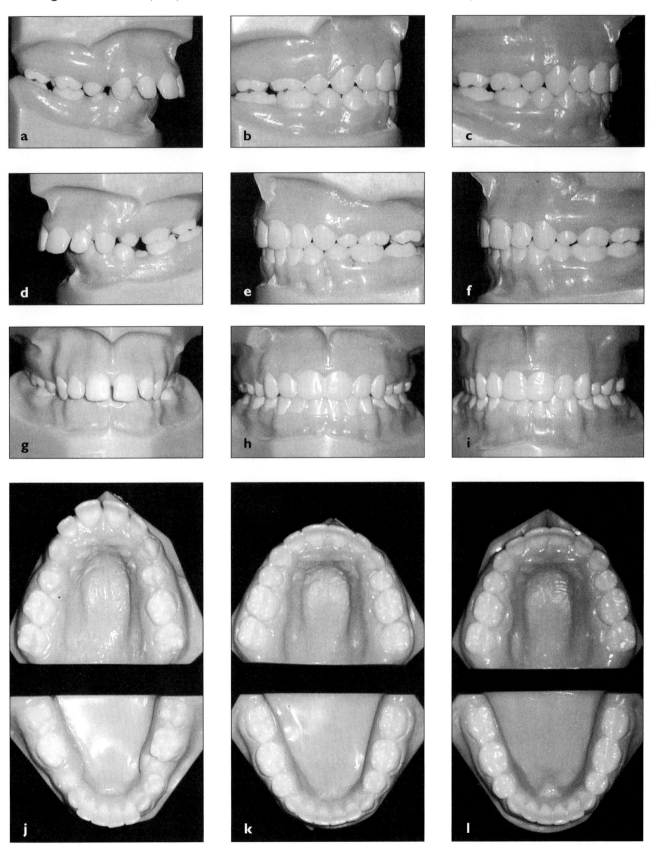

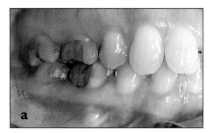 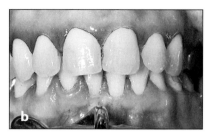 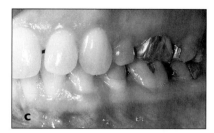

Fig 2-42 Patient L.S. Intraoral photos of occlusion approximately 20 years after orthodontic treatment.

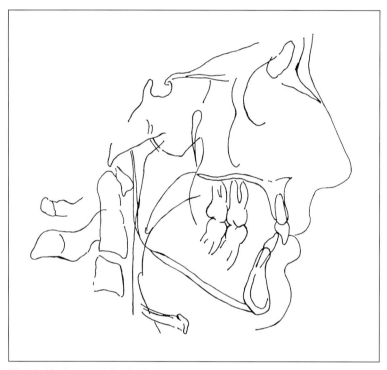

Fig 2-43 Patient L.S. Cephalometric radiograph tracing 20 years after treatment.

mandible, with an overclosure, a large overjet, and a deep bite. Mandibular premolars were extracted to achieve a Class I molar relation. It should have been recognized that the maxilla was slightly retruded (skeletally) and that the mandible was even more retrognathic, but the condition was somewhat masked by the overclosure. If anything, the patient would have been better treated with maxillary premolar extraction alone because one second premolar was already congenitally missing.

References

1. Kopecky GR. Timing of cervical headgear treatment based on skeletal maturation. Am J Orthod Dentofac Orthop 1993;104:162–169.
2. Subtelny JD, Sakuda M. Muscle function, oral malformation, and growth changes. Am J Orthod 1966;52: 495–517.
3. Fishman LS. Radiographic evaluation of skeletal maturation: A clinically oriented study based on hand-wrist films. Angle Orthod 1982;52:88–112.
4. Rosenblum RE. Class II malocclusion. Mandibular retrusion or maxillary protrusion? Angle Orthod 1995;65: 49–62.

Chapter 3

Mandibular Skeletal Retrognathia and Class II Malocclusions

Perhaps the most difficult of the Class II malocclusions to treat are those with mandibular size and/or growth problems: retrognathic mandibular positions, too retruded to be compensated for by reduction in the forward relationship of point A. The maxilla may be in a proper relationship to the forehead or even slightly on the retruded side, but the mandible itself is in poor position relative to the forehead—too far back. This, of course, leads to a considerable AB discrepancy and a large overjet, with point B being too far back because the chin itself is too retrognathic in position. In these instances, utilization of the SNA-SNB difference (ANB) might not be indicative of the skeletal relationship, since point B itself might actually be anterior to the chin. Extraction of maxillary premolars will not be enough to correct the overjet; something may need to be done in the mandible to permit adequate orthodontic correction. In essence, these patients should be started early to control the direction of mandibular growth, doing whatever possible to enhance forward positioning of the chin. Furthermore, comprehensive correction should await later age levels to confirm that adequate growth of the mandible will not take place, in which case alternative approaches might be needed.

Class II Malocclusion with Mandibular Retrognathia

Case presentation: B.B.

This case exemplifies a young male, early in the transitional dentition, with a Class II malocclusion, in whom orthodontic treatment was started in 1962 at an early age but whose mandibular growth was inadequate and unfavorably directed. (Progressive radiographs and photographs will be presented because dental casts do not materially add to the discussion.) The patient was obviously excessively retrognathic with a resultant convex facial profile (Figs 3-1 and 3-2) and had an extensive overjet, despite the fact that there were two congenitally missing maxillary lateral incisors and a missing maxillary left first premolar that had been extracted on the advice of a dentist. Cervical headgear traction was initiated in hopes that the maxillary dentoalveolar process could be prevented from further anterior development and mandibular growth could somewhat reduce the overjet and improve the bony profile. A mandibular lip bumper was used to optimize arch length by preventing forward movement of the mandibular molars; however, this was not enough to pre-

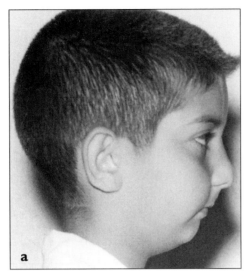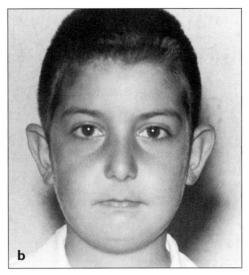

Fig 3-1 Patient B.B. *(a, b)* Facial photographs depicting retrognathic, convex facial characteristics.

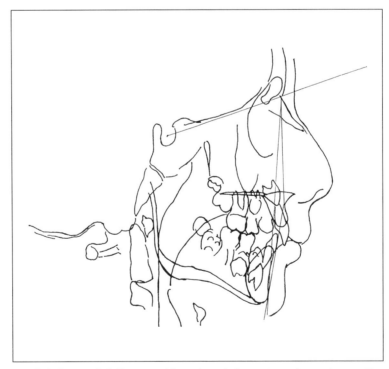

Fig 3-2 Patient B.B. Tracing of lateral cephalometric radiograph revealing underlying dentoskeletal relationships.

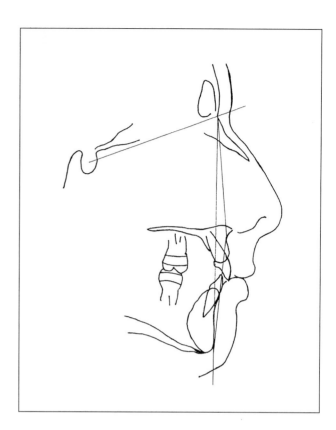

Fig 3-3 Patient B.B. Dentoskeletal profile relationships after orthodontic treatment; a retrognathic mandible and a Class II molar relationship are still evident.

clude extracting mandibular premolars to overcome the severe crowding. Furthermore, at this time it was not realized that the bumper, in uprighting the mandibular molars, could increase vertical height and thereby increase overjet. Some overjet reduction did occur, however, but not enough to improve the facial profile significantly (Fig 3-3). The mandible did not grow sufficiently to achieve a more acceptable occlusal relationship, so overjet was never really eliminated. Facial esthetics was of such great significance to the patient that a sizable Silastic chin implant was placed by a surgeon (on the parents' instructions) that eventually became well "inlayed" into the symphysis, as observed on a 1970 headplate (Fig 3-4). As a note of interest, some degree of scoliosis had been medically diagnosed and was clinically evident in this patient. According to the parents, the child had even been placed in a Milwaukee brace after orthodontic treatment. Many times a Milwaukee brace has been known to reduce lower facial height and position the chin more forward,[1] but even this did not enhance facial appearance, so the parents decided on the implant.

Later (1981), the patient's profile still seemed somewhat convex, but definitively not as retrognathic, because of the chin implant (Fig 3-5). Because of the largeness and position of the implant and the fact that points A and B had been retropositioned, his lips appeared more recessive than seemed desirable for good facial esthetics (nasoplastic surgery had been undertaken prior to the time of the photographs).

The molars were not in a full Class I relationship, but either end-to-end or slightly Class II, with the buccal dentition in a cusp-to-cusp interocclusal relationship (Fig 3-6). Surprisingly, despite the "Class II-ishness," there was no overjet; in fact, he had an almost edge-to-edge interincisal occlusion. An explanation for the minimal overjet was found on the lateral radiograph. The implant was well-imbedded in the symphysis (Fig 3-7) and seemed to have had an influence on the incisor apices: they seemed to be more closely related to the lingual plate of the symphysis while the crowns were considerably more proclined. It was almost as if the lower lip musculature had exerted pressure on the implant, which, in turn, had had a retropositioning

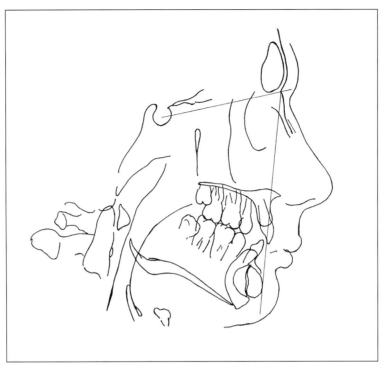

Fig 3-4 Patient B.B. Tracing of lateral cephalometric radiograph depicting Silastic chin implant.

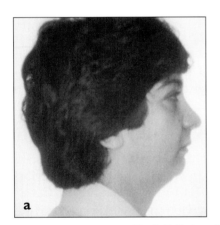 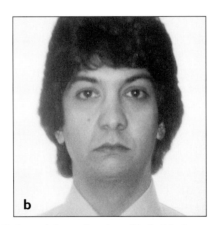 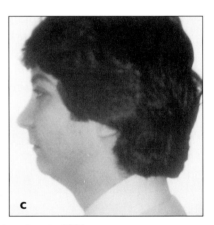

Fig 3-5 Patient B.B. (a to c) Frontal and profile facial photographs taken in 1981.

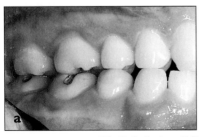 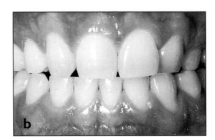 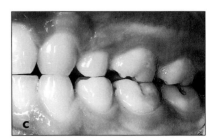

Fig 3-6 Patient B.B. (a to c) Intraoral photographs showing occlusal relationships in 1981.

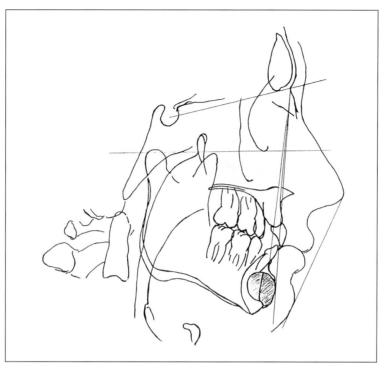

Fig 3-7 Patient B.B. Tracing of cephalometric radiograph revealed a deeper embedment of the Silastic implant in 1981.

effect on the incisor apices. Since the start of treatment, the symphysis during growth had been positioned considerably more downward than forward (Fig 3-8). Growth of the mandible had occurred, but not of the magnitude needed nor in the right direction to materially improve the anteroposterior occlusal relationship. There may have been some asymmetry in the growth of the two sides of the mandible since the midline relationship had altered materially.

The cervical appliance had been effective in controlling the forward positioning of point A, since this landmark had not come forward commensurate with the forward positioning of nasion. To a degree, this was also reflective of congenitally missing maxillary lateral incisors and the premolar extraction. As a consequence, the maxillary complex had ended in a slightly retruded position, which was helpful in its relationship to a retrognathic mandible. However, the severe mandibular retrognathism at an early age could not be overcome by growth nor treatment to reach a satisfactory conclusion.

Mandibular growth, both in direction and amount, had proved a disadvantage for correction of a Class II malocclusion. In this case, early orthodontic treatment could not overcome the severe limitations imposed by size and growth inadequacies.

Significance of mandibular growth in Class II correction

In evaluating treatment response and long-term stability in the correction of Class II malocclusion, it becomes evident that much is contingent on mandibular growth. Although the Class II malocclusion centered in the dentoalveolar relationships and with supporting jaws well related, treatment results usually seem to be well achieved and highly stable; of course, in these instances the mandible is also well related. When maxillary protrusion is evident and the mandible is well related to the cranium, then long-term stability of the correction can be an-

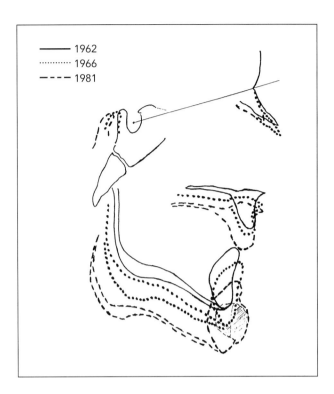

— 1962
········ 1966
---- 1981

Fig 3-8 Patient B.B. Superimposition of three serial cephalometric radiographs indicating predominately downward positioning of the mandibular symphysis from 1962 to 1981; the implant resulted in a more forward relationship of the chin.

ticipated and can usually be achieved by extractions in the maxilla to retroposition point A. Extraction of maxillary premolars will, of course, result in a Class II molar relation, which is preferable to increasing the overjet incident to retraction of mandibular incisors if mandibular premolars are extracted as well. If excessive maxillary protrusion exists, surgical retropositioning might be necessary, but this will still necessitate considerable orthodontic collaboration.

When the Class II malocclusion is the result of excessive mandibular retrognathism because of inadequate or adversely directed growth, the results and stability of orthodontic correction usually are not as good as might be hoped. However, early treatment still seems highly desirable, especially in those patients having aberrant skeletal growth patterns, since such treatment and continual observation can more definitively reveal the direction of mandibular growth. With this information the orthodontist can do whatever possible to prevent adverse mandibular growth from creating an even greater malrelationship and, conversely, enhance more favorably directed growth, potentially reducing the unfavorable skeletal relationship.

In evaluating orthodontically treated Class II malocclusions years out of retention, one gets some distinct impressions. Foremost is that extractions had to be undertaken in patients where the mandible was growing either poorly or asymmetrically. Particular reference is made to patients where it was found necessary to extract four premolars (not solely maxillary premolar extraction cases for maxillary prognathism). Another observation is that, in many Class II patients where extractions were undertaken, a deep bite seemed to develop years after treatment. In other cases, extractions were apparently done where it was subsequently observed that the two sides of the mandible were growing asymmetrically, indicating that not only the amount and direction, but also the symmetry, of mandibular growth seem to be a factor in the development and resolution of the Class II malocclusion.

Reference

1. Alexander RG. The Effects on Tooth Position and Maxillofacial Vertical Growth during Scoliosis Treatment with the Milwaukee Brace [thesis]. Houston: Univ of Texas, 1964.

Chapter 4

One Half of a Class II Malocclusion: Subdivision—Skeletal Maxilla or Mandible or Dental or All?

As diagnostic acumen improves, it is currently perceived that an increasing number of our patients have malocclusions that are related to asymmetrically growing mandibles.[1] These malocclusions exhibit considerable difficulty in orthodontic correction—sometimes never to a desired outcome—and with time appear to deteriorate, rather than improve. In some of these cases, the orthodontist may take refuge in the ego-saving comfort of "poor cooperation" or "failure to wear retainers"; but maybe—just maybe—these cases had unforeseen, undiagnosed, or unanticipated limitations, beyond capacity for a satisfactory result.

It is becoming clearly evident that disparate growth of the mandible can be the cause of myriad problems, sometimes obvious at an early age, sometimes so subtle that they do not become obvious until later, when much of the corrective possibilities have passed, with time compounding any possibility of alteration. It seems pertinent to initiate this discussion by presenting a patient (C.M.) who came into the office with a somewhat typical Class II, division 1, subdivision malocclusion late in the transitional dentition, with a retrognathic, convex facial pattern and considerable overjet (Fig 4-1). Records were taken, and a decision was made to institute headgear therapy to correct the Class II molar relation. The first mistake was a nonperceptive diagnosis, that is, we were not fully cognizant of

asymmetric mandibular growth at that state of the orthodontic art; it was perceived that continued mandibular growth would be helpful in correction of the overjet.

When orthodontic treatment was initiated, it was to correct the occlusion, rather than minimize and/or compensate for the differences in growth patterns between the right and left mandibles. During the course of treatment it became increasingly difficult to achieve a Class I molar relation; inadequate arch length led to four premolar extractions in order to achieve an acceptable occlusion and alignment (Fig 4-2). In retention, a reasonable occlusion was attained but, about 20 years later, facial asymmetry, particular mandibular asymmetry, became obvious (Fig 4-3). Relapse in molar relationship, overjet, and malalignment (with some maxillary and mandibular crowding and a distinct midline deviation) were noted (Fig 4-4). A clearly unsuccessful case. The occlusion was obvious, but what was missed were the telltale signs on the cephalometric radiographs taken prior to treatment: the disparate sizes of the right and left rami, two distinct lower borders of the mandible, and two different occlusal levels of posterior teeth—all clearly observable on the lateral centric headplate. The frontal headplate clearly showed differences in shapes and heights of the rami, as well as the midline deviation.

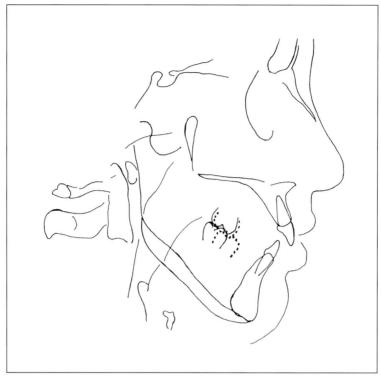

Fig 4-1 Cephalometric tracing of C.M. indicating a unilateral Class II molar relationship and considerable anterior overjet.

What was missed? The mandibular asymmetry and the potential continual disparity in growth of the right and left mandibles, that is, treating the malocclusion and not the malgrowing, disproportionate skeleton. It's "As the jaw grows, the teeth go," and not vice versa. The skeleton must be treated instead of the malocclusion. How should this or a similar patient have been treated? This will be discussed later when the procedures for dealing with asymmetrically growing mandibles are presented.

Class II, Division 1, Subdivision— An "Out-of-Place" Malocclusion

A befuddling problem is the occasional patient with a unilateral Class II malocclusion: the Class II, division 1, subdivision that presents marked difficulty in orthodontic correction, and even at times slowly relapses toward the original occlusal malrelationship after correction. The author has come to the conclusion that a proportion of these patients do not manifest a solely dental or dentoalveolar malocclusion on the Class II side, but demonstrate either a unilateral mandibular growth problem or a unilateral skeletal aberration in form or position. The author has learned to beware the Class II, division 1, subdivision. It may not be dentoalveolar; it may be mandibular asymmetry incident to a unilateral reduction or retardation in growth. Of course, it must be acknowledged that the mandible normally grows asymmetrically and that a certain amount of asymmetry is typical. For example, Melnik[2] has shown that, at early ages (6 to 9 years), the left side of the mandible is usually longer and at adolescence (16 years), the right side is longer. So mandibular asymmetry is normal; but why, in some individuals, is the discrepancy such that it manifests itself as a

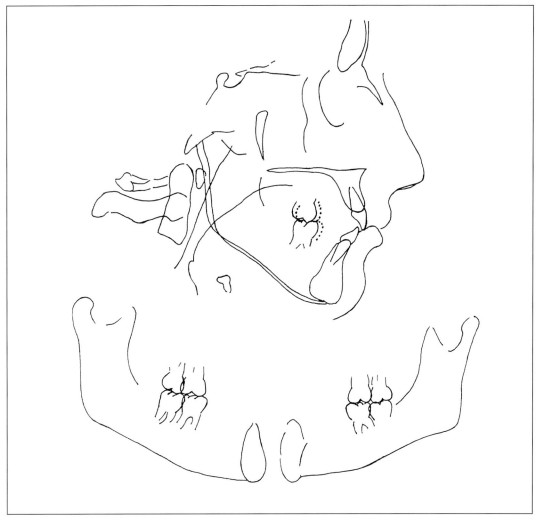

Fig 4-2 Patient C.M. Tracings of lateral and oblique radiographs indicating a Class I (bilateral) molar relationship and reduction of anterior overjet.

Class II subdivision malocclusion? Investigators[3] have studied skeletal and dentoalveolar asymmetry in Class II subdivision subjects. They determined that, on the Class II side, the mandibular first molar was positioned more posteriorly relative to its base (the skeletal mandible) and to the cranium, but the mandible itself was not measurably asymmetric. In a subsequent study of adults with unilateral posterior crossbite, it was found that the mandibular first molar on the side of the crossbite was more lateral and more posterior, as well as posteriorly rotated when compared with the first molar on the noncrossbite side. Again, mandibular asymmetry was not

a recognizable cause nor were the condyles asymmetrically positioned within the temporomandibular fossae, suggesting a more posteriorly positioned glenoid fossa on the crossbite side. It was hypothesized that, during growth and remodeling, the glenoid fossa had become located more posteriorly on the base of the cranium, causing the adult mandible to rotate posteriorly on the crossbite side.

In a longitudinal study conducted by Dibbets et al,[4] which included children with subjective symptoms of TMJ dysfunction, he found that those children shared certain characteristics of craniofacial dysmorphology: the mandibular

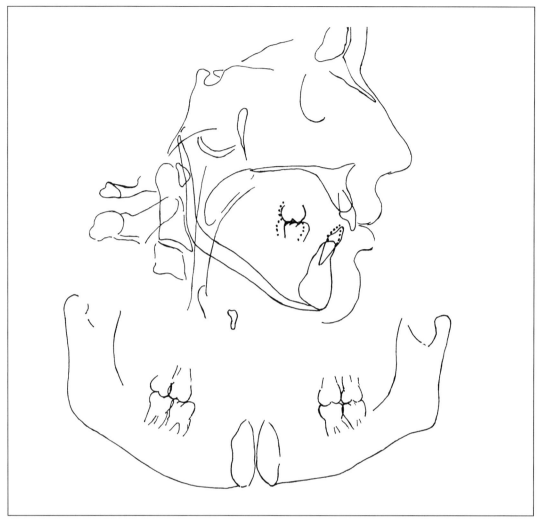

Fig 4-3 Tracings of lateral and oblique radiographs of C.M. about 20 years later, indicating changes that occurred and were observable at the time of recall.

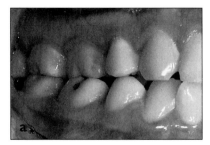 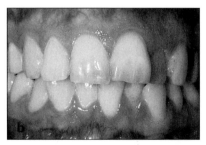 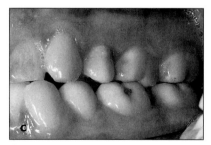

Fig 4-4 Patient C.M. *(a to c)* Relationships of the dentition at the time of recall.

body and the ramus were shorter, the distance from chin to condyle was smaller, and the skeletal profile was more characteristic of Class II when compared with other patients in the study. The assumption is that TMJ dysfunction could reduce the amount of mandibular growth; this reduction or retardation could then be directed toward a "Class II-ish" occlusal relationship and thereby the possibility of a subdivision malocclusion if it is manifested on one side. In fact, in a report[5] on adults undergoing surgery for internal derangement of the TMJ, a small number were shown to have a Class II, division 1, subdivision malocclusion along with small or deformed condyles and a mandibular deviation toward the side of derangement. Half of those in the subdivision group were found to have a Class II malocclusion on the deranged side and a Class I molar relationship with normal condylar and disc morphology on the other side. The others had bilateral internal derangement, but the side with the more advanced derangement exhibited a greater degree of Class II-ishness in molar relation and more condylar deformation or smallness.

One can surmise that a certain proportion of youngsters with Class II, division 1, subdivision malocclusions might be experiencing TMJ dysfunction and internal derangement on the Class II side that could lead to growth disturbance on that side. Although expressed minimally toward Class II while the patient is young, the condition may become more pronounced with growth and age. There may be a growth- and skeletal-related reason for difficulty in correction of the unilateral Class II malocclusion and for its progressive relapse after correction. Thereby the statement: in some cases the Class II, division 1, subdivision may not be solely a dental malocclusion; it might be a skeletal malocclusion, albeit unilateral. Never judge a book by its cover!

In a recent study,[6] utilizing 45-degree oblique as well as lateral and frontal cephalometric radiographs, 29 individuals with Class II, division 1, subdivision malocclusions averaging approximately 12 years of age (range, 7 to 16 years), were evaluated prior to initiating orthodontic treatment. In comparing ramus height on the Class II side with that on the Class I side investigators found that the heights were equal in 48% of the subjects, but the Class II side was

shorter in 31%. In evaluating effective mandibular length, the Class II side was found to be shorter in 48% of the subjects and equal in 35%. Again, an indication that problematic asymmetric growth of the two sides of the mandible may be operative in a number of the Class II, division 1, subdivision malocclusions.

If, in truth, some of these patients have unilateral retardation in growth, then a dilemma in orthodontic treatment presents itself. The unilateral mandibular body and ramus, and possibly the glenoid fossa, must be positioned forward—a formidable task that should be accomplished slowly and during times of greatest residual growth potential. To accomplish unilateral forward positioning of the dentoalveolar process is difficult at best; retropositioning the maxillary buccal dentoalveolar segment may be undesirable because it can create arch asymmetry and an undesirable shifting of the maxillary dental midline. Furthermore, many of the unilateral Class II patients may have a steep mandibular plane incident to the relatively short ramus on the Class II side. Opening the occlusal plane in these cases under the influence of Class II mechanics could lead to an increase in lower facial height with some chin retropositioning. Braun et al[7] showed that, in Class II treatment, for each half millimeter of anteroposterior molar correction, the occlusal plane is opened 1 degree. Correcting a Class II molar relationship to a Class I may require several degrees of occlusal plane opening, which has a tendency to occur during Class II elastic therapy. This could lead to a steeper mandibular plane, opening the anterior vertical dimension more than desired and creating a complication in Class II, division 1, subdivision treatment. Thus, there is an obvious need for an accurate diagnosis and an awareness of the potential asymmetry of mandibular growth, which can become more pronounced with time.

It seems particularly important in a Class II subdivision case that we be cognizant of the fact that the Class II side might be expressing reduced growth. Diagnostic clues include the fact that, first, the maxillary arch is symmetrical but the mandibular arch is back on the subdivision side where the molars are in Class II. Second, the occlusal plane may be tipped cranially from the Class I side toward the Class II side, indicating a concomitant reduction in vertical dentoalveolar development on the Class II side. The maxillary dentoalveolar arch may be compensating vertically for the reduced vertical dimension in the mandible. Once unilateral mandibular growth reduction is recognized, it is important to initiate orthopedic forces to attempt stimulation of mandibular growth on that side. Conventional Class II mechanics cannot be utilized; if a unilateral headgear is placed, we may be moving a symmetrical maxillary arch into an asymmetric relationship with a deviated midline. If light Class II elastics are used on the Class II side, again, some asymmetry may be produced in the maxillary arch while advancing the mandibular dentoalveolar arch. This does not compensate for what may be an asymmetrically growing mandible. In other words, it is particularly pertinent to introduce orthopedic forces on the Class II side. Dental arch movements alone would create asymmetries between the right and left maxillary dentoalveolar segments while we were attempting to improve the mandibular dentoalveolar segment. Additionally, it is important to initiate these forces during young age levels to avail ourselves of the greatest amount of potential growth, which, in turn, could be utilized by the deficient side. If the full permanent dentition is awaited to initiate treatment, then much growth may be lost. A certain number of our Class II, division 1, subdivision cases will be growth problems, possibly related to some TMJ derangement, dysmorphology, or growth disturbance. Orthopedic forces on that side must be initiated at as early an age as possible.

Condylar Degeneration and Class II Skeletal Malocclusion: Rare but Present

Mandibular growth and alteration in mandibular growth patterns can change an occlusion. In fact, it is even logical to assume that a number of bilateral Class II malocclusions are related to condylar problems that lead to a reduction in the amount of mandibular growth, particularly ramal growth; they could also alter the direction of mandibular body growth, which at times may

be expressed as a bending of the mandibular body and an increase in lower facial height. To illustrate, a case will be presented that was determined to be related to condylar degeneration of unknown cause, but presumed to be trauma. The patient was treated as a Class I nonextraction case and retained with an acceptable result. Several years later the patient returned with an open bite and a more severe Class II malocclusion.

Patient A.M.P. The initial records for this 10-year-old patient indicated a nice facial pattern for her age. She was slightly retrognathic and convex, and had well-related denture bases in the transitional dentition. From the radiographs, a well-formed mandible was noted with good width to the rami and the symphysis (Fig 4-5). She had a very acceptable bilateral Class I molar relationship and a small overjet, but a greater-than-desirable overbite. The frontal radiograph showed acceptable skeletal facial symmetry with a small difference in the level of the right and left sides of the nasal floor (Fig 4-6). There was a small discrepancy in midline relationships, the mandibular midline being slightly to the left. Of note, the lateral cephalometric radiograph showed two distinct and separated lower mandibular borders.

The patient was treated to an acceptable occlusion (a full Class I molar relation on the right side and not quite a full Class I on the left) and placed into retention. An acceptable overbite was attained and the midline relationship was much improved, with the mandibular midline slightly to the left. The lateral cephalometric radiograph at the time of retention indicated that a good maxillomandibular relationship had been achieved (Fig 4-7); good balance was noted in the skeletal profile and photographs revealed very pleasing facial characteristics, both in the profile and frontal perspectives.

Six years later, a completely new occlusion, completely new facial characteristics, and completely new skeletal relationships were evident (Fig 4-8). The facial profile had assumed a highly retrognathic, convex appearance. From the frontal perspective (Fig 4-9) the soft tissue chin appeared deviated slightly to the left. Examination of the occlusion revealed a pronounced anterior open bite and a mandibular midline

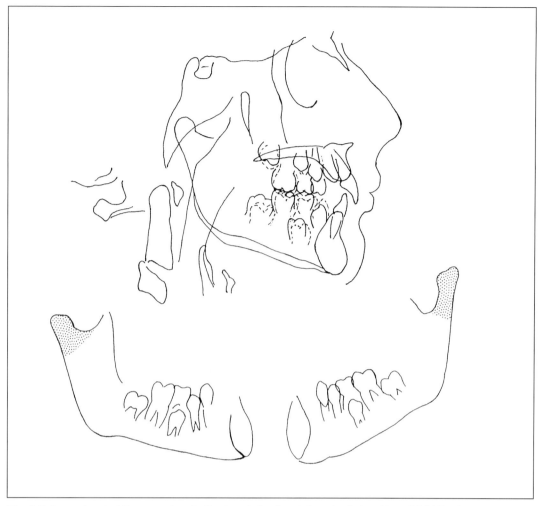

Fig 4-5 Lateral and oblique tracings indicating skeletal and dental relationships of A.M.P. prior to initiation of orthodontic treatment.

noticeably to the left of the maxillary midline. Whereas the left buccal segment was still in Class I, the right buccal segment was now in more of a Class II molar relationship—a complete alteration of the occlusion achieved at retention. The lateral headplate revealed a distinct bending of the body of the mandible anterior to gonion, creating a steep mandibular plane from what had previously been a more flat, acceptable plane. With this change, a marked increase in lower facial height was also noted.

Superimposition of the oblique radiographs (Fig 4-10) taken at each stage—treatment, retention, and final observation—revealed that from treatment to retention there was increment in the heights of the rami (from gonion to the top of the condyle) and in the 6 years from retention to final observation there was a marked reduction in ramal heights. The diagnosis was idiopathic degeneration of the condyles and their necks. There was a history of several traumas, such as falling out of trees, but nothing definitive enough to move it out of the category of idiopathic. Laminagraphs revealed functional movements of the condyles, but there was alteration in form and apparent close contact with the articular eminence when in centric relation. One can only surmise alteration in function and,

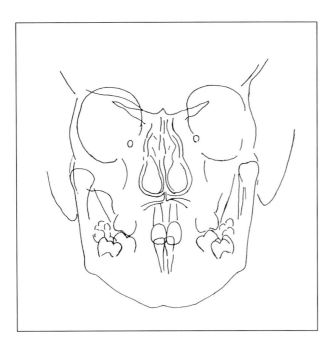

Fig 4-6 Tracing of frontal cephalometric radiograph (A.M.P.) indicating skeletal relationships and anterior dental midline discrepancy.

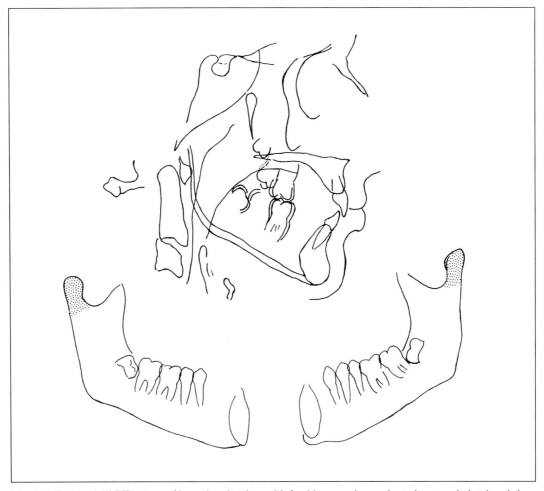

Fig 4-7 Patient A.M.P. Tracings of lateral and right and left oblique radiographs indicating skeletal and dental relationships at time of retention.

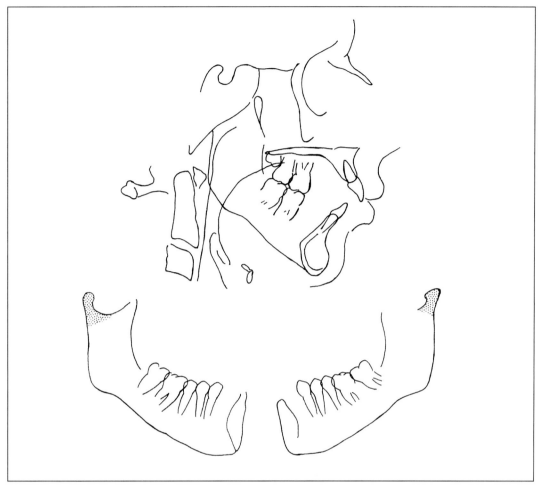

Fig 4-8 Patient A.M.P. Lateral and oblique radiograph tracings revealing marked change in skeletal and dental relationships: now Class II and an anterior open bite.

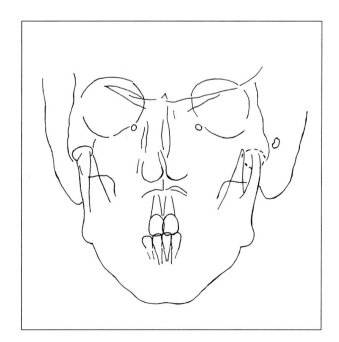

Fig 4-9 Patient A.M.P. Frontal radiograph tracing revealing midline discrepancies and skeletal facial asymmetry.

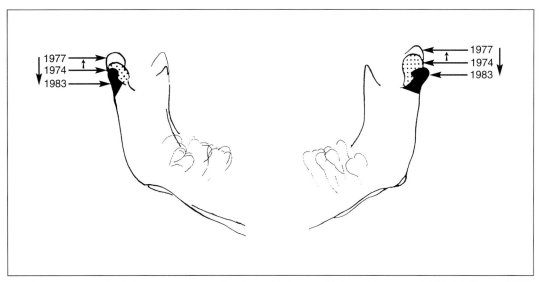

Fig 4-10 Patient A.M.P. Superimposition of right and left mandibular obliques in 1974, 1977, and 1983. Note the change in size and shape of the condyles and the apparent atrophy or reduction from 1977 to 1983.

with that, altered muscle function, an influence causing change in mandibular configuration incident to the condylar degeneration. A dramatic change from a good Class I occlusion to an undesirable Class II subdivision, open bite malocclusion causing an unfavorable alteration of the facial profile.

References

1. Tallents RH, Guay J, Katzberg WR, Murphy W, Proskin H. Angular and linear comparisons with unilateral mandibular asymmetry. J Craniomandib Disord 1991;5:135–142.
2. Melnik AK. A cephalometric study of mandibular asymmetry in a longitudinally followed sample of growing children. Am J Orthod Dentofac Orthop 1992;101: 355–366.
3. Rose JM, Sadowsky C, BeGole EA, Moles R. Mandibular skeletal and dental asymmetry in Class II subdivision malocclusions. Am J Orthod Dentofac Orthop 1994; 105:489–495.
4. Dibbets JMH, Van der Weele LT, Boering G. Craniofacial morphology and temporomandibular joint dysfunction in children. In: Carlson DS, McNamara JA Jr, Ribbens KA (eds). Developmental Aspects of Temporomandibular Joint Disorders, monograph 16, Craniofacial Growth Series. Ann Arbor, MI: Univ of Michigan, 1985:151–182.
5. Schellhas KP, Pollei SR, Wilkes CH. Pediatric internal derangements of the temporomandibular joint: Effect on facial development. Am J Orthod Dentofac Orthop 1993;104:51–59.
6. Sommers EW. Class II division 1 subdivision: A cephalometric study of mandibular asymmetry. Presented at the North Atlantic Component meeting of the Edw H Angle Soc of Orthodontists, Baltimore, May 1995.
7. Braun S, Sjursen RC, Legan HL. On the management of extraction sites. Am J Orthod Dentofac Orthop 1997;112:645–655.

Part II

Mandibular Jaw Malocclusions

Chapter 5

Mandibular Skeletal Malocclusions

Mandibular Retrognathism

Unquestionably, a good many problems in occlusal relationships reside in the size and shape of the mandible as well as in its position. One of the problems, readily noted at an early age, is the continuing development of severe mandibular retrognathism. We are not referring to the mandible that, for all practical purposes, is acceptably retrognathic for the early age levels where facial convexity predominates, but the mandible that is severely retrognathic incident to a genetic predisposition and/or a growth problem.

Patient D.H. This is a clear example of severe retrognathia: an individual with congenital birth defects involving the mandible as well as digits on each hand—pycnodysostosis. The congenital dysmorphology of the mandible involved severe shortness of the rami and the body of the mandible (resulting in severe dental crowding), a severe Class II molar relationship with excessive overjet, bilateral posterior crossbite, and an open bite. Also evident was excessive antegonial bending as well as notching. In many areas severe gingivoalveolar recession was evident. On the lateral cephalometric radiograph, the patient appeared to be literally swallowing his tongue. He had notably reduced and minimal retrolingual airway space and a hyoid bone inferior and posterior to the retruded posi-

tion of the mandibular symphasis. The patient experienced severe respiratory discomfort, not unlike sleep apnea (Figs 5-1 to 5-4). At an early age, as well as in his teens, the patient (and his parents) refused the option of orthognathic surgery because of possible need for blood transfusions. It should also be mentioned that, at that time, distraction osteogenesis was not known relative to the possibilities of lengthening the mandible, which today might be a consideration, especially at early age levels.

The patient desired esthetic improvement in the permanent dentition, so dental alignment and occlusal improvement were undertaken and accomplished with the extraction of four premolars and one mandibular incisor. Esthetic dental alignment was achieved, with some correction of the overjet as well as the maxillary constriction and open bite (Figs 5-5 and 5-6). However, the limitations imposed by the skeletal dysplasia—the severe mandibular retrognathism and malconfiguration—could not be overcome. There could only be minimal improvement in jaw relationships short of orthognathic surgery, conventionally at later age levels. Today, if done earlier, distraction osteogenesis would be a viable consideration, by which to alter the length and, to a degree, the shape of the mandible. It is not likely that the desired improvement in skeletal mandibular configuration and position could have been achieved by conventional

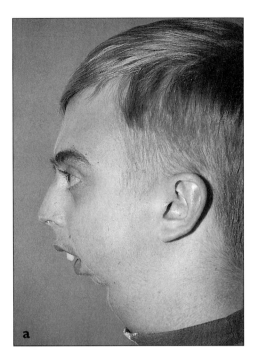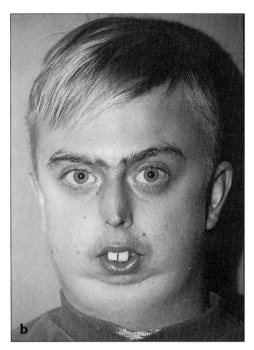

Fig 5-1 Patient D.H. *(a, b)* Photographs of a young male born with excessive congenital mandibular retrognathia.

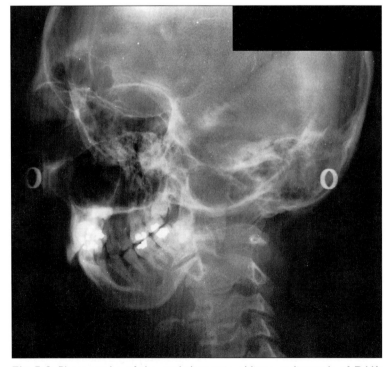

Fig 5-2 Photographs of the cephalometric oblique radiograph of D.H.'s right mandible, revealing short ramal height and excessive antegonial bend.

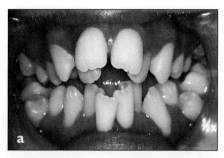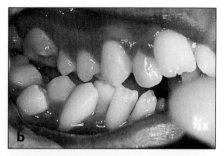

Fig 5-3 *(a, b)* Intraoral photographs of D.H.'s malocclusion revealing the open bite, severe crowding, Class II molar relationship, and the concomitant overjet.

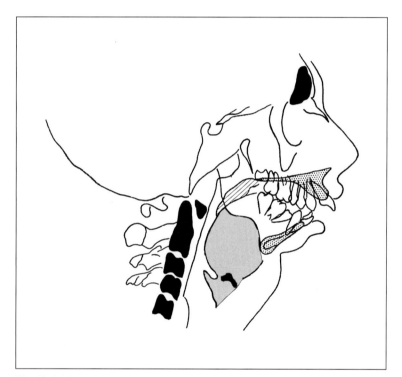

Fig 5-4 Illustrations of the cephalometric lateral radiograph tracing of D.H., indicating skeletal relationships and the posterior posture of the tongue.

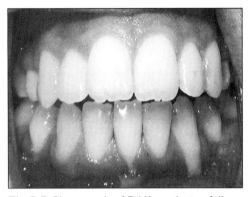

Fig 5-5 Photograph of D.H.'s occlusion following orthodontic correction.

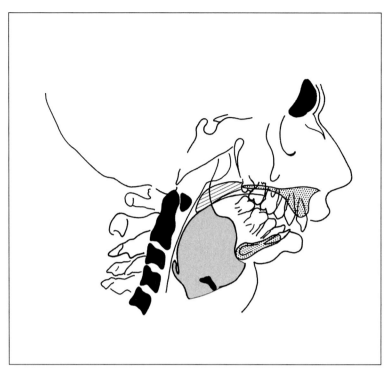

Fig 5-6 Illustrative cephalometric tracing of D.H. following completion of orthodontic treatment. Much of the dentofacioskeletal relations are still evident.

orthodontic/orthopedic influences. In the near past, appliance therapy had been instituted with the distinct hope of stimulating mandibular growth to a greater extent than what would be expected from natural growth processes. Reference is being made to functional appliances. Recent documentation[1-3] has cast considerable doubt whether these appliances are capable of stimulating additional clinically significant mandibular growth, especially in a markedly retrognathic individual who seemed beyond the full expression of mandibular growth that would be needed at the time of appliance application. However, as will be demonstrated later, functional appliance therapy may be usefully applied toward attaining whatever unilateral mandibular growth might be consistent with the patient's genetic potential.

Mandibular Asymmetry

Prelude to mandibular asymmetry

A perplexing problem is the individual whose face appears to become progressively asymmetric, not only in natural development but during treatment as well. There is no question that, generally, the human face is not truly symmetric, but when not beyond certain perceptible limits of asymmetry, the face appears harmonious and pleasing to the eye. In most instances facial asymmetry is so slight that it cannot be readily visualized, but beyond acceptable ranges of variation facial asymmetry becomes readily observable and usually not desirable. Thus a "normal" range of variability in facial asymmetry must be recognized and accepted.

Generally, aside from congenital deformation or malformation of craniofacial skeletal structures—particularly the jaws—when facial asymmetry is perceived, it frequently comes to attention by an observable deviation in the position of the chin away from the facial midline. This leads to the recognition that a significant degree of facial asymmetry may be related to asymmetric mandibular growth or some factor necessitating a mandibular compensating posture. Congenitally or acquired unilateral mandibular growth problems, with the two sides of the mandible growing at different rates, will eventually result in the chin deviating to one side of the facial midline. One can readily assume that, if this deviation is observable in a young patient, it will increase in severity with age and continuous growth. The result may be excessive facial asymmetry, quite undesirable to perceive and which may be difficult, at best, to treat—even with the adjunct of corrective surgery.

The monkey—An illustration of asymmetry

The extent of skeletal facial asymmetry that could be manifest at later age levels is well depicted by the photographs of the skull of a grown monkey that presumably had suffered a fracture or some trauma in the right condylar area at a young age. From the frontal perspective (Fig 5-7), gross facial asymmetry was obvious, with the chin severely deviated to the fracture side. Vertically, the skeletal face on the fracture side was considerably shorter and the lower borders of the mandible were severely tilted cranially, visualizing from the nonfractured side to the fractured side. The occlusal plane deviated to conform to the tilt of the lower mandibular borders. Viewed from the posterior (Fig 5-8), the ramus on the fractured side is obviously shorter. From the lateral perspective (Fig 5-9) of the nonfractured side, the mandible appears well formed and well sized, and it completely prevents the fractured side from being seen. From the fractured side, it is obvious that the shortness of the ramus permits a complete visualization of the gonial region and the lower border of the nonfractured side. It is presumed that, incidental to the trauma, the mandible did not continue to grow symmetrically despite the regeneration of a condyle (bulbous and distorted) on the fractured side (Fig 5-10). When the disarticulated mandible is visualized (Fig 5-11), differences between the two sides are clearly recognized. The development of such problems is not exclusive to an isolated monkey; it has been demonstrated in individual cases under treatment in orthodontic practice.

Unrecognized developing mandibular asymmetry in patients

This can best be exemplified by individual cases where a potential for mandibular growth was present, but something happened along the way to alter it in one of the condylar regions. Incidental to trauma, in some cases, growth has been observed to be retarded or reduced on one side of the mandible. In these instances, it is not unusual to observe that continued full expression of mandibular growth on the nontraumatized side caused the chin to progressively deviate toward the affected side, causing visible facial asymmetry and disfigurements. Thus, mandibular asymmetry might not be readily discernible at an early age but, by the time of completion of mandibular growth, can result in a markedly visible deviation of the chin and mandible toward the affected side. By this time, most of the corrective possibilities are more limited and difficult, as the deviation progresses.

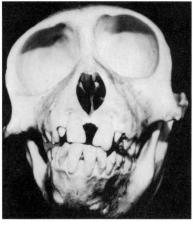

Fig 5-7 Monkey skull revealing gross facial skeletal asymmetry with severe chin deviation to the right. (Courtesy of Dr Al Moore, University of Washington.)

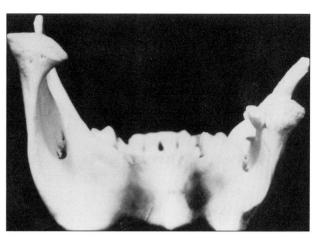

Fig 5-8 Posterior view of the monkey mandible reveals the shorter ramus on the right side. (Courtesy of Dr Al Moore, University of Washington.)

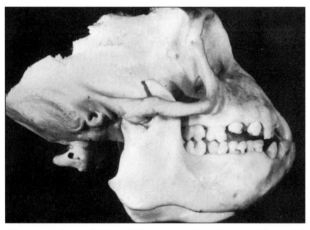

Fig 5-9 The right mandible reveals the shorter ramus and the higher level of the bottom of the right mandibular body. (Courtesy of Dr Al Moore, University of Washington.)

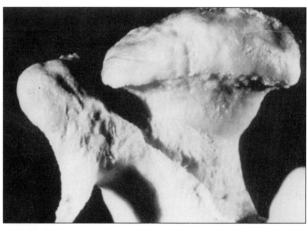

Fig 5-10 Bulbous, distorted condyle on the right side with what appears to be a repaired fracture line at the neck. (Courtesy of Dr Al Moore, University of Washington.)

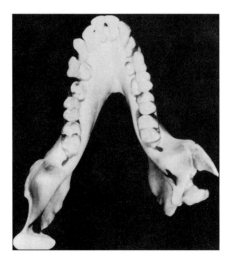

Fig 5-11 Occlusal view of the mandible revealing clear differences at the ramal sites of both sides of the mandible. (Courtesy of Dr Al Moore, University of Washington.)

Case presentations

Patient S.R. Changes in the condylar region have been observed to affect facial appearance, alteration in mandibular growth, and, thereby, occlusal relationships. This is well exemplified by patient S.R., who had a somewhat typical Class II, division 1 malocclusion in the early transitional dentition with considerable overjet, too much overbite, and a retrognathic, convex facial pattern. After records were taken, a decision was made that she was not ready for contemplated headgear therapy in conjunction with a bite plate and lip bumper, so treatment was delayed for 1 year. The following year it became obvious that a serious mistake—as well as a nonperceptive diagnosis—had been made, since the asymmetric mandibular configuration had not been noticed. The occlusion was obvious, but what was missed were the telltale signs on the initial cephalometric radiographs (Fig 5-12): the disparate sizes of the right and left mandibles, two distinct lower and posterior borders, and two different occlusal levels of the posterior teeth—all clearly observable on the radiographs. The midline deviation was evident on the frontal head plate (Fig 5-13), and, in conjunction with the two obliques, clearly showed differences in height and shape between the right and left rami. Facial asymmetry was present on the frontal photographs (Fig 5-14).

When orthodontic treatment was initiated, it was to correct the occlusion, rather than to mini-mize or compensate for the variance in the two mandibles and the differences in their growth patterns. During the course of treatment it became increasingly difficult to achieve a bilateral Class I molar relationship. A midline disparity and, finally, inadequate mandibular arch length (particularly on one side), led to four premolar extractions in order to achieve an adequate occlusion and acceptable alignment (Figs 5-15a and 5-15b). It was during retention that facial asymmetry, particularly mandibular asymmetry (Fig 5-16), became obvious. Orthodontically, a well-aligned dentition with good occlusion was achieved, but unfortunately the maxillary arch was aligned to a skewed mandibular arch on a distorted skeletal base. The smile showed nicely aligned teeth, but the alignment was out of place. In an attempt to improve facial appearance, it was decided to perform a right-sided genioplasty in order to achieve some symmetry (Figs 5-17) and to minimize the skewed position of the occlusion. This was an obvious compromise that aided the appearance but was far from ideal.

What was missed? The mandibular skeletal asymmetry and the continual disparity in growth between the right and left mandibles (Figs 5-18 and 5-19). Again we were treating the malocclusion and not the malgrowing, disproportionate, supporting skeleton. In such cases, the skeleton must be treated instead of the malocclusion to attain the best possible result.

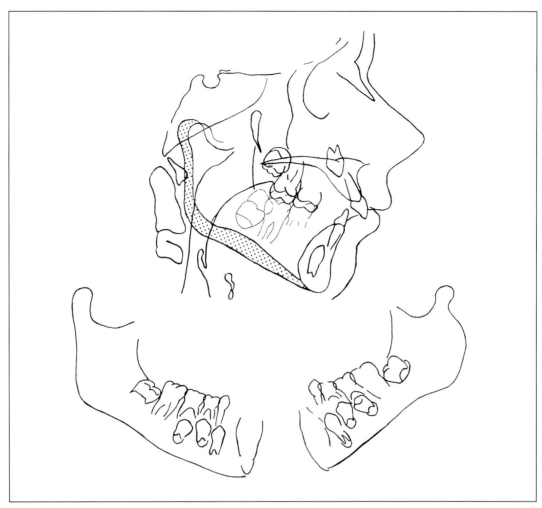

Fig 5-12 Tracings of lateral cephalometric and right and left oblique radiographs of S.R., depicting the disparity in the mandibles and the occlusal levels of the posterior occlusion.

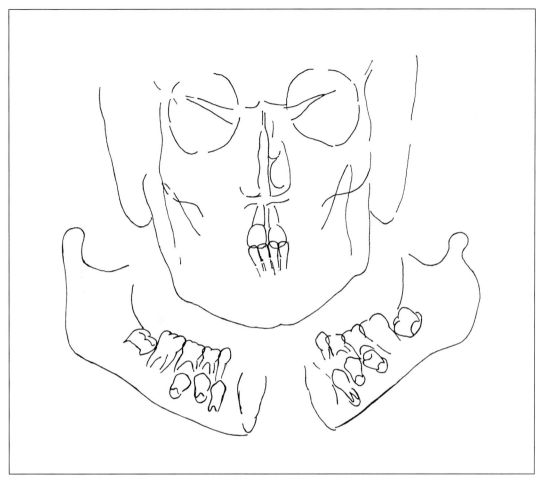

Fig 5-13 Patient S. R. Tracings of the frontal and oblique radiographs, revealing facial asymmetry incident to the asymmetric right and left mandibles.

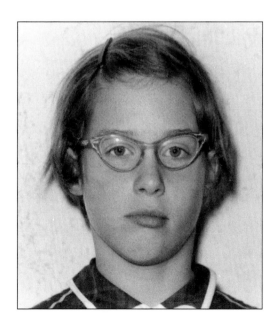

Fig 5-14 Frontal photograph of S.R. Note asymmetry incident to chin position and mandibular heights in the gonial region.

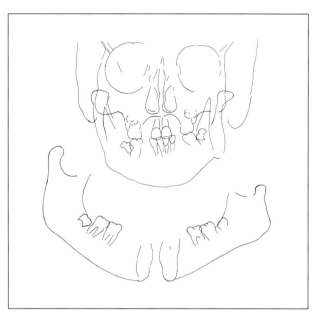

Fig 5-15a Frontal and oblique radiograph tracings of S.R. at the time of retention.

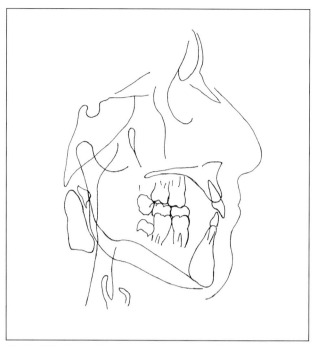

Fig 5-15b Lateral radiograph tracing of S.R. at the time of retention.

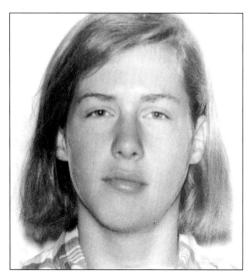

Fig 5-16 Patient S.R. Frontal photograph indicating facial asymmetry at the time it became apparent to the parents as well as the orthodontist.

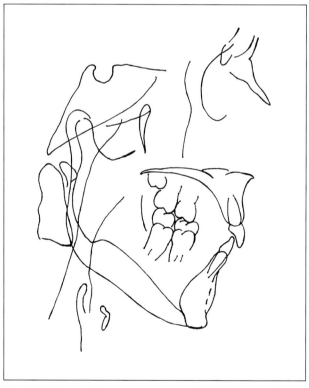

Fig 5-17 Lateral headplate tracing of S.R. following hemimentoplasty; the prominent aspect of the deviated chin was resected.

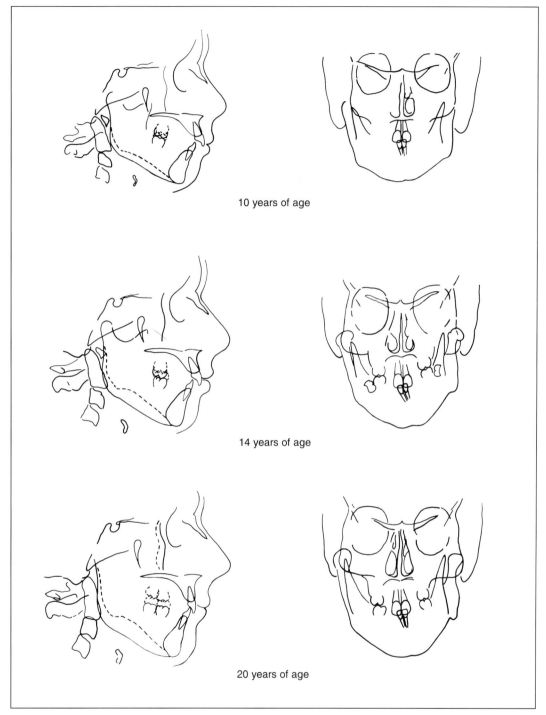

10 years of age

14 years of age

20 years of age

Fig 5-18 Cephalometric tracings of S.R. at three different ages, depicting continued growth of the asymmetric mandible.

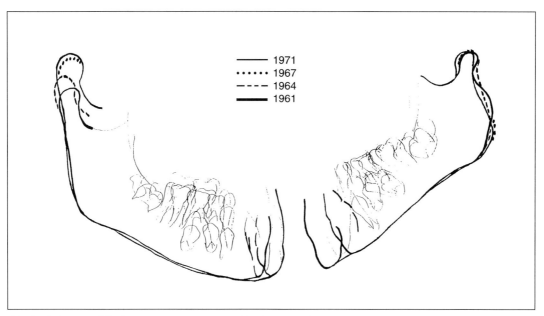

Fig 5-19 Patient S.R. Superimposed tracings of right and left mandibular oblique radiographs at four different years and age levels, revealing differences in extent of ramal growth.

Patient M.C. It seems advisable at this point to present the second case, one with a similar result, but with a definitively different cause. The patient presented at 11 years of age (in the transitional dentition) after initial records (Fig 5-20) had been taken and first premolars had been extracted as part of a serial extraction program at another office. She presented with a mesognathic (straight) facial pattern with lips back, a bilateral Class I molar relation, a deep overbite, and mandibular anterior crowding (Fig 5-21). She exhibited what is sometimes called a "super Class I" on the left side with a resultant midline discrepancy, the mandibular midline to the right. She also presented a temporomandibular joint click on the left side, but no pain. The lateral cephalometric radiograph showed two posterior borders of the rami as well as two distinct gonial regions (Fig 5-22a). The frontal head plate revealed some skeletal facial asymmetry, with the mandibular midline slightly to the right and the vertical position of the right gonial region more cranially located.

At the time of retention approximately 3 years later, she had been treated to a well-aligned, well-configured occlusion, but all the aforementioned characteristics—the super Class I on one side, the asymmetric position of both ramal posterior borders, and the vertical skeletal asymmetry as seen on the frontal cephalogram—were still clearly evident (Fig 5-22b). Facial asymmetry was more obvious and the deviation of the chin to the right was even more evident. It was now clear that the mandible was growing asymmetrically—the left side growing more than the right—placing the lower midline to the right. She stayed in retention for a while as the asymmetry became progressively more pronounced (Fig 5-23).

In an attempt to reduce the asymmetry, we placed her on a functional appliance (Harvold type), to correct the mandibular midline by bringing it to the left in order to achieve more vertical dimension on the right (Fig 5-24); in essence she was brought to a more super Class I molar relationship, somewhat comparable to

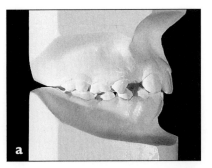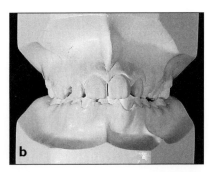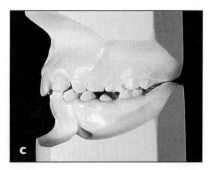

Fig 5-20 Patient M.C. *(a to c)* Casts depicting the occlusion at the time of initial records, preceding extraction of four first premolars.

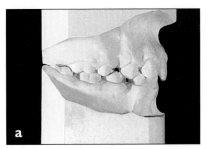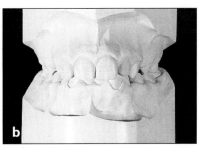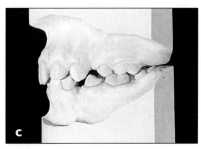

Fig 5-21 Patient M.C. *(a to c)* Casts 1 year later, after extractions had been undertaken at the previous office (before transfer).

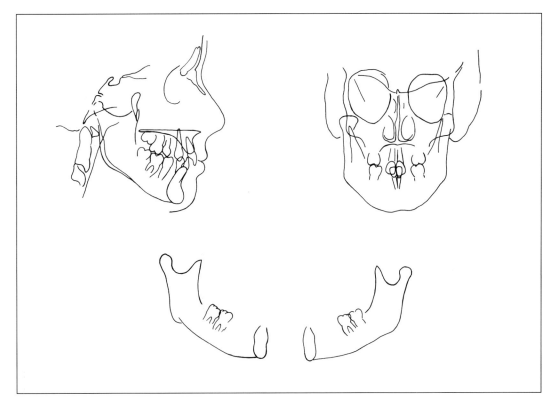

Fig 5-22a M.C. Tracings of lateral, frontal, and oblique radiographs depicting relationship of structures at 11 years of age.

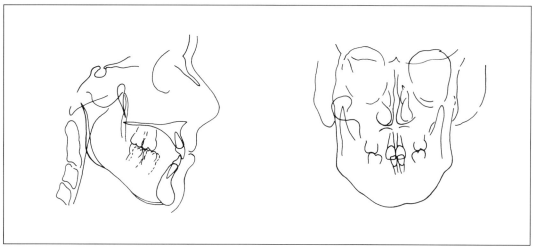

Fig 5-22b Patient M.C.Cephalometric tracings reveal the dental and skeletal relationships at the time of retention (14 years of age).

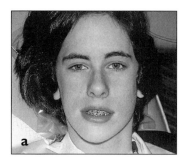 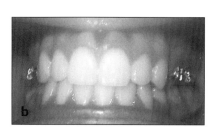 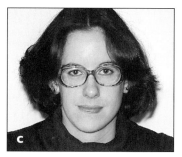

Fig 5-23 Patient M.C. *(a)* Frontal photograph taken 1 year before retention showing asymmetry; *(b)* occlusion shortly after retention; *(c)* frontal photograph 1 year after retention.

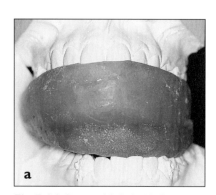 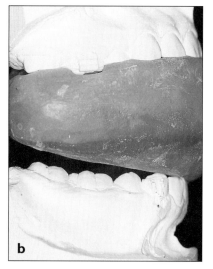

Fig 5-24 Patient M.C. *(a, b)* Casts with the intensive functional appliance, indicating mandibular arch being forced to the left and extent of desired eruption on the right.

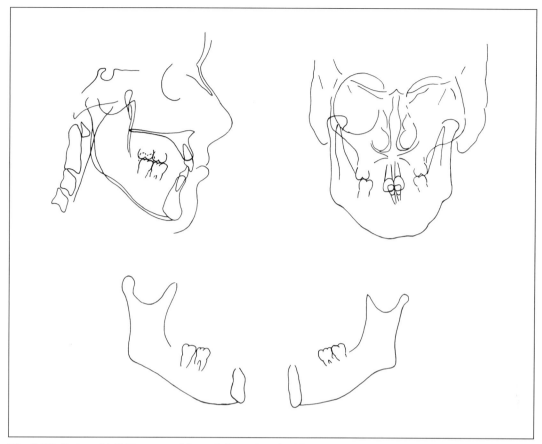

Fig 5-25 Patient M.C. Tracings of lateral, frontal, and oblique radiographs revealing skeletal and dental asymmetries at 20 years of age.

the other side. However, the patient was becoming more asymmetric skeletally (Fig 5-25). Actually, the wrong approach was being used to correct the asymmetry: it was finally diagnosed as hyperplasia of the left condyle and not hypoplasia of the right condyle (Fig 5-26). Two years later she was still noticeably asymmetric facially and the dentition was well aligned, but the midline discrepancy (the mandible to the right) and the Class III relationship of the left molars were clearly evident (Fig 5-27). Fallaciously we were working to make the normal side grow more but that was not the problem. Both hyperplasia and hypoplasia will create a

mandibular midline deviation; thus, whichever side of the mandible is growing more will cause a midline deviation toward the other side. In the case of hypoplasia, the affected side of the mandible is growing less, so the mandibular teeth will fall back into a more Class II occlusal relationship while the midline will deviate toward that side. In the case of hyperplasia, the mandibular midline will deviate away from the hyperplastic side, while the molars on that side will advance anteriorly into a super Class I or a Class III relationship. This of course, assumes that the maxilla is reasonably symmetric anteroposteriorly on both sides.

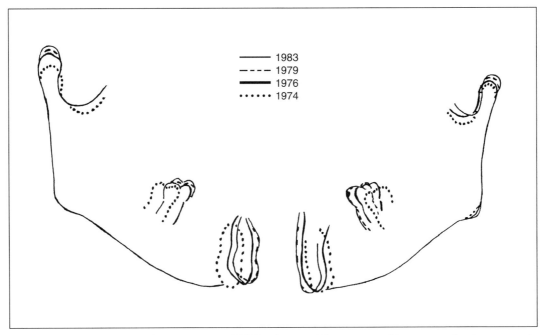

Fig 5-26 Superimposed oblique tracings of M.C. taken at different ages. Note excessive increment in condylar height on left.

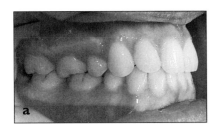

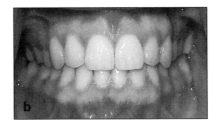

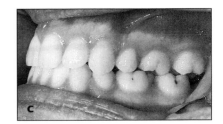

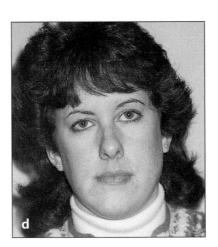

Fig 5-27 Patient M.C. (*a to d*) Intra-oral occlusal and frontal views 2 years later.

Patient A.S. The author's daughter represents another case in which unforeseen growth—unilateral condylar hyperplasia—can lead to undesirable mandibular and facial asymmetry. The patient was treated at a young age to correct a unilateral (right) crossbite of the posterior teeth. Records indicated nothing unusual at the time treatment was initiated in 1961 (Fig 5-28). The crossbite was corrected and new records were obtained in 1963. The mandibular midline, originally to the right, was now overcorrected to the left of the maxillary midline. What was not noticed was the difference between the levels of the lower borders of the right and left mandibles (Fig 5-29).

Once the full permanent dentition, excluding second molars, was in place, orthodontic appliances were placed for further alignment and occlusal refinement. Casts obtained in 1964 and 1966 revealed good occlusion with acceptable midline relationships (Fig 5-30). In 1973 a midline discrepancy became more noticeable, with the mandible deviating to the left. Cephalometric radiographs revealed a greater discrepancy between the right and left lower mandibular borders. Because of the midline discrepancy, some posterior occlusal relationships were less than ideal (Fig 5-31).

By 1980 a marked midline discrepancy, with the mandibular midline to the left, was evident. Malalignment of the incisors was also noticeable. Third molars had been previous extracted, so they could not be considered the culprits causing the malalignment. Cephalometric radiographs taken in 1980 (Fig 5-32) revealed gross discrepancies between the right and left mandibles; oblique radiographs revealed an apparent increase in the neck length of the right condyle. Superimposition of right and left oblique radiograph tracings (Fig 5-33) indicated exaggerated right condylar growth between 1973 and 1980.

In 1984 gross facial asymmetry was clearly evident, marked by a pronounced deviation of the chin to the left. Cephalometric radiographs (Fig 5-34) revealed skeletal chin deviation and mandibular asymmetry: pronounced disparity between the right and left mandible and what appeared to be an elongated neck of the right condyle. Laminagraphs taken in 1984 in an effort

to diagnose the problem seemed to confirm the elongated neck, but a subsequent MRI revealed that it was a hyperplastic "cap" on the superior surface of the right condyle (Fig 5-35). The cause was unknown. A condylar shave was undertaken in 1985 and subsequent occlusal and skeletal relationships seemed reasonably stable. Records obtained in 1996 (Fig 5-36) indicated some, not full, degree of stability, but maintenance of facial and dental asymmetry, though acceptable, has been far from ideal (Fig 5-37).

Midline and other considerations in mandibular asymmetry cases

These cases also serve to emphasize another point. Most often, as part of orthodontic treatment, there seems to be a tendency to treat to the mandibular dental midline; the maxillary dental midline is usually made to conform to the mandibular midline. In mandibular asymmetry cases it should be the reverse. The maxillary jaw is a fixed, stable bone and, aside from congenital maxillary misconfiguration, the midpalatal suture (raphe) is the true midline indicator. Embryologically, the two palatal shelves change from vertical to horizontal, meeting and fusing in the midline. It seems logical that orthodontic treatment at all ages should be focused on the maxillary dental midline as the stable midline, if it aligns with the midpalatal raphe. In patients where the mandible is growing asymmetrically, it would be foolhardy to orthodontically align dental midlines with the mandibular midline. This would create skewed dental arches, particularly the maxillary, on an unskewed maxillary base.

The two aforementioned cases raise another point with respect to an asymmetrically growing mandible. At the present time, it is not possible to restrain the growth of the mandible, or even one side of the mandible. Consequently, it does not seem likely that we can orthopedically or orthodontically slow or reduce growth in the case of condylar hyperplasia. However, there are indications that it may be possible to orthodontically cause one side of a mandible to at least more closely approach its genetic potential. This, of course, would be helpful for patients diagnosed with unilateral hypoplasia.

Fig 5-28 Patient A.S. Records taken at 7 years of age. *(a)* On the lateral headplate tracing, stippling shows difference between lower mandibular borders. On the frontal and oblique views, right mandible is striped. *(b to e)* Cast reproduction of the occlusion reveals the posterior crossbite and anterior midline discrepancy.

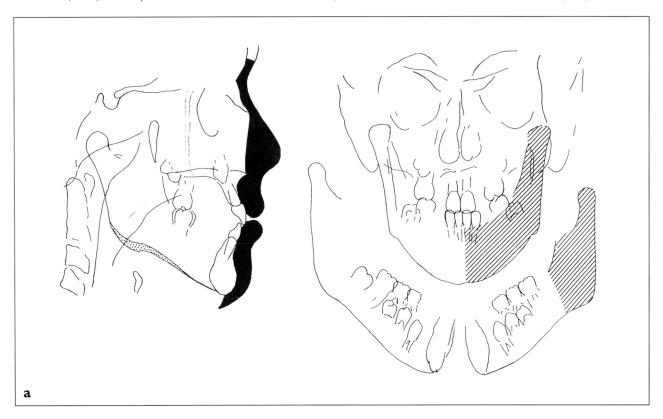

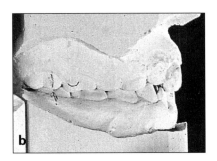
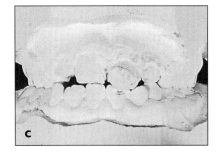
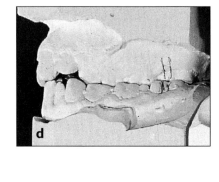
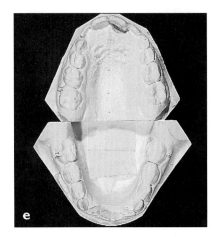

Fig 5-29 Patient A.S. *(a to e)* New records taken in 1963.

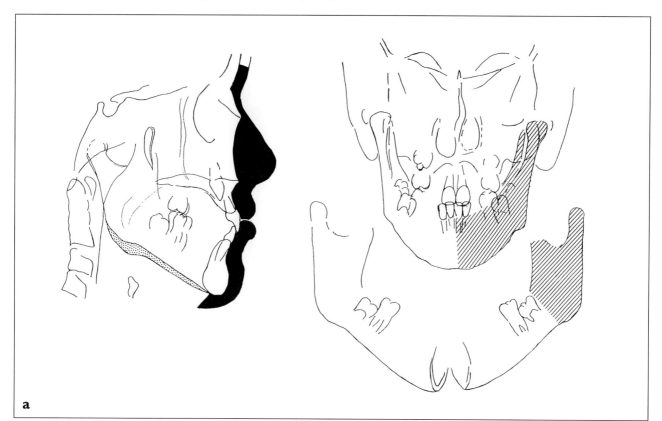

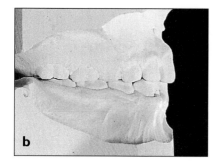
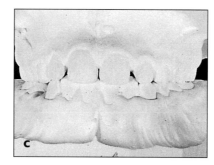
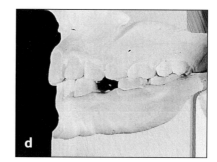

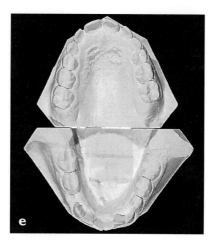

Fig 5-30 Patient A.S. Dental casts obtained in 1964 *(a to d)* and 1966 *(e to h)* indicate acceptable occlusal relationships. Maxillary second molars, still not fully erupted in 1966, are rotated.

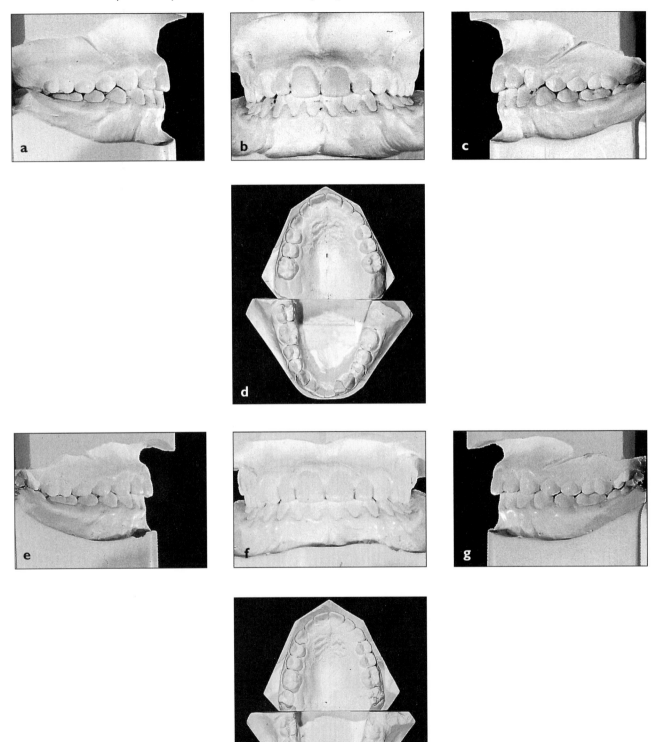

Fig 5-31 Patient A.S. *(a to e)* Records in 1973 reveal changes in occlusal relationships and mandibular lower border disparity.

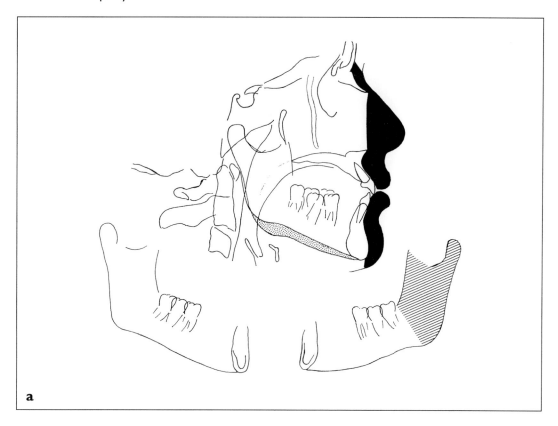

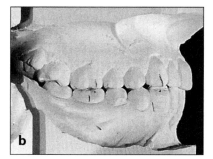

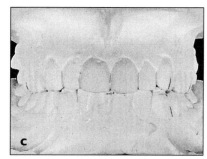

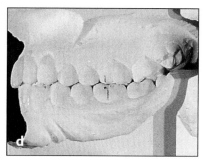

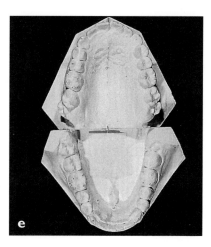

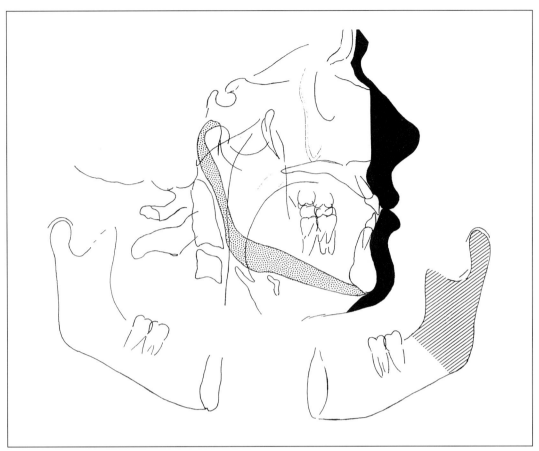

Fig 5-32 Patient A.S. Cephalometric tracings indicating pronounced changes in the mandible.

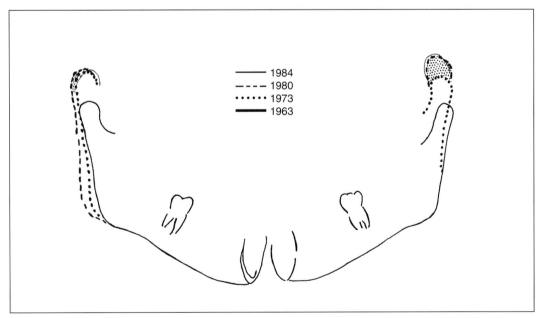

Fig 5-33 Patient A.S. Superimposition of right and left oblique radiographs indicating notable changes over the years. (Stippling indicates exaggerated growth of right condyle.)

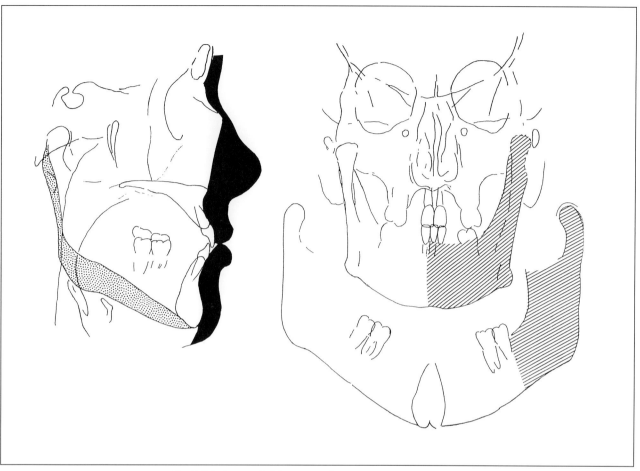

Fig 5-34 Patient A.S. Tracings of radiographs taken in 1984.

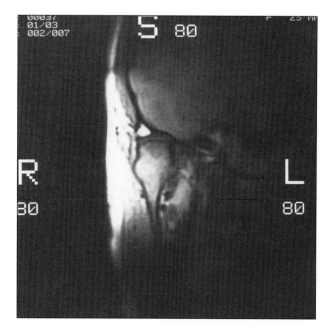

Fig 5-35 Patient A.S. An MRI revealing a hyperplastic cap on the superior surface of the right condyle.

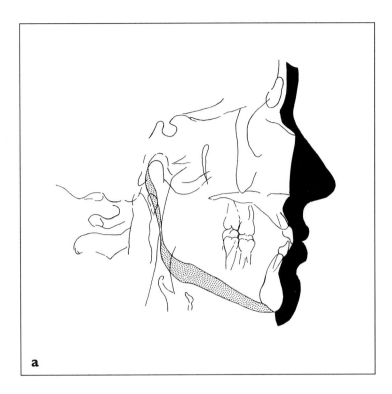

Fig 5-36 Patient A.S. *(a, b)* Tracings of cephalometric radiographs taken in 1996.

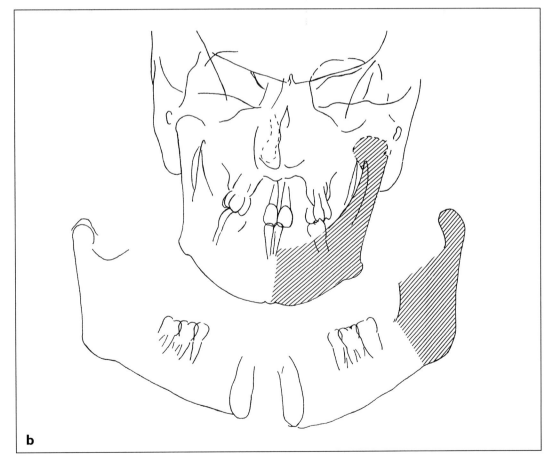

Fig 5-37 Patient A.S. *(a to h)* Frontal photographs and intraoral views of the occlusion indicate relative stability from 1985 to 1996; dental and facial asymmetry has not progressed, but is still evident. The dentition was equilibrated sometime after the condylar shave surgery.

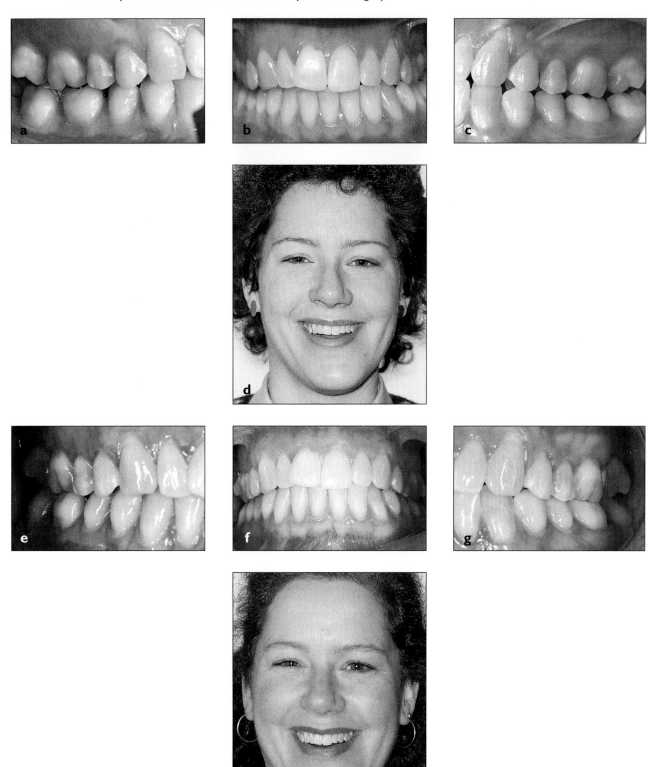

These cases also clearly indicate that asymmetric mandibular growth should be recognized at early age levels; if permitted to continue into the teens, greater mandibular asymmetry will be evident and the occlusion will be more grossly deviated. Thus, asymmetric growth of the mandible must be recognized early so that procedures can be instituted to control mandibular development over as many of the growing years as possible, striving for the greatest possible facial symmetry at later ages. If the severe distortion caused by the asymmetry could be circumvented or minimized, it would be highly desirable esthetically.

A clear perception is growing in our office and clinic that more and more young individuals are manifesting some degree of mandibular asymmetry. Some of the apparent increase may be correlated with increased diagnostic perception on the part of the practitioner; some may be due to the increasing numbers of diagnosed fractures at the vulnerable neck of the condyle; others may be traced back to unrecognized facial trauma that has left its mark; and some may be related to undiscovered temporomandibular joint problems resulting in joint and/or disc degeneration. As a consequence, the need to understand mandibular asymmetry and its diagnosis and possible treatment procedures to preclude extensive malformation and facial asymmetry becomes pertinent to orthodontists, as well as the growing child with the problem.

References

1. Livieratos FA, Johnston LE Jr. A comparison of one-stage and two-stage nonextraction alternatives in matched Class II samples. Am J Orthod Dentofac Orthop 1995;108:118–131.
2. Johnston LE Jr. A comparative analysis of Class II treatments. In: McNamara JA Jr, Carlson DS, Vig PS, Ribbens KA (eds). Science and Clinical Judgment in Orthodontics, monograph 18, Craniofacial Growth Series. Ann Arbor, MI: Univ of Michigan, 1986:103–148.
3. Johnston LE Jr, Paquette DE, Beattie JR, Cassidy DW Jr, McCray JF, Killiany DM. The reduction of susceptibility bias in retrospective comparisons of alternative treatment strategies. In: Dryland Vig K, Vig PS (eds). Clinical Research as the Basis of Clinical Practice, monograph 25, Craniofacial Growth Series. Ann Arbor, MI: Univ of Michigan, 1991:155–177.

Chapter 6

Developing Mandibular Asymmetry

Lessons Learned from Past Cases

In developing an orthodontic approach to the treatment of mandibular asymmetry, especially at young ages, the conclusion has been reached that the inclusion of orofacial function and orthopedic forces is a very important facet of treatment, especially in cases of condylar fracture. As propounded by Harvold et al,[1] we now realize that new condyles can be regenerated when they are congenitally missing or resorbed incident to fracture. Several cases have been instrumental in bringing this fact to recognition—cases from which valuable lessons were learned.

Patient M.M.: A congenitally missing condyle and minimal ramus

First, a young patient (M.M.) was born with a congenital mandibular problem, hemifacial microsomia. Hospital records showed that, on the affected side, he had agenesis of one ramus superior to the gonial region, a diminutive—almost vestigial—coronoid process, and, with the lack of a ramus, no condyle (Fig 6-1). Concomitantly, the patient had microtia and no external auditory meatus. Hospital laminagraphs of the unaffected side revealed a complete ramus with normal condylar and coronoid processes. At the time of referral for orthodontic treatment at age 12, the frontal radiographs clearly revealed facial

asymmetry with tissue deficiency in the ramal region on the affected side and a marked deviation of the chin toward the affected side (Fig 6-2). The lower face, mouth, and jaw were displaced to the left, with considerable depression in the left cheekbone area. Upon opening, the chin deviated severely to the left, indicating mandibular malfunction. In occlusion, the mandibular dental midline deviated to the left while the left maxillary and mandibular posterior teeth were infraerupted, resulting in an upward cant of the occlusal plane from right to left. Radiographically, the left side of the skeletal face appeared underdeveloped in the zygomatic and left ramal region. When compared with the original hospital radiograph, the left ramus was still considerably shorter vertically than the right ramus, but seemed to have grown. The left floor of the nasal cavity, along with the occlusal level of the molars, was higher on the affected side.

With orthodontic treatment, a reasonable occlusion was achieved. Cervical appliance therapy was initially undertaken to retract the protruding maxillary dental arch; subsequently, heavy elastic forces were used to retract the maxillary arch, which concomitantly exerted a forward orthopedic pull on the movable mandibular arch. A maxillary acrylic biteplate was used to disarticulate the maxillary and mandibular dentition, with an occlusal splint on the left side to create interocclusal space on the right. Vertical elastics were

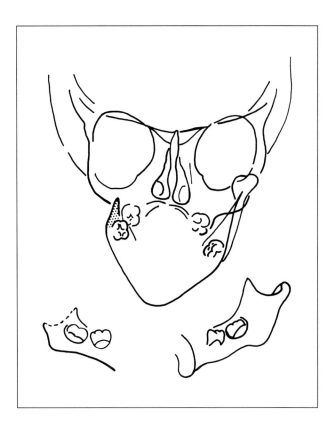

Fig 6-1 Tracings of hospital radiographs taken of M.M. during infancy. Anteroposterior (frontal) radiograph and right and left lateral jaw laminagraphic radiographs indicate lack of ramus and condyle on the left side, where a vestigial coronoid process seems present.

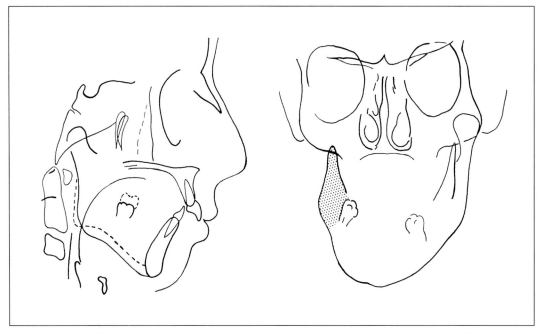

Fig 6-2 Patient M.M. Tracings of lateral and frontal radiographs indicating extent of mandibular skeletal discrepancy at time of referral for orthodontic treatment.

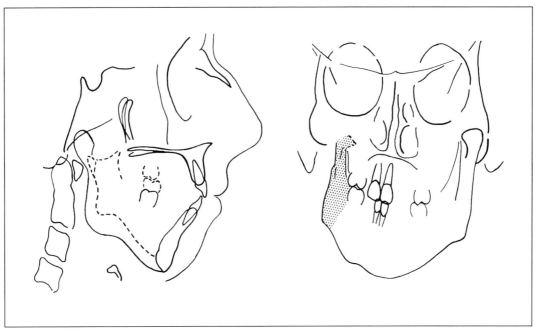

Fig 6-3 Patient M.M. Frontal and lateral cephalometric radiograph tracings, postretention.

used, first on the right and then on the left, in an attempt to level the two sides of the occlusal plane as much as possible.

Cephalometric radiographs following treatment (Fig 6-3) showed that the mandible did not grow on the affected side (compared with the unaffected side), but a recognizable ramus was observed to be developing on the affected side with definitive antegonial notching and a semblance of a condylar process. Since there was no surgical reconstruction of the left ramus with a bone implant, this was an unexpected finding; however, it was definitively smaller than the right ramus. It is assumed that the influence of muscle activity on bone and periosteum during function was instrumental in the new bone development. As mentioned, functional stimulation was also introduced orthopedically by the use of strong Class II elastic orthopedic forces on the affected side. Additionally, the unilateral bite block served to reposition the mandible and perhaps stretch the soft tissues associated with the affected ramus, causing a deposition of new bone.

Although function was probably instrumental in new bone development on the affected side, less-than-ideal functional movements may have resulted in condylar problems on the unaffected side, as shown on the oblique radiographs as a flattening of the head of the condyle (Fig 6-4). Compensatory functional movements on the normal side resulting from aberrant functional movements on the affected side may have altered the configuration of the condyle. However, the point to be stressed is that functional movements, and the generating muscle tension forces, can cause deposition of new bone; this could be materially helpful in the orthodontic treatment of these patients. Today, there is evidence that mandibular growth can be functionally stimulated to approach—and even at times to reach—its potential.

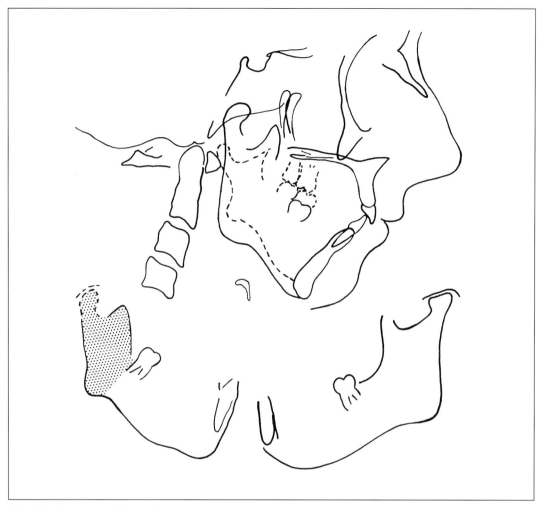

Fig 6-4 Patient M.M. Lateral and oblique tracings revealing the development of a left mandibular ramus and a flattening of the right mandibular condyle.

Trauma, condylar fracture: Muscle function and new condylar development

Patient M.S.: Early and good. The following case is not one with congenital mandibular dysmorphology, but is an example of recognizing a potential problem and functionally treating it to an acceptable facial symmetry and a concomitant reasonable dental occlusion. In this instance, a 6-year-old boy fractured and dislocated a mandibular condyle in a bike accident. The knowledge that a fractured and displaced condyle could regenerate at early age levels and that functional control of mandibular posture could facilitate continued mandibular growth was important in his treatment. Given the

condylar fracture, it was already a foregone conclusion that a growth problem would occur on that side. It was also realized that rapidly instituting function was essential in stimulating continued growth on the fracture side. Harvold et al[1] has postulated that, under functional influences, myoblasts have potential for developing into cells with osteoblastic properties and that muscle function, through tension, is known to instigate new bone formation; thereby, new condyles could be formed. The patient was immediately placed on functional exercises—opening, closing, and increased chewing. In view of the fact that the problem was on the left side (a condylar fracture) (Figs 6-5 and 6-6), functional appliance and Class II elastic therapy

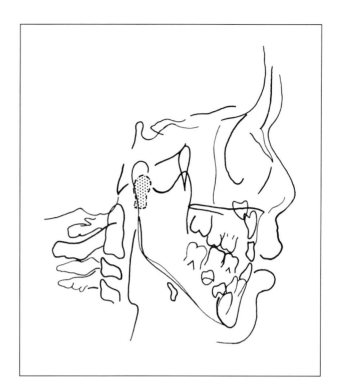

Fig 6-5 Patient M.S. Lateral cephalometric tracing revealing the fractured condyle.

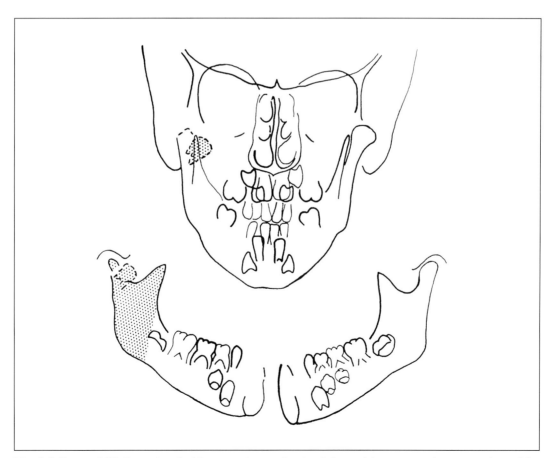

Fig 6-6 Patient M.S. Frontal and oblique tracings indicating left condylar process fracture and condylar displacement.

were undertaken (1970), concentrating forces on the left side. If bilateral elastics were used, they were twice the strength on the left as they were on the nonfracture side. Functional appliances were designed to bring the left side forward and toward the right, correcting midline as well as molar relationships. Several stages of treatment were instituted, but always with the same philosophy: keep stimulating development on the fractured side. In this case, congenitally missing mandibular second premolars were coexistent with arch-length problems, so extractions were undertaken during the course of treatment. Full orthodontic therapy was consistent with maintaining a stimulative force on the fracture side (the potentially poorly growing side) until the patient was ready for retention.

By the approximate time of retention (1977), and following a subsequent placement of a functional appliance–type of retainer (1979), a very acceptable occlusion had been achieved. Considering the continuing potential for malgrowth of the left mandible, excellent facial symmetry had been achieved. Cephalometric radiographs revealed development of very reasonable symmetry of the skeletal mandible (Fig 6-7). It was noted from the oblique films (Fig 6-8) that there had been a regeneration of the fractured condyle. The patient had undergone continued stimulation of mandibular development throughout treatment as well as retention. Throughout treatment there had been periodic use of functional stimulation, when indicated, via Class II mechanics, biteplate therapy, and bite block therapy, as well as orthodontic tooth movement with continual use of heavy unilateral Class II elastics to maintain a reasonably good occlusion and acceptable facial symmetry.

From all indications, mandibular growth (Fig 6-9) incident to the periodic functional stimulation over the years has generally kept the affected side increasing in dimension, although not fully comparable with the unaffected side (Fig 6-10). It is a clear example of how growth can be stimulated to approach its genetic potential; it is possible that it could eventually be made to approach its potential on the affected side. Without therapy it is entirely credible that there would have been retarded growth on the affected side and progressive development of considerable facial asymmetry.

In this case, radiographs (Fig 6-11) revealed the development of a new condyle on the fractured side, albeit not of similar configuration to the normal condyle. Also noted clinically was the development of a TMJ click on the nonfractured side believed to be a functional alteration incident to the presence of the fractured condyle and continued development of the new condyle, creating altered functional demands on the nonfractured side. When the problem is a jaw malocclusion, such as this unilateral condylar growth problem, retention must be sophisticated and geared to skeletal malrelationships, skeletal growth problems, and the soft tissues. It cannot be relegated strictly to the occlusion. When stimulative procedures are used to develop bone, then stimulative processes must continue during retention. Functional-type retainers must be constructed to continue placing developmental functional influences on the affected side.

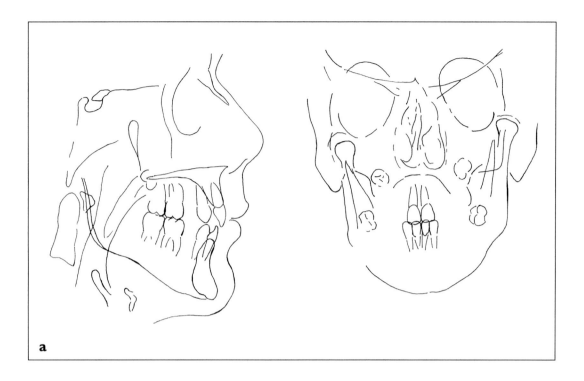

Fig 6-7 Patient M.S. (a) Lateral and frontal cephalometric tracings indicating acceptable facial symmetry and, particularly, mandibular symmetry. (b) Tracing of cephalometric wide-open radiograph indicating reasonably symmetric and adequate mandibular movement.

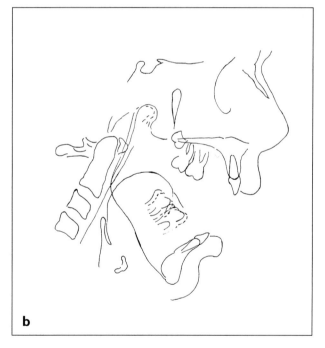

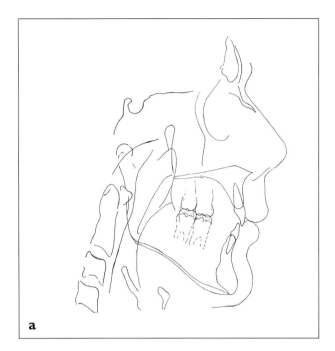
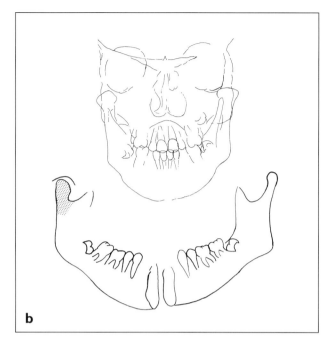

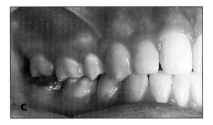
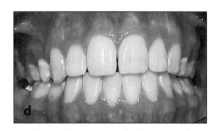
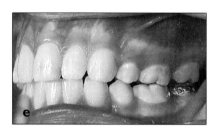

Fig 6-8 Patient M.S. *(a, b)* Tracings of lateral, frontal, and oblique radiographs taken in 1979, when a functional appliance–type of retainer was introduced, since a dental midline discrepancy, a change in the level of the posterior occlusal levels, and a skeletal mandibular asymmetry was becoming noticeable. *(c to e)* By 1981, the asymmetry was clearly evident.

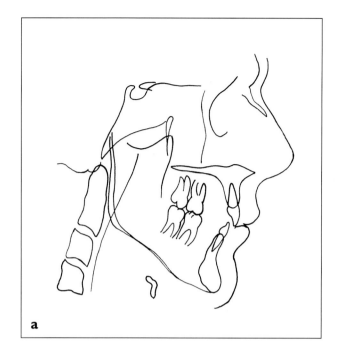

Fig 6-9 Patient M.S. *(a, b)* Lateral and frontal cephalometric tracings, with two oblique tracings (1983), indicating continued growth and reasonable facial symmetry.

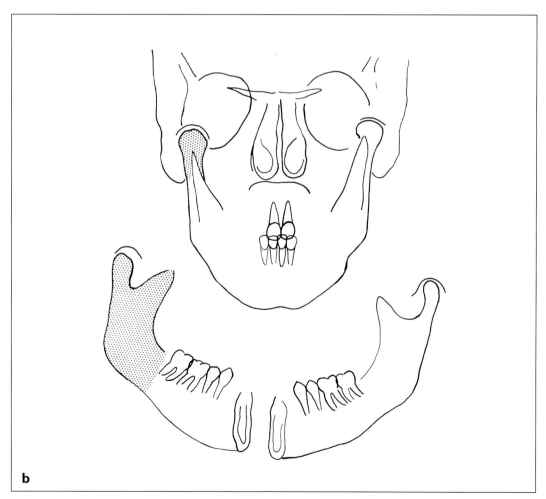

Fig 6-10 Patient M.S. Tracings of lateral and frontal cephalometric radiographs *(a)* at the time of initiation of treatment (1970), *(b)* retention (1977), and *(c)* when the patient reached 19 years of age (1983). *(d to g)* Type of functional retainer used. There is a midline overcorrection.

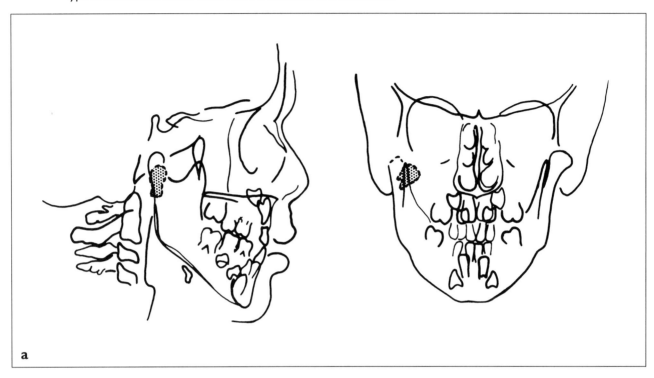

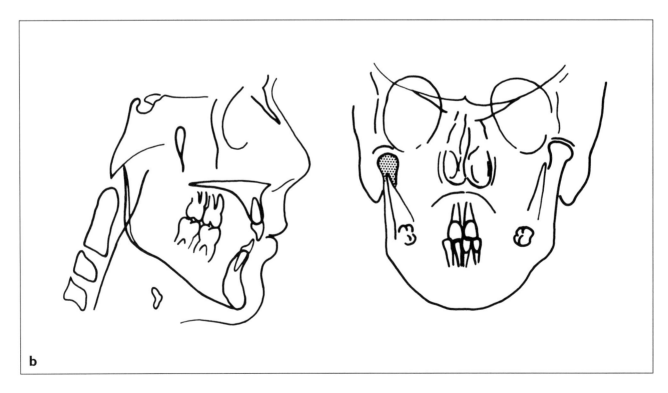

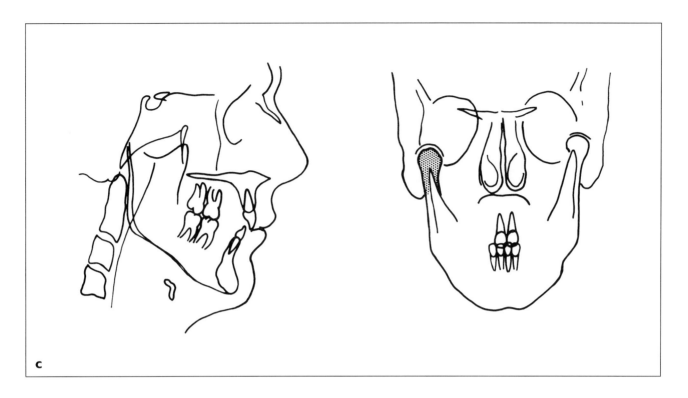

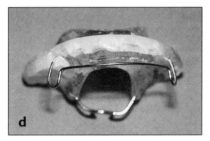

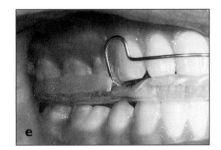
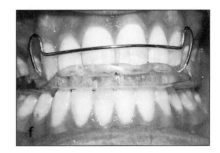
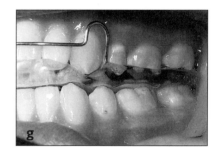

Fig 6-11 Patient M.S. *(a)* Serial tracings of right and left oblique radiographs from 1970 to 1983 depicting changes during treatment and increment in age. *(b)* Tracings of laminagraphic radiographs of the right and left condyle in open position. *(c)* A submental vertex radiograph taken 1984. The dental midline discrepancy is evident, as well as differences in the two temporomandibular joints.

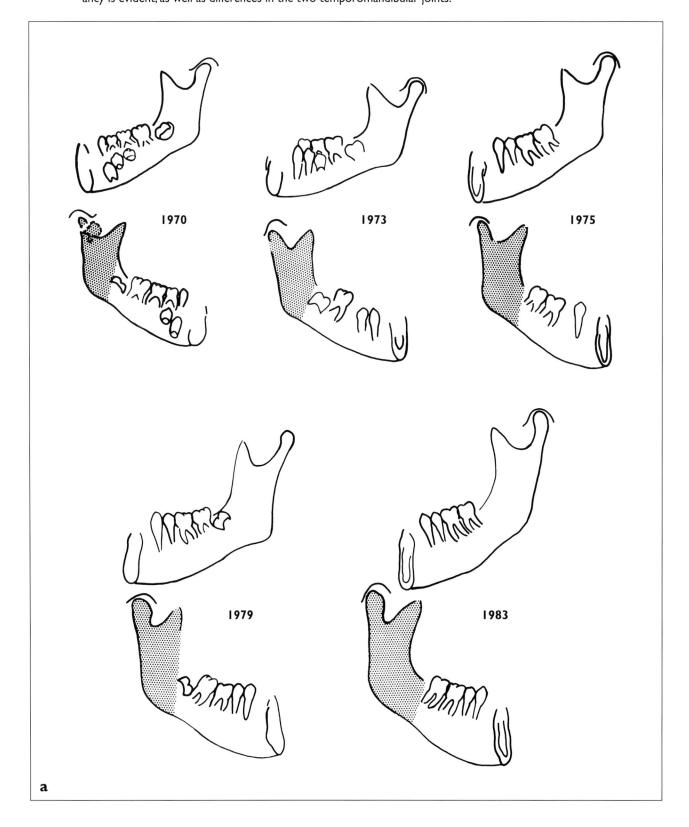

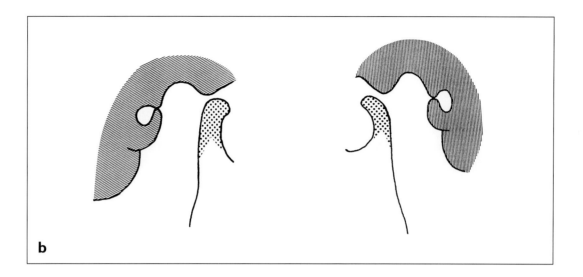

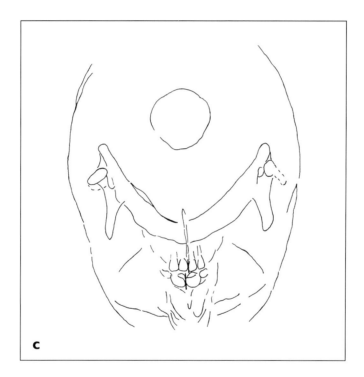

Patient M.S.: Postretention evaluation. Years after retention, the patient appeared reasonably symmetric in facial appearance. At the age of 31 (7 years after dismissal from the office and 25 years after initiation of treatment following fracture of the left condyle), new records were taken. The lateral cephalometric radiograph (Fig 6-12) revealed fairly good jaw relationships and a reasonable straightness to the skeletal profile. The two sides of the mandible appeared fairly symmetric on the head plate, in that one side superimposed reasonably well on the other. Although two distinct and separate images were not evident, one condyle appeared to be slightly more cranial than the other: there were two radiographic images of the condylar superior surfaces. The mandibular plane was not steep and was within acceptable limits. On the lateral head plate there seemed to be comparable heights to the dentoalveolar segments in the premolar and molar regions, and at this time two different occlusal planes were not evident. The discrepancy to be noted on the head plate was the anteroposterior positions of the two buccal segments: the buccal teeth on one side (presumably the left) appeared slightly distal to those on the other side. A slight overjet was evident, indicating a small relapse; however, the overbite relationship had remained acceptable.

On the frontal cephalometric radiograph (Fig 6-12), reasonable skeletal symmetry was evident in the sense that there was not an overall impression of skeletal asymmetry. There was, however, a notable difference in vertical dimensions from the gonial angle to the top of the condyle: the left ramus was shorter than the right. On the left side, a new condyle could be seen; it was rather large and from the frontal perspective appeared to be located directly posterior to the coronoid process. An indentation or notch in the bone was evident at the neck of the new condyle, which can be presumed to be the fracture line. The left ramus was quite acceptable in its width relationship to the maxillary midline. Surprisingly, the skeletal chin was slightly to the right; concomitantly, a definitive antegonial ingression was noted inferior and medial to the right ramus, and the vertical dimension from the gonial angle to the top of the condyle was greater on the right side than on the left. Addi-

tionally, the neck of the right ramus appeared to be bent laterally, causing the condyle to lie more to the lateral of the coronoid process than usual and distinctly different from that on the fractured side. It is felt that this was a progressive functional adaptation to the developing new condyle. On the frontal cephalogram the occlusal plane appeared to be level from right to left, indicating that there were no distinct differences in posterior dentoalveolar heights. The mandibular dental midline was distinctly to the left of the maxillary midline, a defined dental midline discrepancy. Considerable adaptation in mandibular form seemed to have taken place as a result of new functional activity incurred incident to the fracture and progressive development of a new left condyle over the years. This may be an indication that muscle function can modify form and create not only a new bony structure simulating a condyle but also differences in architecture incident to altered functional activity and functional demands.

The lateral oblique radiographs were interesting and quite revealing (Fig 6-12). The right ramus showed a well-defined neck—somewhat elongated, but with acceptable architecture—and a properly configured condyle. Some degree of antegonial notching was evident in conformity to what was observed on the frontal head plate. What appeared to be almost a notching directly posterior to the symphysis on the lower border of the right mandible was noted. Again, this may be an indication of altered muscle function, such as the suprahyoid, the digastric, or the geniohyoid.

When the left ramus and its condylar region were observed on the left oblique radiograph, it was evident that the ramal height from the gonial angle to the superior surface of the new (or simulated) condyle was not very much shorter than that on the right side, indicating that there had been increment in the vertical dimension of the left ramus. The new condylar structure had a rather thick neck and did not seem to have the normal configuration of a condyle; it appeared bulbous and seemed to encroach on the sigmoid notch space. Radiographically, the appearance was of a cap on top of a cap—almost like a condyle superimposed on a condyle. It was most likely layers of new ossification, creating a

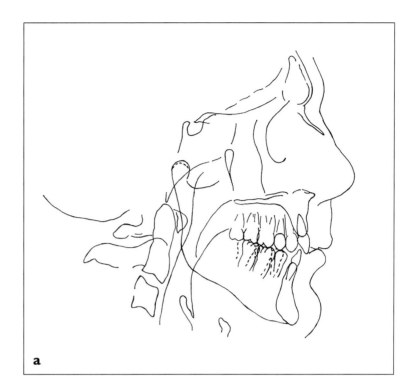

Fig 6-12 *(a, b)* Tracings of lateral, frontal, and oblique radiographs of patient M.S. in 1995, 25 years after the condylar fracture, showing some asymmetry and alteration in occlusion, but reasonable symmetry.

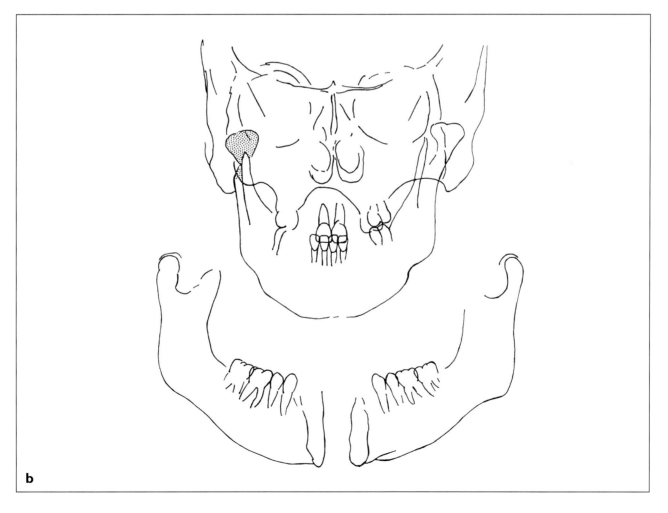

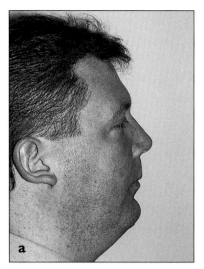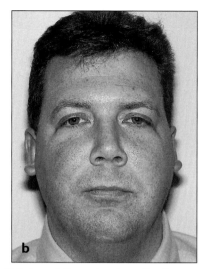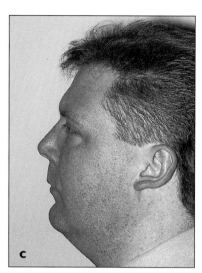

Fig 6-13 Patient M.S. *(a to c)* Frontal and profile photographs taken in 1995.

thick, although curved, superior surface on the new condyle. The left condyle and neck appeared to be closer to the coronoid process than observed on the other side. The left coronoid process seemed wider and more vertically situated relative to the head of the new condyle than was observed on the right side—a definite change in the configuration of the superior aspects of the ramus, in the condylar and coronoid regions.

On the frontal photograph (Fig 6-13) the patient looked fairly symmetric, with a slight deviation of the chin toward the left. In profile, no disparity nor any apparent manifestation of retrognathia incident to the unilateral condylar fracture were noted. He did have a chin button and a relatively straight profile. The occlusion had held up very acceptably: from the frontal perspective the appearance was very pleasing, with teeth well aligned (Fig 6-14). Deviation of the mandibular dental midline toward the left was apparent upon close examination, but the alignment of the anterior dentition masked it very nicely. As for the occlusion, the right buccal segment, as well as the canines, were in an excellent Class I relationship. On the left side, the occlusion left something to be desired; relapse in interocclusal relationships on the affected side had resulted in the mandibular molars and premolars being positioned a little more distally

than desirable: not a full Class II relationship but more end-to-end. Nor were the left canines in a Class I relationship; they were almost cusp-to-cusp. The cusp of the maxillary left canine appeared to be considerably attrited to the point where a flatness or slight concavity appeared where the mandibular canine had functioned against it.

Significant changes could not be noted in the follow-up records obtained at 34 years of age (1998). The result seems to be stable and, esthetically and functionally, highly adequate. Considering the condylar fracture, the potential growth disturbance on the left, and the minimal facial asymmetry—not to mention the new functionally incurred condylar structure—one must say that this is a very acceptable result. Obviously, at 34 years of age, very little growth can be anticipated, especially in the mandibular region; so it can be anticipated that there will be comparably little change in the occlusion. Continuing to wear the functional retainer would have been helpful, but he seemed to have tired of it and had not worn it for approximately 12 years as of the last date of records. Also, one might surmise that much of the functional adaptation incident to the fracture and to the orthopedic effects to overcome possible adverse sequelae had taken place; so it could be speculated that the occlusion will probably stay put.

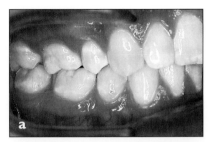 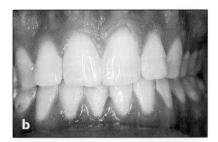 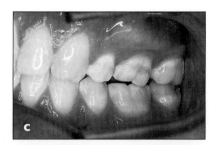

Fig 6-14 Patient M.S. *(a to c)* Intraoral photographs of the occlusion in 1995.

The functional demands on the mandible, as well as the functioning of the mandible itself, has probably reached a stage of adapted stability. It is hoped that the occlusion and facial appearance have also reached a relatively stable point.

Notably, the occlusion on the fracture side is slightly Class II. One wonders if this is not the basis for some Class II, division 1, subdivision malocclusions; can some of them be the result of unilateral condylar trauma or a TMJ problem on one side? It is difficult to perceive how a patient can develop a one-sided Class II malocclusion. There may be an underlying skeletal growth problem so that the unilateral maldevelopment of the mandible develops into a Class II, division 1, subdivision malocclusion.

Timing significance of early functional muscle action after condylar fractures

Patient S.M. The importance of stimulating continuing functional control of mandibular posture and growth has been pointed out. Function is important in the treatment of a fractured condyle and should be instituted as soon as possible after the fracture. The significance of timing can be readily demonstrated by the case of an 8-year-old girl who had suffered a fracture of the neck of her left condyle incident to an ac-

cident in the schoolyard. She fell from a jungle gym and hit her chin. She experienced pain and several lacerations, so was sent to a hospital for examination and possible treatment (1978). According to the hospital note, she had difficulty and pain upon opening. A panoramic radiograph indicated a distinct fracture at the neck of the left mandibular condyle, which was displaced anteriorly out of its fossa, revealing a distorted radiographic picture. The condyle was probably somewhat medial to the ramus and to the fossa itself. In the panoramic view it appeared as though the radiologist were observing the superior, rather than the lateral, surface of the condyle. The ramus and condyle on the right side had a very normal appearance.

The child was in the early transitional dentition and had not experienced eruption of the permanent lateral incisors at the time of the accident. None of the dentition appeared fractured or displaced, and no structures aside from the left condyle appeared altered. Hospital records further revealed that no surgical procedure had been undertaken in the condylar region, but that interocclusal wiring had been placed to stabilize the occlusion. The wiring was removed after an undisclosed period, and the case was followed radiographically with panoramic films. Seven months after the accident, the panoramic radiograph clearly indicated a

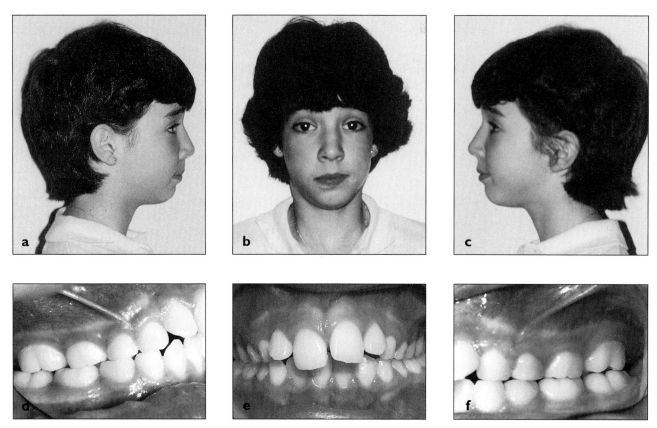

Fig 6-15 Patient S.M. *(a to f)* Frontal, profile, and occlusal photographs taken at time of referral.

displaced left condyle, distinctly forward of the fossa and not readily recognizable (having the appearance of a nubble instead of a condyle), apparently undergoing distortion as well as atrophy. No fracture line was obvious incident to healing, and a distinct condylar neck and head were not discernible. The condyle had probably been pulled forward, medially, and inferiorly and was atrophying in a position medial to the ramus and considerably inferior and anterior to the temporomandibular fossa. The panoramic film also indicated that the molar occlusion was Class I on the right, but on the side of the fracture there was a more forward maxillary molar relationship—possibly the beginning of a Class II relationship. The panoramic radiograph taken at the time of the accident indicated a bilateral Class I molar relationship, despite the presence of a condylar fracture. Two years after the frac-

ture, the condyle was barely visible radiographically. The bony tissue had more of the configuration of a spicule, distinctly forward of the temporomandibular fossa and the articular eminence. The neck of the condyle appeared rounded, with an anterior fingerlike projection where the old condyle seemed to be. The occlusion, as interpreted from the panoramic radiograph, appeared to be a well-defined Class I on the right side but a distinct end-to-end molar relationship on the left (fractured) side. On the fractured side, radiographic differences indicated a shorter ramus, a lack of condylar definition, and a somewhat elongated coronoid process when compared with the nonfractured side.

Three years after the accident, the patient, now 11, was referred for orthodontic treatment and records were taken (Figs 6-15a to 6-15j).

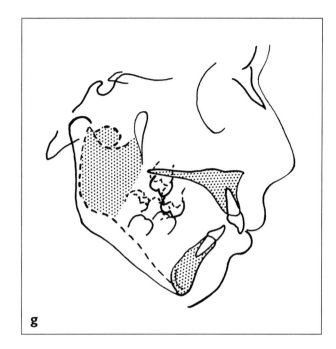

Fig 6-15 Patient S.M. *(g, h)* Tracings of cephalometric and oblique radiographs taken at time of referral.

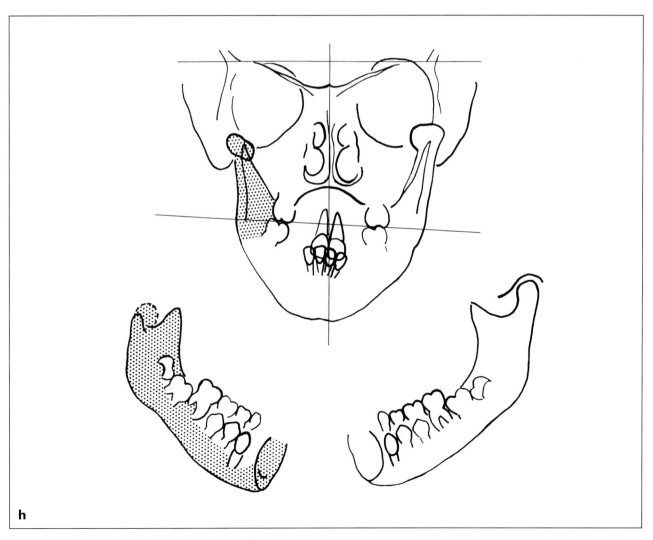

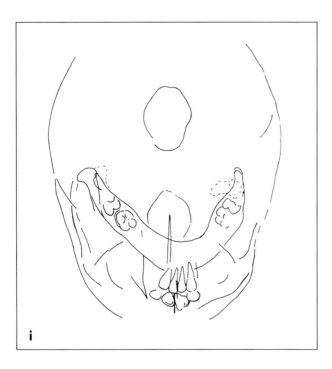

Fig 6-15 Patient S.M. *(i, j)* Tracings of submental vertex radiograph and laminagraphs taken in centric and wide-open positions of the mandible on both sides.

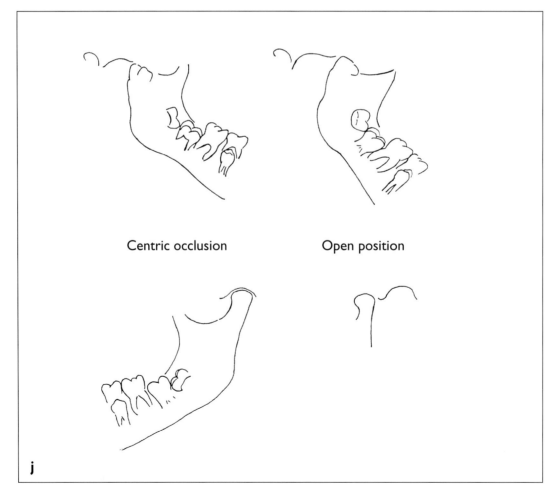

Centric occlusion   Open position

During the 3-year interval, no functional exercises had been prescribed, except that normal function had been reinstituted after the removal of fixation. Frontal photographs and the frontal cephalometric radiograph revealed facial asymmetry. The chin was deviated to the left and, on the frontal radiograph, the left gonial region seemed more cranially positioned than on the right. On the facial photographs a distinct tilt of the lips was noted, with the left corner of the mouth more cranially positioned than the right. The mandibular dental midline was notably to the left of the maxillary midline. Her buccal occlusion, still in the transitional dentition, exhibited a well-defined right Class I molar relationship. On the left side, the molars were in a more end-to-end relationship, approaching Class II, with the maxillary molar somewhat forward of the mandibular. On the lateral cephalometric radiograph, the posterior surfaces of the two rami indicated that the shorter ramus (the left) was forward in relation to the right. The gonial region of the left mandible was considerably higher than the right, indicating less vertical development of the left ramus. This caused the lower border of the body of the left mandible to appear more cranially positioned on the lateral cephalometric radiograph.

The frontal cephalometric radiograph revealed considerable skeletal facial asymmetry, especially mandibular asymmetry, with the left ramus more medially positioned. The skeletal chin deviated considerably to the left (fracture) side. The maxillary dentition was well related to the skeletal facial midline, but the mandibular dental midline was notably to the left; the mandibular incisors seemed to be axially inclined toward the right. On the oblique radiographs, the right ramus and body of the mandible were well defined and of acceptable dimensions. The left mandible exhibited a much shorter vertical dimension to the ramus than the right, and there was no condylar head nor well-defined neck on the left oblique. The radiographs in all perspectives and dimensions indicated skeletal facial asymmetry. Two different levels of the occlusal surfaces of the molars were evident on both the frontal and lateral head plates. On the frontal head plate, the left occlusal level was more cranially disposed, giving a

decided tilt to the occlusal plane from that perspective. On the lateral cephalogram, two occlusal planes could be visualized, and it was presumed that the left occlusal plane was the higher (more cranial) of the two. Additionally, anteroposterior asymmetry with respect to the mandibular molars was observed, with the higher (more cranially positioned) molars being more distal than the other (presumably nonfractured) side. There was also indication of inadequate vertical dentoalveolar development on the fractured side, in both the mandibular and maxillary buccal regions.

Clinically, the chin, upon wide opening, deviated very obviously to the left. The amount of mouth opening seemed to be somewhat restricted for a youngster this age. Knowing function to be important to treatment, we initially placed bite blocks to increase the extent of mouth opening. The patient was also instructed to initiate exaggerated functional activity to the greatest possible extent in opening and closing the mouth. These were followed with functional appliances to specifically increase mouth opening and reposition the mandible toward the right, bringing the mandibular midline closer to the maxillary, based on the assumption that increasing muscle tension on bone would stimulate some degree of bony mandibular development. This was pursued for a considerable time in an attempt to work toward greater skeletal and facial symmetry. After a greater degree of opening was achieved, orthodontic appliances were placed on the maxillary and mandibular arches to initiate tooth alignment and further stimulate the left mandibular region. Although not symmetric (Figs 6-16a and 6-16b), facial appearance from the frontal perspective seemed improved. It is acknowledged that growth had been taking place during treatment to this point. The subject also seemed to be able to open much wider than initially, although a distinct deviation of the mandible toward the left was still discernible. When a lateral head plate was taken in the wide-open position, it was observed that there was considerable movement of the right mandible and markedly less movement of the left mandible (Figs 6-16c and 6-16d). Additionally, the right gonial region was seen to be more anteriorly positioned than the

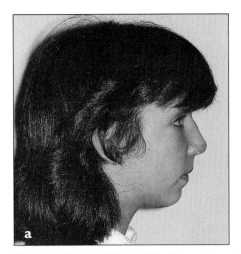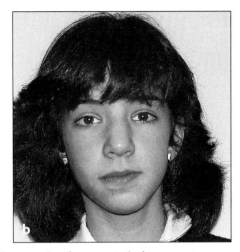

Fig 6-16 Patient S.M. *(a, b)* Profile and frontal photographs after a period of treatment (1984).

left in the fully open position. After several years of orthodontic treatment with full appliance therapy and periodic utilization of bite blocks and functional appliances, as well as Class II orthopedic forces on the left side, a new panoramic radiograph was taken at age 16. This film indicated the formation of a new condyle, although having an unusual configuration. Frontal, lateral, and oblique radiographs also indicated new condylar development, but small and differently formed compared with the right condyle; coexistent was apparent new ramal growth. Although there was evidence of increased height of the left ramus, dimensions comparable to the nonfractured side were not achieved, possibly due to the delay before functional activity and orthodontic stimulation were initiated—approximately 3 years. From the frontal perspective there was still the upward tilt of the occlusal plane from right to left, a distinct positioning of the chin to the left, and a mandibular dental midline shift to that side. The mandibular central incisors were tilted to the right, while the maxillary central incisors were tilted somewhat toward the left. The

same relationships were evident when she was placed into retention a year later. However, greater soft tissue facial symmetry was evident, with improved vertical dimension in the left ramal region.

A new left condyle was radiographically observable when final records were obtained in 1990 (Fig 6-17). The new left condyle seemed to be more anteriorly directed than the right condyle, seemingly more related to the infratemporal fossa rather than the glenoid fossa. The discrepancies in ramal height were improved, but, notably, more antegonial notching was observable on the left side. Of special interest, asymmetry in width dimensions seemed more pronounced in that the left ramus appeared more closely related to the cranial facial midline than did the right side. Because of this, it was also apparent on the frontal photograph that the left cheek was more "fallen in" (concave), that is, more closely related to the facial midline, adding to the visualized facial asymmetry (Fig 6-18). Obviously, whereas some growth was stimulated vertically and anteroposteriorly and the position of the left body of the

Fig 6-16 Patient S.M. *(c, d)* Centric relation and wide-opening of the mandible. Tracings of frontal and right and left oblique radiographs taken after a period of functional and orthodontic treatment.

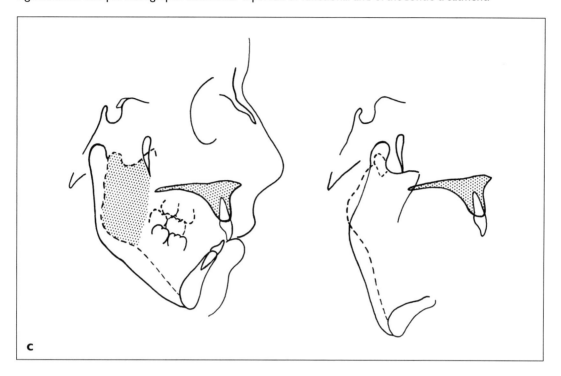

c

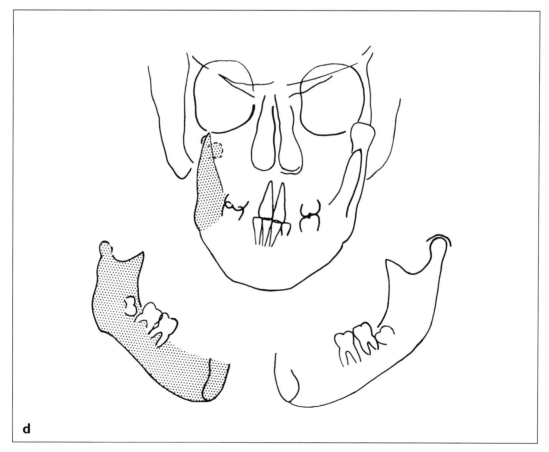

d

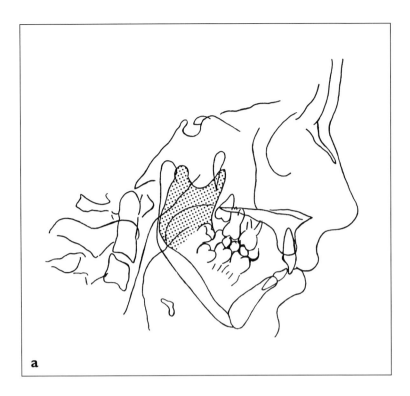

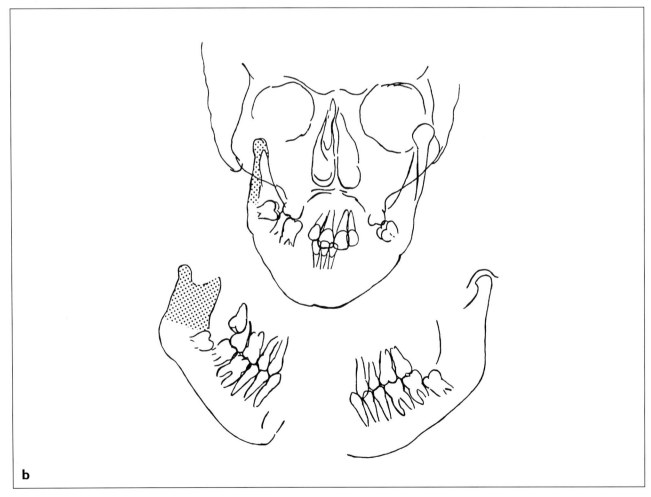

Fig 6-17 Patient S.M. *(a, b)* Tracings of lateral, frontal, and oblique radiographs obtained in 1990, indicating skeletal configurations and relationships observable at that time.

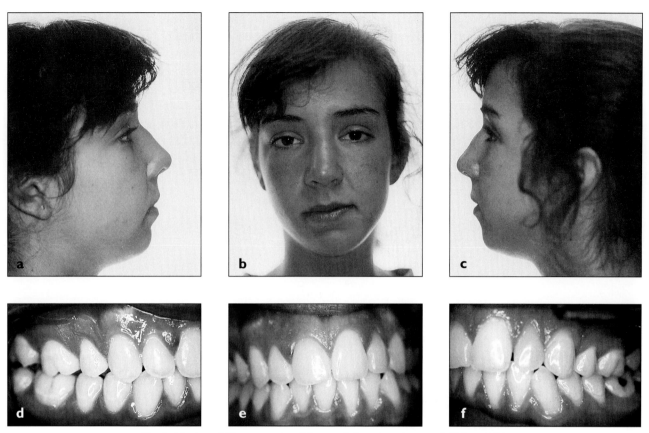

Fig 6-18 *(a to f)* Photographs of face and dental occlusion of S.M. in 1990.

mandible and ramus was improved, inadequate lateral facial growth precluded achieving greater facial asymmetry. The lateral head plate clearly defined two occlusal planes, as well as two lower mandibular borders, indicating shorter dentoalveolar heights on one side. The anteroposterior discrepancy in molar positions was still evident, with a more defined Class II-ishness on the left side, although somewhat improved from the initial relationship. During the late stages of treatment, a buccal shield was used on the fractured side in conjunction with the functional appliance to buccally distend the cheek in hopes of improving soft tissue symmetry in width and masking the degree of skeletal asymmetry. To a degree, this seemed helpful, but facial symmetry was never fully achieved in the lateral dimensions.

Function and skeletal growth: A synopsis

It seems obvious that mandibular function is essential for the full expression of growth and development of that bone. It is surmised that muscle function and the influence of muscular activity on bone and periosteum is instrumental in new bony development. In the latter case (S.M.), a new condyle and an increment in ramal height, as well as anteroposterior dimensions, seem to have been achieved in addition to improved occlusal arrangement, albeit discrepancy in occlusal levels remained. The unfortunate aspect of this case, compared with the previous one (M.S.), where functional activity had been introduced very early after the fracture, is that this patient did not show comparable favorable development of bone and condyle, very possibly due to the considerable discrepancy in the time of initiating function. In the second case there was a 3-year hiatus during the development of this child where stimulatory influences were not initiated; in essence, time was lost, along with some of the potential for improvement in skeletal development. Of course, it can be argued that the fracture occurred at a later age in the second patient, a girl, and that girls usually mature much earlier than boys. However, both were in the transitional dentition at the time of fracture, both had left condylar fractures, and both expressed considerable facial growth; but one achieved a better result with

time than the other. It is stressed that function—in these cases articular function—is important and should be initiated as soon as possible after a condylar fracture is diagnosed. Waiting introduces considerable risk, since time without function as an integral part of treatment potentially loses bone that could have been developed during that period, bone that could have helped mask a developing facial asymmetry.

Reference

1. Harvold EP, Vargervik K, Chierici G (eds). Treatment of Hemifacial Microsomia. New York: Alan R Liss, 1983.

Chapter 7

Mandibular Asymmetry: Diagnosis and Treatment

Clinical Diagnosis of Developing Mandibular Asymmetry

The important fact to note from the aforementioned cases is that, to a degree, mandibular dimension and configuration can be controlled to maintain some semblance of facial symmetry, provided, of course, that treatment can be instituted at early age levels, when a good degree of growth potential is still available. Developing mandibular asymmetries and growth retardation can frequently be noted at young ages and should be treated then. At the present time it seems that more and more mandibular asymmetry is being noted in young, growing children. Whether the problem is now being more readily diagnosed, or whether an increase in causative factors is the reason, is open to question; however, in our clinical population it seems that there is an ever-increasing recognition of developing facial asymmetry. Of crucial significance is the facility of being able to differentiate, at young age levels, normal asymmetry from potentially abnormal—particularly mandibular—facial asymmetry. A sufficiently accurate diagnosis is the key to the game. Looking at the extremes of excessively abnormal asymmetry affords clues, enabling the diagnostician to differentiate developing abnormality in facial symmetry. A young individual with hemifacial microsomia is an example of extreme mandibular asymmetry, well beyond the range of normal, revealing characteristics that may be helpful in recognizing the features of this deformity. Immediately, differences in configuration and dimensions of the right and left sides of the mandible are noted and recorded as facial asymmetry. Of course, the obvious will be seen almost immediately: an overall impression of a definite difference between one side of the face and the other. In recognizable facial asymmetry, one most frequently sees a pronounced deviation of the chin relative to the facial midline.

A chin deviating toward one side of the face compels an examination of the occlusion, to evaluate midline relationships. If observed, it should trigger a search for a skeletal discrepancy in symmetry. Midline discrepancies, in the sense that the mandibular dental midline deviates relative to the maxillary, may be an indication that one side of the mandible is growing less, or excessively more, than the other, more normally growing side. Of course, if a midline deviation is noted, it is incumbent upon the diagnostician to determine whether it is due to a lateral mandibular shift incident to the occlusion (as might be the case with a unilateral crossbite) or whether there is a distinct difference in the size and/or growth of the two sides of the mandible. If it is determined that the midline discrepancy is not correlated with a mandibular shift from rest to occlusion, then the posterior occlusion itself should be an added indication as to whether asymmetric growth of the mandible and/or maxilla is taking place. If a Class II molar relationship exists on one side coincidental with a midline deviation toward that side, it may be an indication that, on that side, the mandible is growing insufficiently compared with the other side. If a Class III molar relationship exists and it is not on the same side as the midline deviation and seemingly normal maxillary structure is evident, then it is credible that overgrowth of the mandible is occurring on that side. In either situation, the mandible is probably growing asymmetrically, and more pronounced mandibular asymmetry will be evident at later age levels. Hypoplasia seems to occur much more frequently than hyperplasia, so that, in most cases of mandibular asymmetry, it will be observed that there is a Class II molar relationship on the side of the shorter mandible.

Cephalometric Evaluation of Mandibular Asymmetry

To a great extent, reliance can be placed on cephalometric radiographs to diagnose early stages of developing facial asymmetry. Characteristics can be readily noted on the frontal head plate as well as the lateral cephalometric radiograph (Fig 7-1), and confirmation of some of the observations can be ascertained from oblique films (Fig 7-2). If oblique films are not taken, some information can be gleaned from panoramic radiographs. The panoramic and oblique radiographs may reveal information relative to the configuration of the condyles and may direct attention to dysmorphology, if present: for example, fractures, a "mushroom" condyle, etc. Certain characteristics on the lateral cephalometric radiograph should initiate a careful evaluation of possible developing mandibular asymmetry. If the two lower borders of the body of the mandible are separated and do not intersect at or near the gonial region, one can ascertain the possibilities of developing mandibular asymmetry. If other craniofacial structures superimpose reasonably well on the

radiograph and two distinct and separate lower borders of the mandible are observed, then it can be surmised that one lower border is closer to the cranium than the other. This may be indicative of shorter ramal height on one side, or it may indicate a shorter posterior dentoalveolar height on that side. Coexistent with this, one would notice on the lateral head plate that there are two posterior occlusal planes, indicating that the occlusal surfaces of the premolars and molars on one side are in contact with the opposing dentition at a higher level, or more cranially, than the other side. Most frequently the higher occlusal plane will be correlated with the lower border of the mandible that is at the more cranial position; many times there is a shorter ramus on the less-than-adequately developing side of the mandible. These characteristics could be corroborated on the frontal cephalometric radiograph.

In examining the frontal cephalometric head plate, one will see that the skeletal chin and the mandibular dental midline are deviated toward the side, revealing an apparent shortness of the ramus. Also notable on the frontal head plate, coexistent with the shorter ramal height, will be an occlusal plane situated more cranially on that side: a tipping of the posterior occlusal plane from right to left. The tip may be correlated with a shortness in the maxillary vertical dimension compensating for the limited posterior mandibular dentoalveolar height (caused by the stunted ramus). A word of caution when utilizing the frontal head plate: if there is a tipping of the posterior occlusal plane, it should be confirmed that the shorter maxillary vertical dentoalveolar height is not due to unilateral vertical nasomaxillary asymmetry. The mandible may be positioning itself at a higher level on that side in order to make occlusal contact. What must be looked for are two different levels of the two nasal cavity floors (Fig 7-3). If there is vertical skeletal nasomaxillary shortness on one side, the floor of the nasal cavity will be more cranial on that side. This would indicate unilateral vertical shortness in the nasomaxillary complex rather than a compensatory shortness in the maxillary posterior dentoalveolar process, where the floors of the nasal cavity would be more approximate in levels. When this right-to-left tip in the occlusal

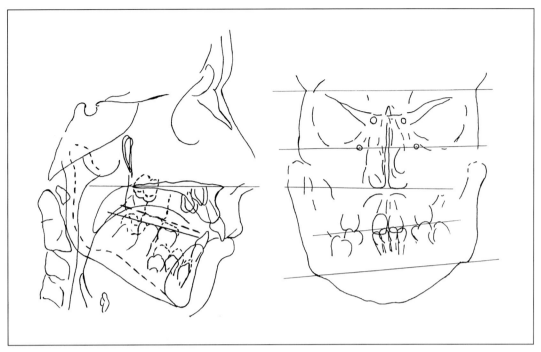

Fig 7-1 Tracings of the lateral and frontal cephalometric radiographs of a young patient with facial asymmetry.

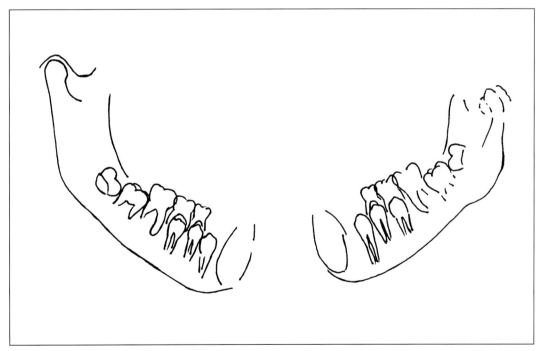

Fig 7-2 Tracings of oblique films of patient illustrated in Fig 7-1.

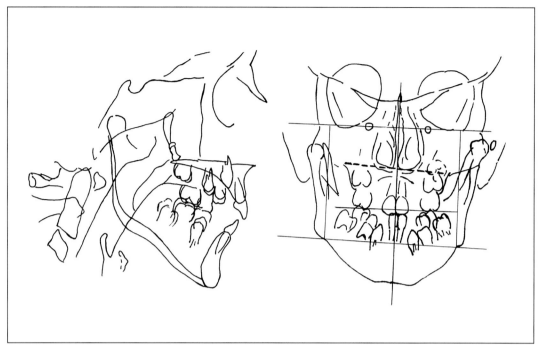

Fig 7-3 Tracings of lateral and frontal cephalometric radiographs of a young patient with vertical maxillary asymmetry. Dashed line on frontal view indicates shortness on one side of floor of the nasal cavity and adaptive increment of posterior dentoalveolar height on that side.

plane is noticed, it will usually be reflective of a vertical growth discrepancy in the ramus on the short side. The oblique radiographs may also reveal shortness of the ramus, because one side can be compared with the other. Even if a dysmorphology is not seen in the condyle, one can ascertain that there has been a reduction in growth on that side and it will lead to mandibular asymmetry.

Another observation in using the lateral cephalometric radiograph to diagnose developing mandibular asymmetry would be two distinct and separate posterior surfaces of the two rami (Fig 7-4). Concomitant with this anteroposterior discrepancy would be the observation that the mandibular molar position on one side is distinctly more distal and somewhat distantly removed from the molar position on the other side. The obvious anteroposterior discrepancy in the position of the molars would indicate that one side of the mandibular arch is farther distal.

This might be an indication that the bodies of the mandible are not growing anteroposteriorly sufficiently equally to maintain symmetry. Again, it might be correlated with some growth retardation or inadequacy in position on the side where the molar is more distal, resulting in a Class II relationship. It is further possible that the mandibular fossa on that side is more posterior than the other side, resulting in a discrepancy in the positions of the condyles, the rami, and the mandibular bodies, creating a facial asymmetry and a unilateral Class II molar relationship.

To reiterate: characteristics of developing facial asymmetry should be recognized early so treatment can be initiated early. It is becoming more recognizable in anteroposterior jaw relations and in width relations having a noticeable chin deviation and malrelated dentition. What does not seem to be as readily recognized is a frequently concomitant vertical asymmetry on the affected side.

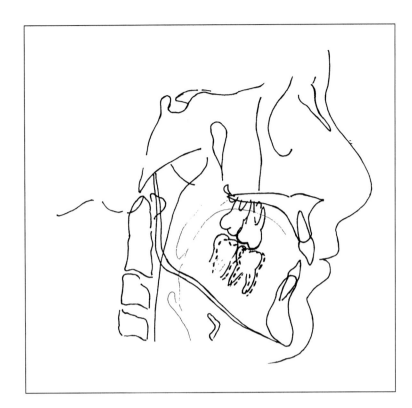

Fig 7-4 Tracing of lateral cephalometric radiograph of a young patient with mandibular asymmetry. Two posterior borders of the rami and a concomitant discrepancy in the anteroposterior positions of the right and left mandibular molars are evident.

Orthopedic-Orthodontic Treatment of Mandibular Asymmetry

The unilateral bite block

The advantages of using unilateral bite blocks for the treatment of developing mandibular asymmetry became apparent by happenstance. Considerable difficulty was being encountered in attaining prolonged wearing of functional appliances, which were being used to correct mandibular discrepancies; specifically, cooperation from many youngsters was lacking. As a consequence, limited results were being achieved with functional appliance use. In a case where the patient refused to wear the appliance, a bite block was substituted. It was noted that, when the patient closed with the bite block in place, the dental midline relationships immediately changed. It was further noted that, if the

mandibular bite block was high on one side with occlusal contact on that side, the mandibular dental midline deviated toward the side of occlusal contact. In essence, the appliance was functioning as a unilateral bite block. After reduction of the bite block on the high side, only enough to permit contact on the other side, it was noted that, again, the mandibular dental midline deviated toward the side of occlusal contact with the block. To determine whether this could be an applicable phenomenon, a study was conducted in the Department of Orthodontics at Eastman Dental Center to validate this observation. Orthodontic students and other personnel not under orthodontic treatment were included in the study. Double-thickness wafers of mouth guard material were placed on the occlusal surfaces of one side of the mandibular posterior dentition to evaluate mandibular-to-maxillary dental midline relationships, since the maxilla is, in essence, a fixed

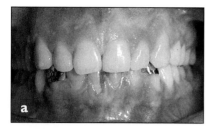
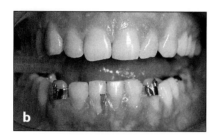
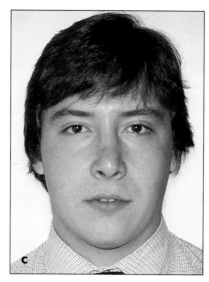
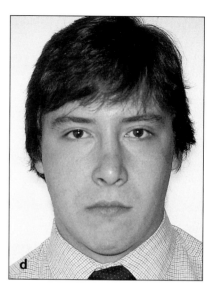

Fig 7-5 *(a to d)* Frontal and facial photographs of an orthodontic student with and without a right unilateral bite block composed of two wafers 5 mm thick. Note change in chin and mandibular midline (demarked) position.

dental midline. First, the wafers were placed on the occlusal surfaces between the posterior teeth on one side and the midline relationship was photographically recorded; then the wafers were placed on the other side and midline relationships were photographed again. In each instance midline relationships were also observed clinically and recorded. It was found that the introduction of the unilateral bite block wafers between the posterior teeth caused the mandibular midline to move toward the side of occlusal contact (Fig 7-5). Subjects with evident mandibular asymmetry, as well as subjects with definitive midline discrepancies, were also studied utilizing unilateral bite block wafers. In each

instance, the chin and the mandibular midline moved toward the side of the simulated unilateral bite block. Frontal cephalometric radiographs were taken on the same subjects with and without the bite block in place. Superimposition of the tracings indicated that the mandibular dental midline moved toward the side of the unilateral bite block (Fig 7-6). Of course, concomitantly the occlusion was disarticulated incident to the bite block positioning. Cephalometric laminagraphs taken on a selected number of subjects showed that when a bite block was in place, condylar position more closely approximated rest position; possibly a result of disarticulating the occlusion.

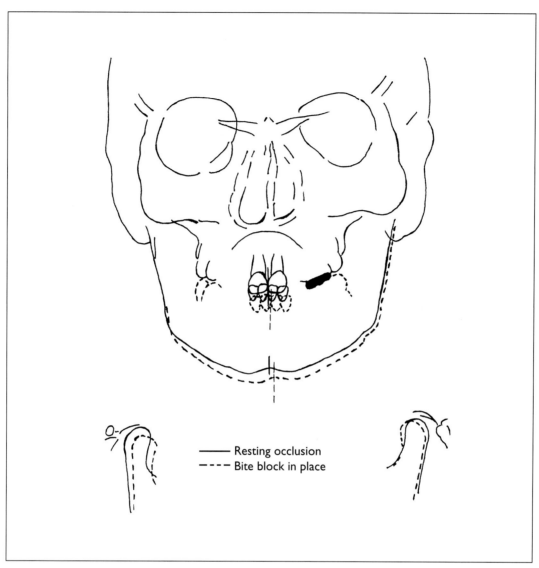

———— Resting occlusion
- - - - Bite block in place

Fig 7-6 Superimposed frontal radiographs taken with and without a right unilateral bite block in place. Note shift in mandibular midline to the side of the bite block. Laminagraph tracings indicate change in condylar position.

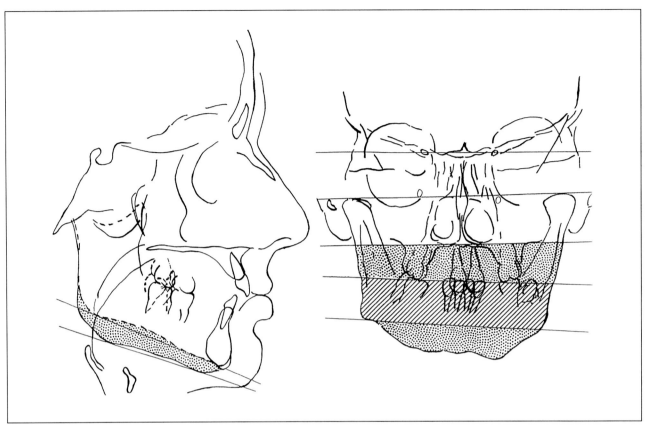

Fig 7-7 Lateral and frontal cephalometric tracings of an individual with facial asymmetry, depicting midline discrepancy, shortness of left ramus, left maxillary and mandibular posterior alveolar heights, and occlusal plane disparity.

The unilateral bite block and orthodontic therapy

These studies initiated the use of unilateral bite blocks in orthodontic correction of mandibular asymmetry (Fig 7-7). The unilateral bite block was used on the so-called "normal" side, usually the well-growing side, to cause a dental midline swing toward the side of the bite block. Utilization of the unilateral bite block on the nonaffected side causes a disarticulation of the occlusion, which results in an interocclusal opening on the non–bite block side (Fig 7-8). This opens the interocclusal space, posturing the mandible downward and literally moving the condyles down from the fossa and opening an interocclusal dimension on the affected side, thus serving to stretch the postural muscles on both the affected and unaffected sides. The rationale is

that this will permit vertical dentoalveolar growth on the affected side (Fig 7-9a), while preventing such occurrence on the nonaffected side, since the bite block prevents eruption of the buccal teeth. Furthermore, it can facilitate vertical development of the dentoalveolar processes, via orthodontic influences, on the side with an open interocclusal space (Fig 7-9a). Posterior teeth could be supraerupted to occupy the interocclusal space. Where desired, light vertical elastics could be employed to increase maxillary and mandibular posterior dentoalveolar heights on the vertically shortened side. Also, a class II vector could be incorporated with the vertical elastics to facilitate correction of anteroposterior molar relationships.

It is readily observed that the anterior occlusal plane, that is, the level of the maxillary incisors, is also affected in the facial skeletal

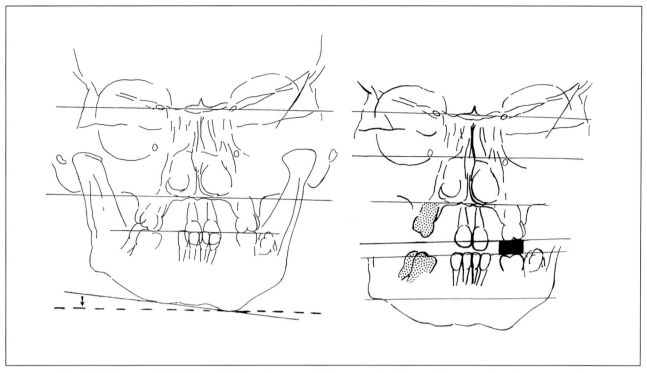

Fig 7-8 Tracings of Fig 7-7 modified to show need of moving the left gonial region inferiorly to approach skeletal facial symmetry (left) and placement of bite block (black) on the nonaffected side to correct midline relationship.

asymmetry problem. The incisal occlusal plane on the left (affected) side, in the case described above, is more cranially positioned than the right side and must be corrected to level the full occlusal plane. An archwire, incorporating a helical "shoe" loop mesial and distal to the left canine, is constructed to place depressive action on the canine, moderate eruptive action on the left posterior teeth, greater eruptive forces on the left incisors, and lesser forces on the right incisors (Fig 7-9b). Eruption of the canine is more easily achieved than depression because of its long root; this will aid in flattening the occlusal plane. After vertical repositioning of the mandible on the affected side, the teeth are permitted to erupt into occlusion on the unaffected side by removal of the unilateral bite block. It is hoped that vertical eruption of the posterior teeth will hold the

vertical repositioning of the mandible on the affected side and will permit adaptive growth changes in the condylar region to help maintain the result.

It should also be noted that, in some cases, the basic problem of skeletal asymmetry may be manifested in the maxillary complex rather than in the mandible. Inadequate vertical skeletal development on one side of the maxilla may cause the mandible to shift unilaterally and vertically, simulating a torquing into occlusion. This appears the same as mandibular asymmetry, but in reality is the result of an asymmetric vertical repositioning of the mandible to achieve full occlusal contact. Overtly, facial appearance may be the same, but the causative mechanism differs: we are developing maxillary skeletal asymmetry rather than mandibular asymmetry. Here, treatment is similar, in that mandibular unilateral

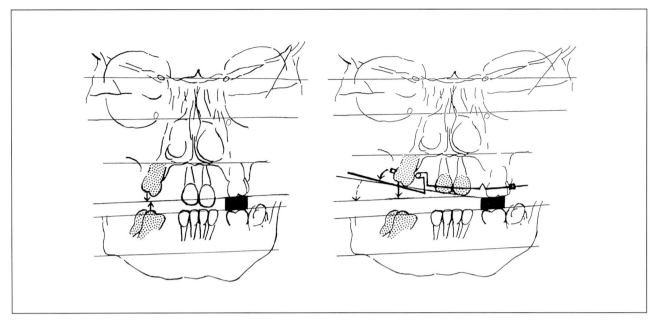

Fig 7-9a A unilateral bite block is placed on the right side to prevent eruption on that side and permit eruption of posterior teeth on the left side incident to occlusal disarticulation. Archwire therapy is initiated to orthodontically erupt the left posterior teeth; the double helical shoe loop is placed distal to the left canine.

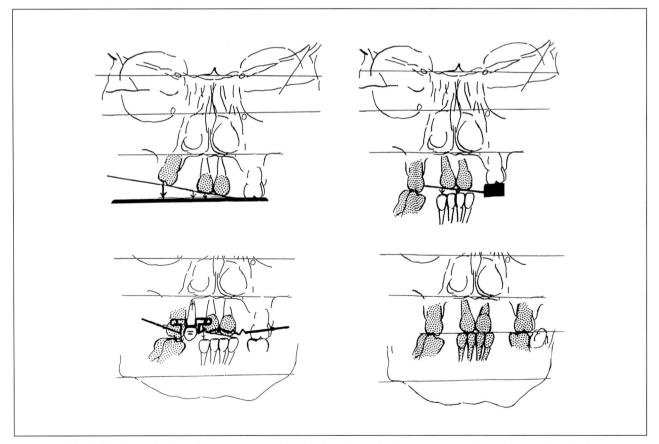

Fig 7-9b The right buccal segments are maintained, and eruptive forces are placed on the anterior dentition to align with the plane of occlusion.

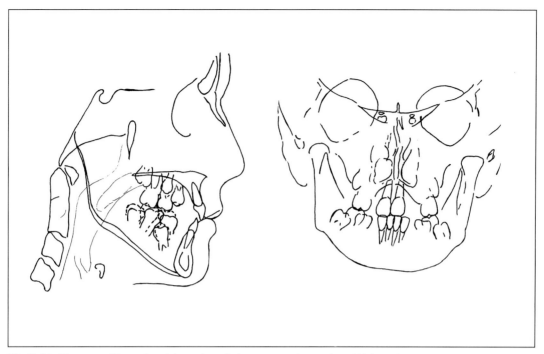

Fig 7-10 Tracings of lateral and frontal cephalometric radiographs of K.A. in the transitional stage of dental development with mandibular and facial skeletal asymmetry.

bite block therapy is instituted in an attempt to anchor the mandibular arch. In addition, vertical elastic and/or archwire therapy is instituted to increase maxillary posterior dentoalveolar height on the affected side in an effort to prevent the mandible from having to unilaterally shift into vertical malposition in order to achieve full occlusal contact. Again, this condition should be orthodontically treated as early as possible to preclude its developing into more severe facial asymmetry and malocclusions.

Patient K.A.: Camouflage of mandibular asymmetric development

K.A. is an example of a young female patient in whom facial and occlusal asymmetry was noted during the transitional dentition period. After treatment was instituted to correct the occlusion, the potential advantages of unilateral bite block use became evident. The facial asymmetry is readily noted on the frontal radiogram (Fig 7-10) and photographs (Fig 7-11), while the aberrant dental midline relationship can be seen on

the radiograph as well as the facial and occlusal photos. In 1984 a left unilateral bite block was incorporated into the orthodontic treatment procedures (Fig 7-12). Tracings of progressive frontal radiographs during the treatment and retention periods indicate improved dental midline relationships and skeletal mandibular position, in the sense that chin position is improved (Fig 7-13). Frontal photographs indicate improvement in facial symmetry (Fig 7-14). These improvements were reasonably maintained after dismissal from treatment and retention (Fig 7-15). It is reasonable to hypothesize that, if treatment had not been directed toward improving mandibular position, primarily chin position and occlusion, the young lady would probably have appeared more facially asymmetric with progressive growth into the late teen years. The use of unilateral bite blocks is encouraging in concept; they should be used when the greatest changes are occurring incident to growth. It should also be recognized that treatment may have to be reinstituted periodically over prolonged periods in order to achieve the desired, acceptable result in facial symmetry and occlusal relationships.

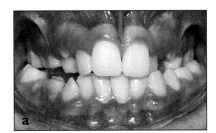
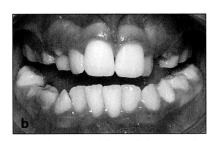
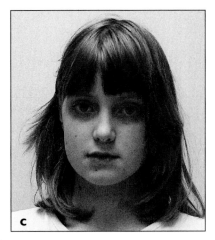

Fig 7-11 Patient K.A. *(a to c)* Facial and frontal photographs indicating asymmetry.

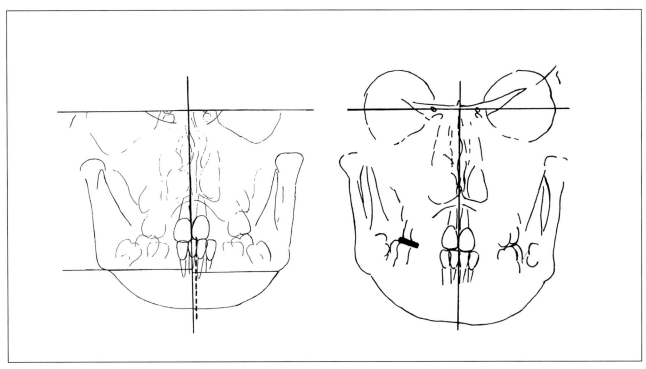

Fig 7-12 Cephalometric tracings of frontal radiographs of K.A., depicting midline discrepancy concomitant with mandibular asymmetry (1982) *(left)* and improvement in midline relationships after initial orthodontic treatment and placement of a unilateral (left) bite block (1984) *(right)*.

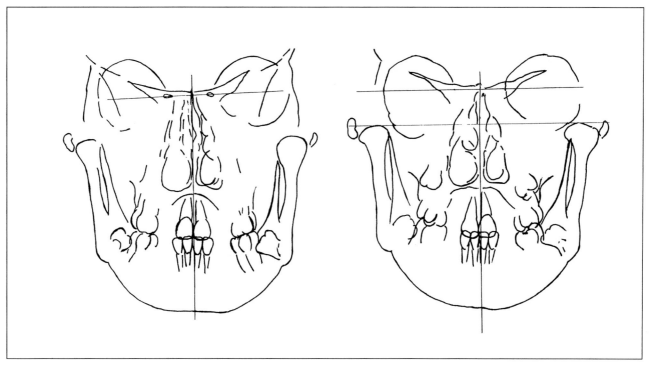

Fig 7-13 Tracings of frontal radiographs taken of K.A. at the time of preparation for retention (1988) *(left)* and after a period of retention (1989) *(right)*.

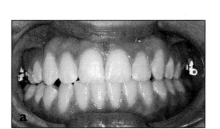
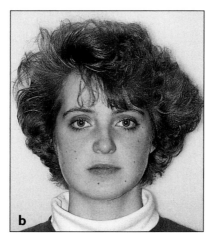
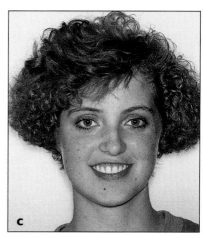

Fig 7-14 Patient K.A. Frontal and facial photographs taken in 1988 *(a, b)* and frontal photograph taken in 1990 *(c)*.

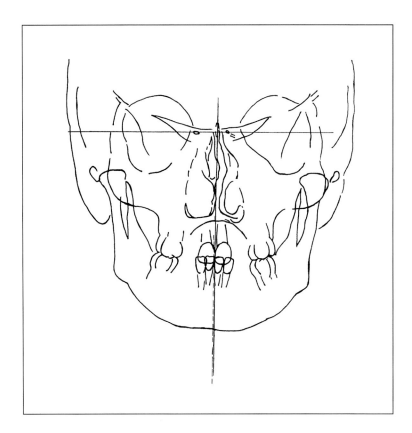

Fig 7-15 Cephalometric tracing of frontal radiograph of K.A. approximately 5 years after retention. The midlines have remained relatively stable, with the mandibular midline now slightly to the left (dashed vertical line). The patient appears acceptably symmetric in the sense that facial asymmetry is no longer readily observable.

In the treatment of mandibular asymmetry, there are several principles that should be kept in mind. First, there must be a repositioning of the mandible in the direction of achieving better symmetric relationships by stretching muscle fibers and stimulating new bony development in the condylar region. Of course, the importance of function should not override the genetic potential for that particular structure and individual. It is further suggested that this new development be incrementally attained during early age and growth levels to take advantage of the greatest possible amount of potential growth. As a consequence, it is important that facial asymmetry be diagnosed early enough to facilitate the greatest possible reduction of asymmetric relationships by means of functional improvement. Much of the correction of mandibular asymmetry is contingent on muscle function and the muscle tension that causes bone development and repositioning of the mandible into new spatial relationships with the teeth in occlusion. This new mandibular position, which is directed toward improved facial symmetry, is maintained by the increased posterior height of the dentoalveolar process and the movement of teeth correcting disparate occlusal planes, most frequently achieved by the correction of posterior dentoalveolar height.

Significant increase in dentoalveolar height is more achievable on a side of the mandible where there is inadequate or reduced growth (hypoplasia) and not where the mandible is growing excessively (hyperplasia). Excessive unilateral growth of the mandible will lead toward visual asymmetry, which is usually correlated with too much growth, and is virtually impossible to control via the usual orthodontic or orthopedic measures. In cases of hypoplasia, unilateral bite blocks are helpful if placed on the nonaffected side to create a significant opening of the interocclusal dimension on the affected side. Placement of a unilateral posterior bite block on the nonaffected side will preclude the eruption of teeth on that side and will permit eruption of occlusal levels on the shorter (affected) side. This can be facilitated with the use of orthodontic archwires and/or elastics to increase maxillary and/or mandibular posterior dentoalveolar heights. Note that the placement of a unilateral bite block establishes a new mandibular position that causes the mandibular dental midline, as well as the chin, to shift toward the side of the bite block. It is observed that the orthodontic increase in heights of the posterior dentoalveolar processes on the affected side—other than the side of bite block placement—aids in maintaining the improvement in the dental midline. In essence, it is hoped that the occlusal interdigitation will be helpful in maintaining the position of the mandibular body and thereby increase facial symmetry. The assumption is that new bony development has occurred on that side of the mandible and that the newly created occlusion will help to maintain it. What we are trying to do is correct the anteroposterior discrepancy in mandibular position by repositioning the shorter side of the mandible forward via functional appliances, while approaching proper midline alignment. To a degree, improvement in vertical and anteroposterior relationships on the affected (shorter) side should lead to better chin positioning, which will, in turn, greatly enhance facial symmetry.

The longer the asymmetry is permitted to develop without orthodontic intervention, the greater will be the problem needing correction; and the greater the magnitude of required correction, the less the probability of improving facial asymmetry without the intervention of orthognathic surgery. The sooner the orthodontic correction of the asymmetry is attempted during the early growing years—the rapidly growing years—the greater the potential for correction and the lesser the magnitude of correction required at later age levels.

Chapter 8

Mandibular Skeletal Prognathism

Some individuals have inherited the potential to develop a jaw dimension problem, manifested as mandibular prognathism. It is commonly thought that a Class III molar relationship is indicative of excessive length of the mandible. A Class III malocclusion may indeed be indicative of a prognathic mandible, but it may also be indicative of a retrusive maxilla, or even a combination of the two. The frequency of Class III malocclusion in the Caucasian population of the United States has been found to be approximately 5%.[1,2] It is much higher in Central America and some of the Scandinavian countries and is reported to be as high as one third of the orthodontic patients in Japan.[3] In roughly 51% of that Class III population, maxillary retrusion or deficiency was observed to be the prevalent feature of the malocclusion. Maxillary retrusion is reported to be present in 62% to 63% of the Class III population, in combination with various sizes of mandibles.[4] However, it should likewise be pointed out that, in another study of 149 patients with Class III malocclusions, it was found that the most common Class III pattern occurred when the maxilla was within the "normal range of prognathism," while the mandible extended beyond this range[5]; only about 25% of the Class III malocclusions could be categorized as maxillary skeletal retrusion. In seeking differences between mandibular prognathism and the normal position, investigators came to the conclusion that it was more a difference of mandibular morphology and position than of size. The gonial angle was larger than normal; the glenoid fossa and condylar head were more anteriorly positioned in the cranial base than normal. Furthermore, 60% of the children with Class III molar relationships exhibited the normal range of dimensions in prognathism, and it was only later growth that significantly increased the proportion of adults having Class III prognathism.

Such observations are pertinent to the present discussion because, where mandibular prognathism is concerned, we must recognize possible skeletal facial changes through periods of childhood, adolescence, and then adulthood to determine the type and timing of treatment. It is imperative to know where growth occurs, in what direction, when growth will most express itself, how much growth is remaining, and how we can influence these factors to achieve optimal results. To our mind, at present, very little can be done orthodontically to significantly control the amount of mandibular growth to be expressed or to significantly inhibit that growth. At present, it seems that the only potential for orthodontically influencing a developing mandibular prognathism, short of orthognathic surgery, is to orthopedically alter the direction of mandibular growth. A redirection of mandibular growth, to position the mandible more downward than forward, is, in reality, minimizing the anteriorly directed component of mandibular growth as much as possible. Directing the chin downward as it grows increases lower anterior facial height and, at the same time, minimizes the forward positioning of the chin relative to the forehead and upper face. When a reasonable possibility for success is evident, this course of action should be seriously considered.

Chin-cup therapy has been initiated at early age levels to redirect mandibular growth while the patient has not yet exhibited definitive mandibular prognathism nor is obviously posturing the mandible into an overclosed position. The chin cup is used in conjunction with a high-pull headcap to reposture the chin into a more downward and backward position, increasing lower anterior facial height and posterior interocclusal opening. The purpose of mandibular repositioning is to permit further eruption of the molars into the increased interocclusal space. Increased eruption of the posterior teeth will, of course, further increase lower anterior facial height as the chin postures more downward and somewhat backward when the molars are brought into occlusion. Chin-cup therapy is undertaken for varying periods of time until, if so indicated, the patient is ready for more comprehensive treatment.

Mandibular Prognathism: Early or Late Treatment?

It must be stressed that, in selected cases where the discrepancy between the jaws is not excessive and where eruption of posterior teeth is desirable, the mandible can be repositioned to reduce prognathism. This approach to the treatment of potential mandibular prognathism must be undertaken with the knowledge that it will be long term and time consuming; however, in certain cases it might circumvent the necessity for surgery. It also involves a pretty fair "guessing game" as to the amount of future mandibular growth as well as the judgment to determine whether it can be adequately redirected. It must be re-emphasized that this type of treatment should be undertaken at comparatively early age levels when the greatest chance for success in redirecting mandibular growth can be anticipated.

There are those who believe that, at early ages, orthodontic preparation should be geared toward the inevitability of orthognathic surgery. During this time, the dentition is periodically evaluated, adjusted, and prepared for the eventuality of mandibular surgical retropositioning on the assumption that surgical correction is inevitable. If this assumption is based on molar relationships at a young age, it may be fallacious; it requires a great deal of predictive assumption because mandibular shifts, overclosure, and other factors might be involved. Others think it advisable not to initiate any orthodontic treatment whatsoever until the later growing ages, so that surgery can be undertaken expeditiously without the concern of additional surgical intervention to compensate for continuing growth. This, too, may serve to the disadvantage of the patient since it doesn't allow for the possibility of mandibular repositioning or altering the direction of mandibular growth. Then again, the discrepancies could be adequately camouflaged in some cases. It could also be rationalized that, if the patient does require surgery, much has already been done orthodontically, so that surgical corrective procedures can be readily initiated.

The question arises as to how to recognize, at an early age, a developing skeletal mandibular prognathism and to differentiate the case from one of apparent mandibular prognathism (in reality a maxillary skeletal retrusion). Lozman[6] retrospectively studied a longitudinal radiographic series of untreated Class III malocclusions available at the Burlington Growth Center in Ontario, Canada. Summarily, at early maturational stages, the maxillary retrusive group exhibited mandibles that were actually decreased in body length and ramal height. The chin was acceptably related to the forehead, albeit the mandibular denture base was surprisingly retrusive. In contradistinction, the patients with future true skeletal mandibular prognathism exhibited maxillas of average length but protrusive, with a protrusive denture base; their mandibles tended to be prognathic and have a protrusive denture base, although its body length fell within the mean. The latter patients had true mandibular skeletal prognathism at later stages of maturation.

In the maxillary retrusive Class III cases, the maxilla was deficient anteroposteriorly; likewise, the mandible was usually deficient in body length to some degree, despite the fact that it was positioned forward relative to the maxilla. In the mandibular prognathism cases, the mandible was anterior to the maxilla, despite the maxilla being protrusive and the mandible being only approximately average in length. It may be surmised that, in a developing mandibular prognathism, the condyle and glenoid fossa are relatively forward and, in some way, must be incorporated into our skeletal analysis.

References

1. Mermingos J, Full CA, Andreasen G. Protraction of the maxillofacial complex. Am J Orthod Dentofac Orthop 1990;98:47–55.
2. Turley PK. Orthopedic correction of Class III malocclusions with palatal expansion and custom protraction headgear. J Clin Orthod 1988;22:314–325.
3. Ishii H, Morita S, Takeuchi Y, Nakamura S. Treatment effect of combined maxillary protraction and chincup appliance in severe skeletal Class III cases. Am J Orthod Dentofac Orthop 1981;92:304–312.
4. Guyer EC, Ellis EE, McNamara JA Jr, Behrents RG. Components of Class III malocclusion in juveniles and adolescents. Angle Orthod 1986;56:7–30.
5. Jacobson A, Evans W, Preston CB, Sadowsky PL. Mandibular prognathism. Am J Orthod 1974;66:140–171.
6. Lozman RN. The Longitudinal Evaluation of Dentofacial Maturation in Untreated Class III Malocclusions Based on Indicators of Skeletal Maturational Development during Infancy and Childhood [senior research]. Rochester, NY: Eastman Dental Center, 1997.

Part III

Vertical Jaw Malocclusions: Vertical Skeletal and Dentoalveolar Malocclusions

In years past, consideration of early orthodontic treatment was usually relegated to, and formulated in terms of, appliance therapy such as headgears, biteplates, expansion appliances, and functional appliances, to control anteroposterior and buccolingual dentoalveolar relationships. Strong consideration was given to achieving a Class I molar relationship. For a long time, little consideration was given to vertical dentoalveolar relationships and the effect of those changes on the anteroposterior relationships of the occlusion. Today it is acknowledged that changes in the posterior regions could affect the postural relationship of the mandible, thus altering interrelationship of skeletal jaw structures; this could lead to an increasing tendency toward a Class II or Class III molar relationship and two common orthodontic problems recognizable at early ages—the excessive overbite (deep bite) and, conversely, the inadequate overbite (open bite).

Chapter 9

The Deep Bite: Excessive Anterior Overbite

Malocclusions manifested by a deep dental overbite pose a significant problem to the orthodontist, in that long-term stability of overbite correction is questionable at best. Strong relapse tendencies, although variable in occurrence, have been noted. This creates food for thought: are all deep bites alike? For example, Class II, division I malocclusions are frequently known to have deep overbites, as are Class II, division 2 malocclusions. Both have deep overbites but differ in the characteristics of their Class II malocclusions. Actually, there may be skeletal differences in their malocclusions. Differences in mandibular morphology have been noted between these two malocclusions in that the Class II, division 2 mandible was observed to have a more acute gonial angle and, generally, less steepness to the mandibular plane[1]—differences that could lead to differences in orthodontic correction, stability, and relapse. Wasilewsky,[2] in his study of overbite relapse, which evaluated patients 10 years or longer postretention, noted that, although there was an overall 22.5% correction, there was a dramatic relapse in 44.9% of the overbite correction that had been achieved at the time of retention. Individual variation was noted, of course, but this figure represented a significant degree of unwanted relapse.

Skeletal and Dental Characteristics of Deep Bite: Treatment Correlations

An evaluation of morphologic characteristics associated with deep overbites, skeletal and dental, was undertaken in an attempt to find the causes of deep overbite and of mechanisms to minimize relapse.[2] In this sample, the subjects were not differentiated or evaluated on the basis of Angle molar classification, but were subdivided according to the extent of overbite. The skeletal characteristics found to be associated with deep bite were a greater degree of mandibular retrognathism and a shorter posterior aspect of the ramus when measured from the palatal plane to the antegonial and gonial regions. Additionally, when the mandibular skeletal base in the canine region was significantly narrower than the corresponding width of the maxillary skeletal base, a characteristically deep overbite was noted. When the premaxillary region was more tipped down, or inferiorly positioned, than the posterior aspect of the maxilla, then it was considered to be another morphologic characteristic of deep overbite. Dentally, it was noted that deep overbites were generally not correlated with excessive eruption of the incisors, but more with the axial inclination of these teeth. Notably, the maxillary incisors were significantly more retroclined, as were the mandibular incisors, in deep overbites.

It was also noted that, as a result of orthodontic treatment, the maxillary molars were more erupted and were instrumental in the overbite correction at the time of retention; but relapse of the overbite seemed to be correlated with subsequent intrusion of these teeth, possibly caused by an intrusive effect of the extruded maxillary molars on the mandibular molars. Forward positioning of the mandibular molars as part of orthodontic treatment was also found to be a factor in overbite relapse. The lesson to be learned seems to be, keep or move molars posteriorly to preclude overbite increment or relapse in deep bite cases. Finally, the observation was made that treatment changes resulting in more harmonious skeletal relationships lead to improved correction of deep overbites with notably less relapse at later age levels; this was correlated with greater forward positioning of the mandible with growth and with greater vertical growth in the posterior aspect of the oral cavity. Assumedly greater overbite correction seemed to be correlated with growth increase in posterior dentoalveolar height. Again, growth seems to be a factor in correction and, possibly, long-term stability.

An earlier cephalometric study was undertaken on successfully treated deep bite cases, where orthodontic treatment was initiated at the transitional dentition stage of development.[3] Forty subjects were selected from the inactive files of an orthodontic department and a private practice. The criteria were: a deep overbite prior to treatment, a successful result at the time of retention, and follow-up records available for 2 to 5 years out of retention. Cases were deemed to have been successfully treated when retention models showed a satisfactory correction of the overbite and when molars and canines had been corrected to a Class I relationship. The subjects were divided into three groups, based upon the angulation of the mandibular plane as ascertained from pretreatment cephalometric radiographs. The first group (13 subjects) exhibited a relatively flat mandibular plane of 25 degrees or less; the sec-

ond group (15 subjects) exhibited more average mandibular plane angulations for early ages, ranging from 25.5 to 30 degrees; the third group (12 subjects) exhibited greater steepness in mandibular plane angulations, exceeding 30.5 degrees. Thus, an attempt was made to divide the subjects according to possible differences in mandibular growth patterns.

The degree of overbite, as perceived on the cephalometric radiographs, was measured as the percentage of mandibular central incisor crown that was overlapped by the maxillary central incisor crown. Overall, there was a significant reduction in the overbite depth from a pretreatment average of 71% to an average of 29% at the time of retention. In the postretention evaluation, significant relapse in overbite was not evident; the total sample exhibited only about 4% relapse. However, the extent of correction and relapse seemed to differ somewhat in the three groups subdivided according to their mandibular plane angles. In the subjects with a low or flat mandibular plane, the average overbite was corrected from a depth of 68% to an average depth of 32% at the time of retention; at the postretention level, an average relapse of 4% was noted. In the subjects with more average mandibular plane angles (ranging from 25.5 to 30 degrees), the overbite was corrected from an average depth of 72% before treatment to 25% at retention and exhibited a relapse of 6%, to an average value of 31% at postretention. Subjects with more steepness to the mandibular plane showed an average reduction in incisal overlap of from 75% to 32% at retention and exhibited a minimal average relapse of only 1% at postretention. From all indications, the pattern of mandibular growth direction, as represented by the mandibular plane angulation, could have an influence on overbite correction and stability; patients with the more vertical positioning of the anterior aspect of the growing mandibles demonstrated a smaller percentage of postretention overbite relapse.

Further evaluation of the 40 successfully treated subjects indicated that both maxillary and mandibular anterior dentoalveolar heights increased during the periods studied, with the mandibular region showing the greater increment, seemingly indicating that overbite correction was not necessarily a result of depressing mandibular anterior teeth. Concomitantly, there was an increase in anterior facial height with a discernibly greater increment in lower facial height. Posterior lower facial height (below the level of the palate) increased during all the time periods studied with concomitant increases in both maxillary and mandibular molar dentoalveolar heights, the greatest increase of eruption being noted in the maxillary molar region. Increment in maxillary molar dentoalveolar height was observed to be greater than the vertical growth of the posterior aspect of the nasomaxillary complex, while the reverse was observed in the mandibular region: increase in ramal height exceeded the accompanying mandibular molar dentoalveolar vertical increment. Maxillary molar height in all cases was observed to continue increasing significantly from retention to postretention, whereas this was not true in the mandible. The interpretation is drawn that, in many cases, overbite correction was at least partially dependent on increased posterior dentoalveolar height, that is, in the molar region. Increments in both maxillary and mandibular molar heights aided in the correction of the overbite problem; maxillary molar increase, again, seemed influential in maintaining correction of the anterior vertical problem in the postretention period. Incident to orthodontic correction of the deep bite, the mandibular incisor was found to become more proclined during treatment and was not observed to upright significantly out of retention. The increased proclination was not considered the mechanism of overbite correction, but possibly a prerequisite for long-term maintenance of the correction.

Interpreting these studies clinically, one can hypothesize that the treatment of deep overbites at early ages can readily establish more correct skeletal relationships and, perhaps with growth, maintain the more desirable relationship achieved. Furthermore, since such little relapse was noted incident to early treatment, one can assume a greater probability of a more positive muscular adaptation to the induced changes in skeletal posture and dentoalveolar form. It might also be hypothesized that mandibular growth needs to occur anteroposteriorly to position the chin in a more forward pos-

ture; vertical increment in mandibular posterior dentoalveolar height is likewise highly desirable. Additionally, orthodontic correction, correlated with the increment in mandibular posterior oral cavity height, might necessarily be geared toward increased mandibular molar eruption more than that in the maxillary, since it was shown that, at later age levels, excessive extrusion of maxillary molars under muscle influences might have an intrusive effect on mandibular molars, thereby increasing potential for overbite relapse. Treatment efforts should also be geared toward precluding anterior movement of the mandibular molar.

Anterior Overbites: Treatment Considerations for Dual Occlusal Levels

At this point, it seems desirable to indicate treatment procedures for increasing posterior dentoalveolar height at an early age to correct the deep bite. In evaluating deep bite cases with favorable skeletal features such as a flat mandibular plane, one must differentiate between lack of vertical development of the posterior dentoalveolar process and excessive eruption of the anterior occlusion. Both of these will have differing influences on mandibular position and, of necessity, will require differing therapeutic procedures. An excessive posterior freeway space and an undesirably shortened lower facial height, in conjunction with a deep overbite, is an indication of an overclosed mandible, indicating the probable need for increased posterior dentoalveolar height. In these cases, what can be called a two-step occlusion may be manifested in the mandibular arch: the occlusal level of the premolars and molars are at a definitively lower level (Fig 9-1) than the anterior dentition from canine to canine. The reduced mandibular posterior dentoalveolar height, of course, causes a greater movement of the mandible to achieve closure into full occlusion, resulting in increased depth of the anterior overbite. In this type of case, treatment should be directed toward orthodontic eruption of the posterior occlusion, be it maxillary, mandibular, or both, to correct the

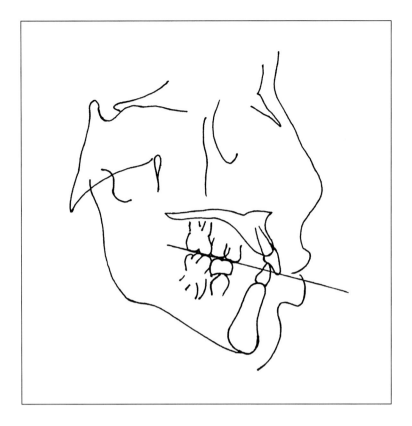

Fig 9-1 Lateral headplate tracing of a young individual with a deep bite and a two-step mandibular occlusion.

deep overbite by eliciting postural changes in the vertical position of the mandible. Of course, concomitant vertical growth of the ramal area would be helpful in physiologically maintaining the increment in dentoalveolar height.

Various mechanisms of treatment can be used to increase molar height. In Class II cases, maxillary headgear can be used favorably to rotate and retract maxillary molars. Additionally, its ability to erupt maxillary molars has been shown to increase lower posterior facial height at early age levels. Achieving mandibular molar eruption, however, especially in correcting an excessive curve of Spee (two-step occlusion), may be more difficult to accomplish but possibly essential.

Archwire design

In a two-step occlusion, whether it be in the transitional dentition or more advanced dental age, utilization of a shoe loop rectangular arch-wire has been found to be effective (Fig 9-2). The shoe loop is placed distal to the mandibular canines with the "toe" of the loop facing distally. The archwire incorporates labial root torque in the incisors, serving to prevent their tipping forward and maintaining them at the original occlusal level. In the posterior region, the archwire is brought down into the bracket of the deciduous first molar or first premolar, thereby activating the loop. The loop acts to raise the teeth in the mandibular buccal segments upward and backward, effectively elevating the first premolars (or primary first molars) more than the permanent first molars—in essence, raising the mesial aspect of the first permanent molars more than the distal, uprighting them. The anterior aspect of the depressed mandibular buccal segments in a two-step occlusion is raised more than the posterior aspect, correcting the occlusal level of the mandibular arch by bringing the posterior teeth to the level of the anterior occlusal plane. This differs dra-

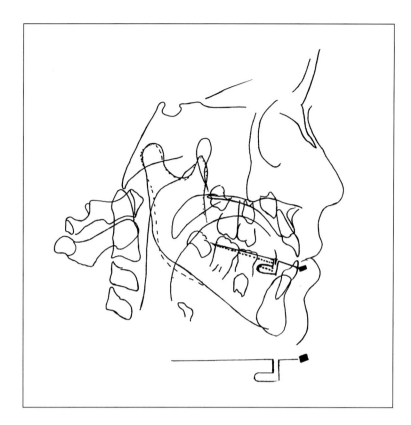

Fig 9-2 Preferred arch wire construction to correct two-step occlusal levels in the mandibular arch.

matically from correcting a deep curve of Spee by incorporating a reverse curve into the archwire, which serves to procline the anterior teeth. Some additional arch length is achieved as well. More important, posterior mandibular dentoalveolar height is selectively achieved while leveling the arch, thus decreasing the overbite.

Musculature, appliances, and deep bite correction

Lip bumpers are effective in achieving added arch length in the mandibular arch, especially in patients having tight lower lip musculature. Using the lip bumper as an intermediary, muscle forces of the lower lip can effect a distal uprighting movement of the mandibular molars and/or a forward movement of the mandibular incisors. When used in conjunction with a biteplate to open the posterior interocclusal dimension, the lip bumper has been shown to effectively erupt as well as upright the more posterior mandibu-

lar molars.[4] When this occurs at early age levels (when advantage can be taken of the natural eruptive process of the mandibular molars), the increment in mandibular posterior dentoalveolar height can reposition the mandible away from the maxilla, causing an increase in lower anterior facial height that can be instrumental in reducing overbite. Furthermore, any physiologic proclination of the mandibular anterior dentition under normal tongue influence, but with reduced mentalis muscle influence, can improve stability, again, as suggested in the findings of the aforementioned treated deep-bite cases.

At times the mandible itself should be repositioned so that teeth can erupt into as favorable a position as possible during early growth spurts, to correct excessive depth of overbite. Orthodontists, by applying forces on the dentition, are able to favorably modify mandibular posture—in the case of the deep bite, into a more open position. Of particular importance in these malocclusions is the vertical growth of the

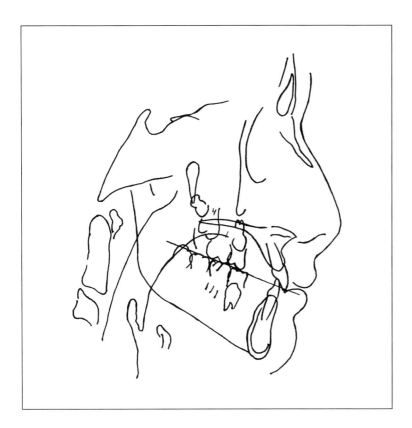

Fig 9-3 Headplate tracing of patient D.M. at time of treatment start. The patient had a deep overbite and a two-step occlusion in the mandibular arch.

ramus to allow for the eruption and maintenance of the positions of the erupted posterior teeth. Correction of the two-step occlusion is most advantageously achieved at early age levels, especially in cases of well-formed, adequately growing mandibles, although at young ages, growth of the mandible periodically expresses inactive phases of growth. In severe mandibular overclosure cases, continued natural eruption of posterior teeth and continued vertical growth of the posterior alveolus is frequently desirable. In such instances, a high-pull chin cup can be used at night, with or without conjunctive use of a lip bumper. Cephalometric evidence has shown that this type of chin cap can reposition the chin downward. This appliance can be particularly useful in cases with excessive freeway space where the occlusion is manifested as an anterior crossbite, with the mandible functioning into an excessively forward, overclosed position, when achieving posterior occlusion. In this position, the patient is sometimes erroneously diagnosed as developing

mandibular prognathism. Mechanically repositioning the mandible and permitting vertical posterior dentoalveolar development not only aids in the correction of excessive overbite, but also achieves better skeletal relationships of the jaws, improving facial appearance.

Case presentations

Patient D.M. This patient is an example of correcting a deep overbite that was documented over a considerable period of time. The patient, a male, presented with dentition in the transitional stage. Initial cephalometric radiographs (Fig 9-3) indicated a good skeletal profile, albeit slightly retrognathic, with a small degree of facial convexity, but acceptable for his stage of development, and an acceptable, low mandibular plane angle. Concomitant with the low mandibular plane angle, the patient had an undesirably short lower anterior facial height. As for the dentition, a Class I molar relationship was evident and a coexistent deep overbite,

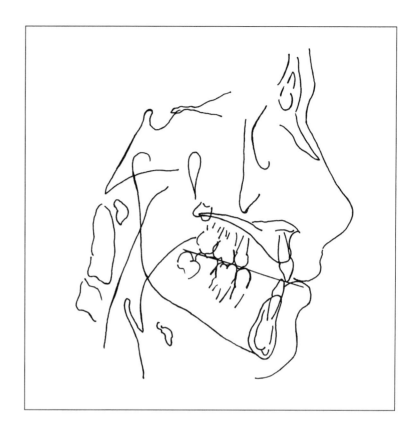

Fig 9-4 Lateral headplate tracing of D.M. at time of retention. Note the overbite correction.

with approximately 50% to 60% of the mandibular incisors covered by the maxillary incisors. The occlusal plane, representing the occlusal surfaces of the mandibular permanent and second deciduous molars, was drawn from the lateral cephalometric radiograph and was found to approximate the incisal edges of the maxillary incisors, but to definitively pass through the approximate midlevel of the mandibular incisors. It was a two-step occlusion with two occlusal planes: the functional occlusal plane along the occlusal surfaces of the posterior teeth being at a distinctly lower level than the occlusal plane represented by the incisal edges of the incisors and canines. Concomitantly, the mandibular incisor was found to be somewhat retroclined relative to the mandibular plane as well as to the "jaw profile," the A-pogonion line. In contradistinction, the maxillary incisor seemed both well proclined and properly positioned relative to the jaw profile. On the rest cephalogram, as a result of the two-step occlusion, there appeared to be an excessive freeway space in the posterior of the occlusion, indicating the possibility of mandibular overclosure—a probable reason for the reduced lower anterior facial height. A significant finding on the cephalometric radiograph was that the premaxilla was slightly tipped down relative to the palatal plane—a skeletal characteristic of deep overbite.

D.M. was treated with a cervical headgear to rotate and erupt the maxillary molars; conjunctively, a lip bumper was used to upright and erupt the mandibular molars. This was followed by full-banded, edgewise therapy. The deep overbite was treated to an acceptable relationship (Fig 9-4), but it was not corrected by depressing the mandibular incisors; actually, they erupted slightly during treatment. The deep overbite was corrected by raising the mandibular posterior functional occlusal plane, more in the premolar than in the molar region, so that the occlusal plane was caused to pass close to the incisal edges of the mandibular incisors (Fig 9-5). Overbite correction, in essence, occurred incident to a change in the level of the func-

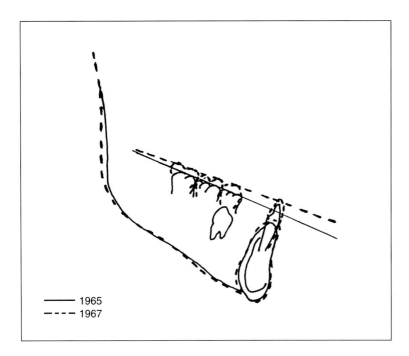

Fig 9-5 Superimposition of D.M.'s mandible on the lingual table of the symphysis and best fit of the mandibular canal in 1965 and at time of retention in 1967, indicating change in mandibular occlusal plane.

tional occlusal plane distal to the mandibular canines, bringing the occlusal plane closer to the mandibular incisal edges. In other words, posterior teeth were differentially brought occlusally to decrease the overbite without depressing the mandibular incisors. These changes in the occlusal plane and overbite were observable when progressive tracings were superimposed on the inner aspect of the mandibular symphysis and the best fit of the mandibular canal in the third molar region. The whole mandibular posterior occlusal level was raised while a small dentoalveolar increment in the incisor region occurred. Throughout treatment the maxillary molars, although positioned more occlusally and mesially, were not erupted excessively to treat the overbite; their occlusal levels were maintained at the same functional occlusal level as the incisal edges of the maxillary incisors.

Growth appreciably aided in correcting the overbite. When progressive cephalometric tracings were superimposed on the palatal plane registering on the posterior nasal spine and pterygomaxillary fissure, increment in the posterior oral cavity height was evident, concomitant with a slightly greater increase anteriorly. Thus,

with growth, there was both anterior and posterior vertical increment in the oral cavity accommodating the elevation of the posterior functional occlusal plane (Fig 9-6). When the headplates were superimposed on sella-nasion registering on the anterior surface of the fossa, increment in nasomaxillary height, both anteriorly and posteriorly, was evident, concomitant with the considerable mandibular growth (Fig 9-6). Although vertical increment in the ramal region was considerably greater than what occurred in the posterior nasomaxillary region, the mandibular plane maintained near parallelism from initiation to completion of treatment; there was only a slight increase in mandibular steepness, resulting in a slightly greater increment in lower anterior facial height.

Evaluating the patient 15 years postretention (Fig 9-7) revealed that much of what had been attained during treatment had maintained itself. The mandible had continued to grow, but the mandibular plane was still nearly parallel to the original plane (Fig 9-8). The palatal plane had continued to progress vertically, and Point A had come slightly forward. The chin had progressed downward and slightly forward; consid-

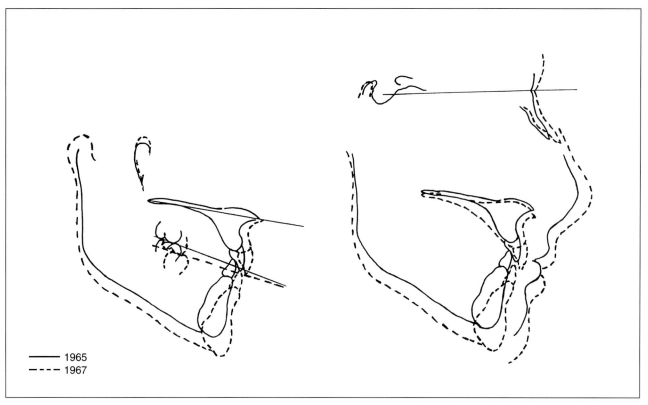

Fig 9-6 Superimposition of tracings on palatal plane of D.M. in 1965 and 1967, showing vertical increment in oral cavity height *(left)* and vertical increment in nasomaxillary height and ramal height *(right)*.

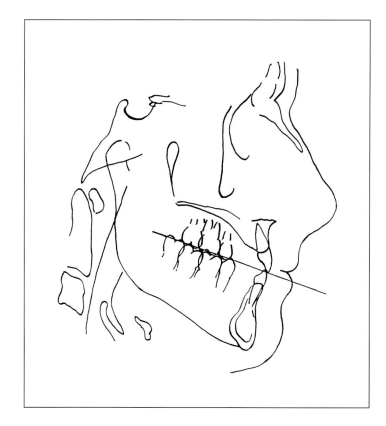

Fig 9-7 Cephalometric tracing of D.M. taken 15 years after initiation of treatment and 13 years after retention.

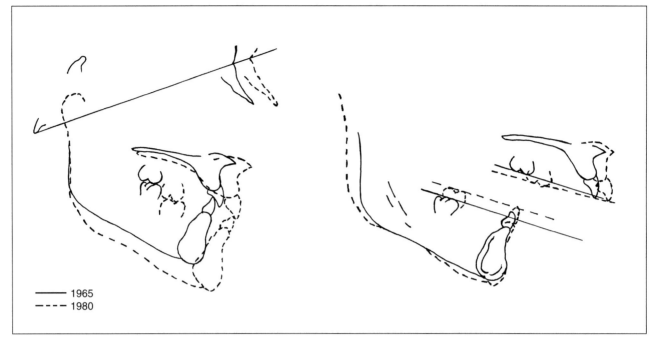

Fig 9-8 Patient D.M. Superimpositions of tracings of lateral headplates taken at start of treatment and at last evaluation in 1980, indicating general pattern of growth of the nasomaxillary and the mandibular areas as well as dental changes incident to correction of the two-step mandibular occlusion.

erable favorable growth was expressed in both the ramal and the mandibular body regions. The Class I molar relationship had maintained itself satisfactorily; acceptable dental interdigitation was evident (Fig 9-9). The one feature that might be subject to criticism was attrition on the cusps of the maxillary canines. Of particular note was the observation that the overbite correction was well maintained. This is particularly pertinent in light of the fact that depression of the anterior teeth, either maxillary or mandibular, did not take place as part of orthodontic treatment. Instead, vertical dentoalveolar growth in the posterior region and concomitant vertical growth at the back of the oral cavity (with increase in ramal height) helped maintain the posterior teeth at a proper functional level. In this instance, correction of the two-step occlusion, commensurate with posterior vertical mandibular growth, resulted in a lasting overbite correction. In fact, sufficient mandibular growth had occurred to accommodate the third molars, resulting in a full complement of teeth that interdigitated well and appeared relatively stable.

The anterior dentition, the maxillary and mandibular incisors, were also very pleasantly positioned and inclined; the mandibular incisors were slightly more proclined than at the start of treatment, but this seemed helpful in maintaining the overbite correction. As the patient matured, he developed a very slightly retrognathic mandible with slight facial convexity, so that a pleasant profile was achieved, as well as an acceptable occlusion that lasted over the years.

D.M. is an example of a patient in whom growth was advantageous and was taken advantage of in order to correct a deep overbite. This was achieved orthodontically by correcting the two-step occlusion, raising the level of the posterior functional occlusal plane; it definitely did not result incident to depression of the anterior teeth. Fortunate in this case, as well, was the fact that extractions were not needed to achieve proper dental alignment. As a consequence, the molars were not moved mesially, serving to emphasize contemporary observations that, if at all possible, extractions should not be undertaken in overbite cases. Additionally, there was less

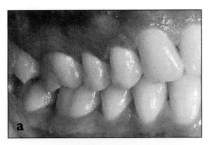 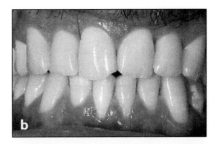 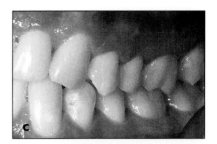

Fig 9-9 *(a to c)* Dental occlusion of D.M. nearly 15 years after orthodontic correction, showing maintenance of overbite correction.

eruption of the maxillary molar incident to treatment than was noted in the mandibular molar region; this, too, may have added to the stability, since, during postretention, the maxillary molar did not have a depressive action on the mandibular molar. Wasilewsky[2] has noted that overeruption of the maxillary molar can cause subsequent depression of the mandibular molar, which could be instrumental in a return of a two-step occlusion.

Patient L.T. This patient presented in the early transitional dentition with deciduous molars present and all premolars and permanent canines unerupted. Observable was a Class I (edge-to-edge) molar relationship with a deep overbite. The mandibular incisors were approximate to the cingula of the maxillary incisors—close to a 100% overbite. Clinically and radiographically, a large posterior freeway space was recorded (Fig 9-10). On the lateral cephalometric radiograph, a somewhat retrognathic, convex skeletal facial profile was noted, but it was not exceptional for the age and stage of development. Some steepness to the mandibular plane was also noted, but acceptable posterior vertical oral cavity height was evident, again not abnormal for the age. On the lateral cephalogram, the maxillary incisors were somewhat proclined, with the incisal edges positioned considerably forward of the jaw profile (A-Po) line. The maxillary molar was observed to be distally inclined. A definite mandibular two-step occlusion was ap-

parent, with the mandibular incisors well above the posterior functional occlusal plane. The maxillary incisal edge was superior to the occlusal plane but was inclined forward, and, if properly angulated, would probably have approximated the occlusal plane. The mandibular incisors were upright and somewhat retroclined relative to the mandibular plane. The rest headplate revealed an excessive freeway space.

Skeletally, a fairly level palatal plane was evident and the premaxilla tipped neither up nor down. Lower anterior facial height was less than ideal; some increment in lower facial height seemed needed.

The patient was treated with a headgear to rotate and slightly retract the maxillary molars, a biteplate to open the bite, and a mandibular lip bumper. Eventually the four first premolars were extracted, the dentition was aligned, and the patient was placed in retention (Fig 9-11) with a Hawley retainer and a mandibular G-wire from second molar to second molar. The mandibular lingual retainer was a mistake because it is now known that these arches prevent eruption of molars; the patient should have been retained with a canine-to-canine G-wire to allow the mandibular posterior dentition to erupt, or, at the minimum, to maintain occlusal levels.

During treatment (Fig 9-12), the noted mandibular two-step occlusion was never corrected. In essence, the mandibular incisors were at the same level above the posterior functional

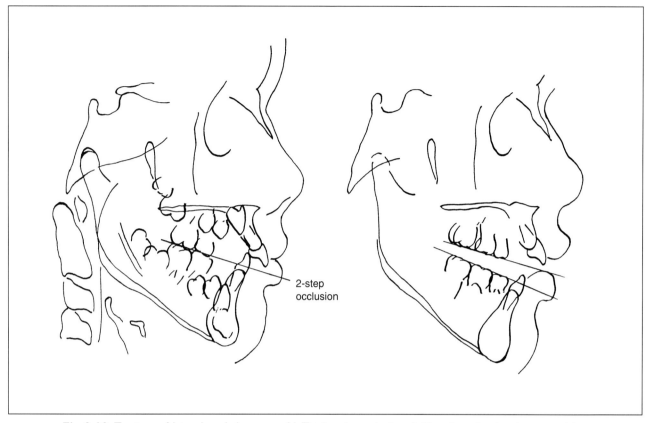

2-step
occlusion

Fig 9-10 Tracings of lateral cephalograms of L.T. taken in occlusion *(left)* and at simulated rest position *(right)*. Dentoskeletal relationships at start of treatment are defined.

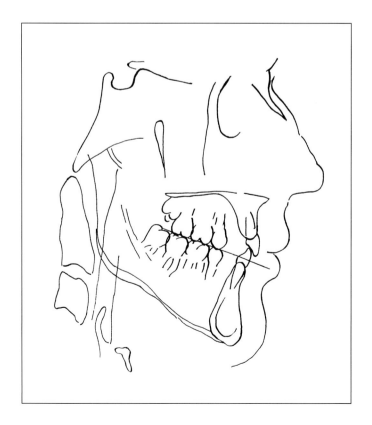

Fig 9-11 Patient L.T. Lateral headplate tracing obtained after completion of active orthodontic treatment.

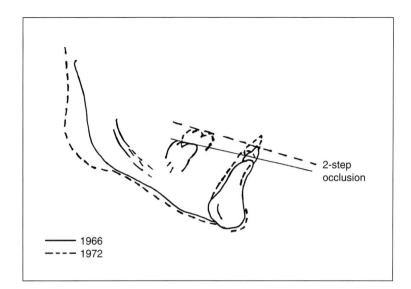

Fig 9-12 Patient L.T. Superimposed cephalometric tracings of the mandible taken at the start of treatment and at retention. Superimposition is on the lingual aspect and trabeculae of the symphysis and best fit of the mandibular canal. The functional posterior occlusal plane was never brought up toward the occlusal plane of the mandibular anterior dentition.

2-step occlusion

—— 1966
---- 1972

occlusal plane after treatment as they were prior. When the before-and-after treatment and the 15-year postretention (Fig 9-13) lateral cephalometric mandibular tracings were superimposed on the inner aspect of the symphysis and bony trabeculae as well as the best fit of the mandibular canal, it was noted that, despite considerable growth, the mandibular incisors were still erupted above the level of the occlusal plane. Mandibular molars had erupted during treatment, but not enough to alter the occlusal plane relative to the incisors (Fig 9-14). The two-step occlusion was not corrected. Additionally, it was observed that, although the mandibular molars were erupted to a degree, they had been positioned mesially away from the hinge area as a result of the extractions, essentially minimizing any benefits of eruption. The mandible still had to overclose to achieve occlusion, hindering overbite correction.

From the beginning of treatment to 15 years postretention, the mandible had continued to grow. Superimposing progress head films on S-N registering on the anterior surface of sella turcica (Fig 9-15) indicated that Point A was held back significantly while progressing downward. Concomitantly, the chin was moving downward

and, to a lesser degree, in a forward direction—which should have been favorable to overbite correction. Much had occurred during treatment and retention but, during postretention, there appeared to have been minimal maxillary and mandibular growth. When the lateral cephalometric radiographs were superimposed on S-N, registering on nasion (Fig 9-15), it became apparent that there had been some increment in lower facial height, along with a continuance of slight mandibular retrognathism and minimal change in skeletal facial convexity. As for the profile, the skeletal positioning of the chin was more vertical than horizontal, with proportional increment in lower facial height.

Appreciable increase in posterior oral cavity height was evident, but the mandibular molars had not erupted commensurate with this change. Also evident was the fact that the maxillary molars had erupted more than the mandibular. During postretention, the maxillary molar had become even more mesially positioned and slightly more erupted. The mandibular molar remained at the same functional level during the 15-year postretention period and, as well, was observed to have moved mesially. The maxillary molars had been erupted and brought

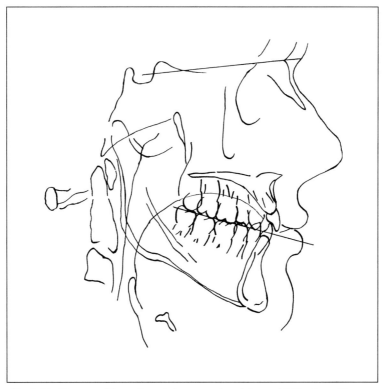

Fig 9-13 Tracing of lateral cephalometric headplate of L.T. taken 15 years postretention.

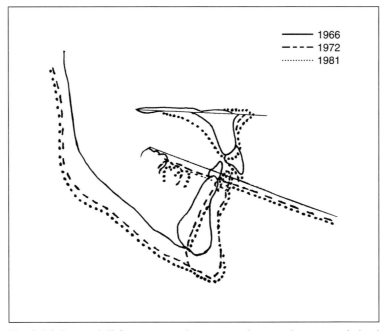

Fig 9-14 Patient L.T. Superimposed tracings indicating changes in skeletal relationships, but lack of correction of the two-step occlusion in the mandibular arch.

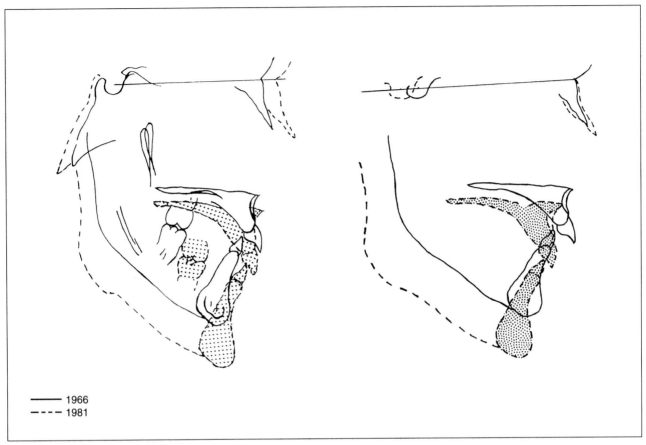

Fig 9-15 Superimposition of lateral cephalometric radiographs of L.T. taken at the initiation of treatment and 15 years later. *(left)* Registration on the anterior surface of sella turcica. *(right)* Registration on nasion along the S-N plane.

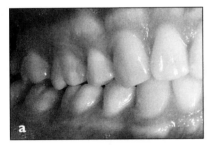 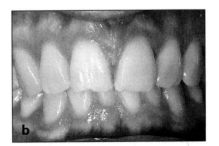 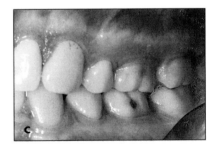

Fig 9-16 *(a to c)* Photographs of the occlusion of L.T. in 1981. The deep overbite is obvious.

mesially after the extractions, creating a possible additional explanation for the deep overbite relapse.

There was minimal reduction in the overbite. Orthodontically, there was inadequate increment in mandibular posterior dentoalveolar height in proportion to the increase in posterior oral cavity height; at the same time, there was too large an increment in maxillary posterior dentoalveolar height and, of course, no depression of the anteriors. Consequently, the two-step occlusion was never corrected, and one of the goals of orthodontic therapy, correction of the deep overbite, was never achieved (Fig 9-16).

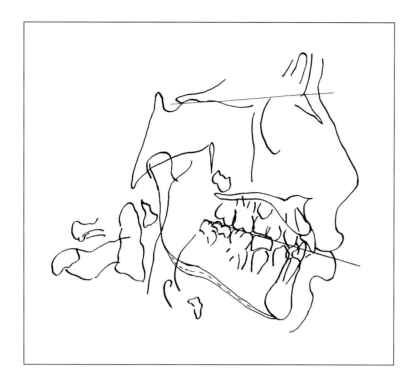

Fig 9-17 Tracing of lateral cephalometric radiograph of R.H. at initiation of treatment.

Patient R.H. Here is another example of failure to correct a mandibular two-step occlusion; the mandibular posterior occlusion was not erupted orthodontically to a good functional level and thereby did not take advantage of the favorable posterior vertical oral cavity growth. At the time of the late transitional dentition, it was obvious that the mandibular posterior functional occlusal plane was considerably lower than that of the anteriors. Concurrently, when the functional occlusal plane was extended anteriorly, it approximated the incisal edges of the maxillary incisors (Fig 9-17). Consequently, when the dentition was in occlusion, the deep overbite became manifested. Posterior occlusal contact resulted in the mandibular incisors being cranially positioned relative to the level of the incisal edges of the maxillary incisors, resulting in a considerable portion of the mandibular incisors becoming overlapped by the maxillary incisors—a deep overbite. Superimposition of headplate tracings obtained at the initiation of treatment and as well at removal of retention (Fig 9-18), in-

dicated that considerable growth had taken place during this interval, with demonstrable vertical increment in the posterior as well as the anterior aspect of the oral cavity (Fig 9-19). The cephalometric headplate taken approximately 15 years postretention (Fig 9-20) revealed that growth in the oral cavity had continued in the same direction, although proportionately less than the amount of craniofacial growth. The postretention records clearly revealed that a deep overbite still existed. It was further obvious that the mandibular two-step occlusion had not been corrected (Fig 9-21) and that the maxillary molar had been caused to or allowed to erupt significantly more compared with the mandibular molar, almost twice as much. In the case of R.H., it was apparent that growth of the mandible was favorable both in amount and direction as well as timing during the treatment years. Growth was downward and forward, positioning the chin favorably and increasing height of the rami and particularly the posterior of the oral cavity. The deep overbite was never fully

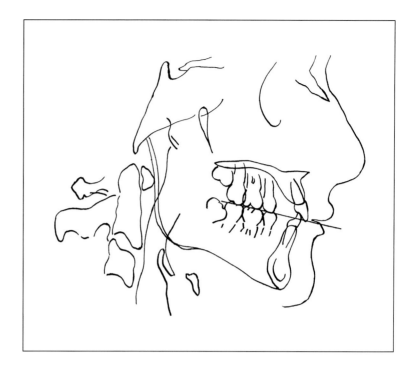

Fig 9-18 Cephalometric tracing of R.H. taken at time of retention removal.

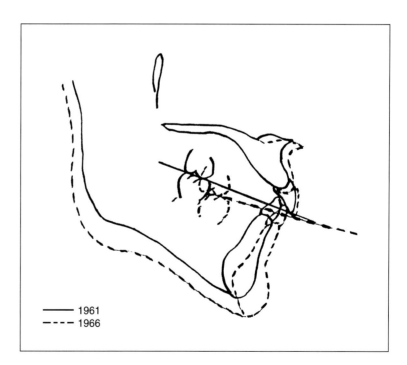

—— 1961
---- 1966

Fig 9-19 Superimposed tracings of R.H., registering on the posterior aspect of the palate, indicate increment of vertical growth of oral cavity.

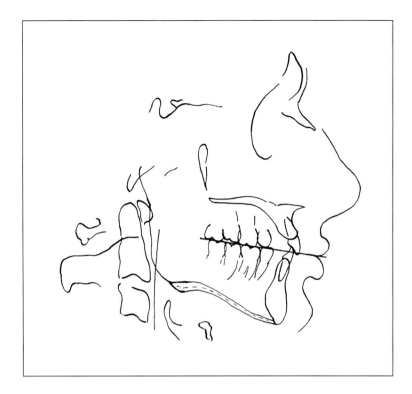

Fig 9-20 Tracing of lateral cephalometric radiograph of R.H. taken in 1979.

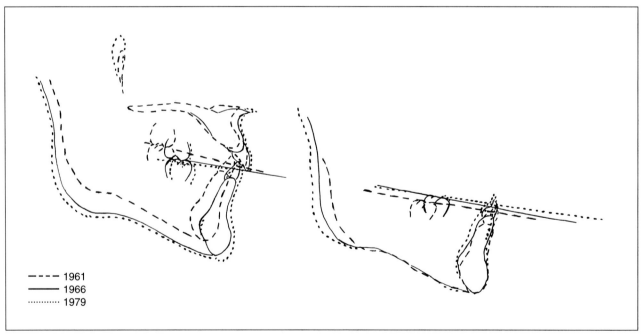

- - - - 1961
——— 1966
·········· 1979

Fig 9-21 Superimposed tracings of R.H. from lateral cephalometric radiographs taken in 1961, 1966, and 1979. Time, treatment, and growth changes in the jaw and dental relationships are readily recognizable.

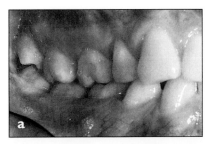 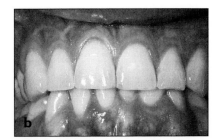 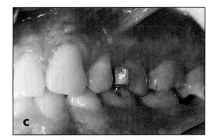

Fig 9-22 *(a to c)* Patient R.H.'s occlusion in 1979; the deep overbite is still evident.

corrected by the time of retention and was still present 15 years postretention (Fig 9-22). Unfortunately, the maxillary posterior dentition had been erupted orthodontically more than had the mandibular. The suggestion readily arises that, in deep overbite cases when a two-step mandibular occlusion is observed, correction should be achieved by erupting the mandibular molars to raise the functional occlusal plane and by limiting eruption of the maxillary molars. It is further suggested that, in the treatment of deep overbites where a two-step mandibular occlusion exists, rather than a supraeruption of the mandibular incisors, vertical growth in the posterior of the oral cavity be used to achieve vertical increment in the mandibular posterior dentoalveolar process.

Mandibular Growth, Deep Bite, and Mandibular Anterior Crowding

It is conceivable that correction of many deep overbites is much more dependent on what is done in the posterior occlusion rather than what is done anteriorly. To paraphrase an old cigarette ad, it's what's in *back* that counts; what's in front is what the orthodontist visualizes. If deep bites are to be orthodontically corrected by ver-

tical increment in the posterior dentoalveolar processes, then it seems important to take advantage of periods of active mandibular growth to accommodate that vertical dentoalveolar growth. One might better anticipate long-term correction of a deep overbite. R.H. exemplifies this observation, since considerable craniofacial growth had occurred during active treatment and much less was expressed in the 15-year postretention period.

It is the pattern of mandibular growth, especially at later age levels, that might bring about relapse in overbite depth and subsequent mandibular incisor malalignment and apparent crowding. The form of the mandible, condylar angulation, and vertical growth of the ramus could all be instrumental in later incisal crowding and bite deepening. The mandibular incisors are noted for their propensity toward crowding in early adulthood, with or without earlier orthodontic intervention. Long-term records obtained as part of an orthodontic-periodontic study at Eastman Dental Center were evaluated to identify factors that might contribute to later mandibular incisor misalignment.[5] The manner in which the mandible grew was as important as the amount of growth. In those subjects demonstrating adverse changes, there were decreases in the gonial angles and mandibular plane angles with significant increases in ramal height,

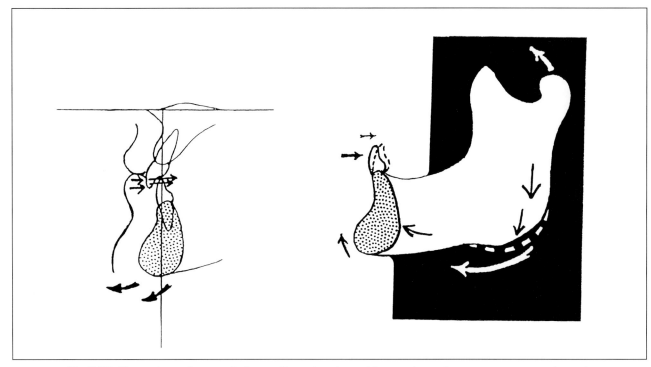

Fig 9-23 Illustrations of a mandibular configuration that, with growth, tends to express proportionately greater horizontal than vertical positioning of the symphysis. Compressive forces of the lips may hold back the maxillary incisors, which in turn may create compressive lingual forces on the mandibular incisors, resulting in mandibular incisor uprighting and possible malalignment.

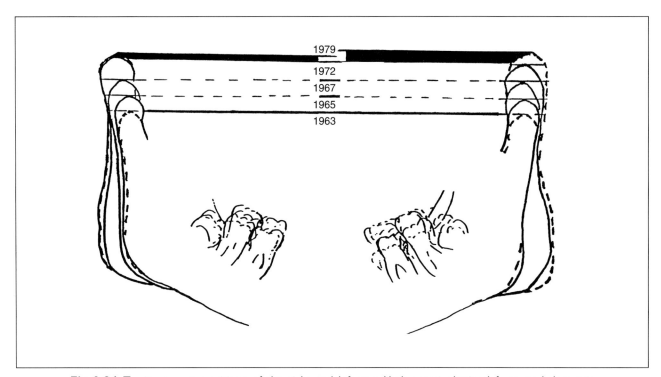

Fig 9-24 Tracing superimpositions of the right and left mandibular rami obtained from cephalometric oblique radiographs of D.G.S. The increment in ramal height from the condylar to the gonial angle regions considerably exceeds the increment in the mandibular molar dentoalveolar height.

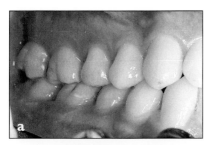 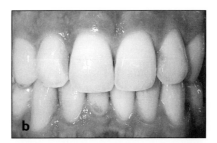 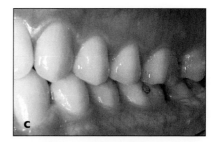

Fig 9-25 *(a to c)* Intraoral photographs of D.G.S. depicting the occlusion 14 years after retention. Note the undesirable relapse into an anterior deep bite.

causing counterclockwise rotation of the mandible. The maxillary and mandibular molars were perceived to erupt, but not of a magnitude to keep pace with the ramal height increment. In subjects exhibiting counterclockwise mandibular growth rotation, concomitant mandibular incisor uprighting was noted. The sequence of these occurrences is depicted in Fig 9-23. It could be rationalized that a mandible with a relatively forward-facing condyle, a wide ramus, a well-formed symphysis, a relatively flat mandibular plane, a somewhat acute gonial angle, and an anteroposteriorly directed growth tendency combined with significant vertical ramal growth and a cessation or diminution of maxillary forward growth could, with ensuing time, cause a retroclination of the mandibular incisors. These features, without the needed concurrent molar eruption, can result in further deepening of the bite as well as possible mandibular anterior crowding. This is depicted in superimposed oblique radiograph tracings of a male (D.G.S.) treated for a deep bite (Fig 9-24) and with photographs of his occlusion 14 years after retention (Fig 9-25). The oblique radiographs show the large increment in ramal height from 1963 to 1979 compared with mandibular molar eruption during the same period. There was more of an increase on the right side compared with the left, which would explain the midline discrepancy in the anterior occlusion at the time of last

records. To be noted in the occlusion photographs is the relapse into a deep bite, as well as evidence of change in incisal alignment. The Class I molar correction and posterior dental alignment had held well anteroposteriorly, illustrating the significance of retention in such cases. It would seem advisable to use some sort of biteplate during retention when there is a possibility of counterclockwise mandibular growth; the interocclusal disarticulation would permit molar eruption in concord with increase in ramal height. Furthermore, it helps assure long-term retention observation and control until completion of mandibular growth.

References

1. Blair ES. A cephalometric roentgenographic appraisal of the skeletal morphology of Class I, Class II division 1 and Class II division 2 (Angle) malocclusions. Angle Orthod 1954;24:106–119.
2. Wasilewsky H. Three Dimensional Evaluation of Overbite Relapse [thesis]. Rochester, NY: Univ of Rochester, 1985.
3. Francis K. Cephalometric Analysis of Early Treatment of Deep Overbite and 2–5 Years after Retention [senior research]. Rochester, NY: Eastman Dental Center, 1971.
4. Subtelny JD, Sakuda M. Muscle function, oral malformation, and growth changes. Am J Orthod 1966;52: 495–517.
5. Raineri W. Late Lower Anterior Crowding: Growth and Orthodontic Treatment [senior research]. Rochester, NY: Eastman Dental Center, 1982.

Chapter 10

The Open Bite

Growth Direction and Open Bites

Indications are that the direction of mandibular growth can influence anterior vertical relationships. In fact, in the deep-bite study, those malocclusions having more vertically growing mandibles demonstrated a smaller percentage of postretention relapse in depth of overbite. Many orthodontists have had the experience of successfully treating a deep bite at one age level, then being disappointed to see their correction develop into an open bite at a later age level. In all probability, this alteration in form was related to excessive vertical mandibular growth and/or excessive eruption of posterior teeth.

Patient J.D. This is an example of a patient initially having a deep overbite that grew into an anterior open bite malocclusion. At the time of presentation—the early transitional dentition—all deciduous molars were present, with premolars and permanent canines exhibiting one-fourth to one-half root formation. Also evident was a Class I (end-to-end) molar relationship and a deep overbite, with the mandibular incisors occluding into the cingula of the maxillary incisors—about 60% overlap. Cephalometric appraisal (Fig 10-1) revealed a somewhat retrognathic facial pattern with slight maxillary retrusion, causing lack of facial convexity, specifically for the age. The premaxilla, or anterior aspect of the hard palate, tipped cranially; also

observable were a short ramal height and posterior oral cavity height. There was excess anterior lower facial height with concomitant steepness to the mandibular plane. Proclination and anterior positioning of the maxillary and mandibular incisors relative to the facial profile were likewise evident. The deep overbite was coexistent with a two-step occlusion; the functional occlusal plane was found to approximate the incisal edge of the maxillary incisor, but to cut through the mandibular incisor crown. Initial treatment started with a biteplate and a cervical headgear, followed by full appliance nonextraction therapy.

Incident to treatment the deep overbite had been reduced. On the lateral cephalogram (Fig 10-2), the maxillary incisor overlapped the mandibular incisor about 10% to 15%. The two-step mandibular occlusion had not been corrected, as evidenced by the functional occlusal plane passing through approximately 50% of the mandibular incisor crown. Incident to therapy, point A and the maxillary incisors had been retracted; the maxillary molars had been erupted and were more mesially positioned. Mandibular molars had been erupted and were more mesially positioned. Mandibular molars had been erupted but not to the same extent as the maxillary. The incisal edges of the maxillary incisors were now above the functional occlusal plane incident to excessive eruption of the maxillary molars.

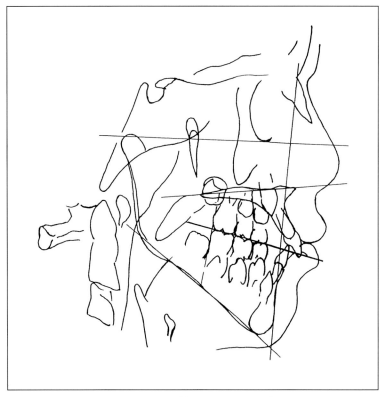

Fig 10-1 Cephalometric tracing of J.D. at the time of initial presentation.

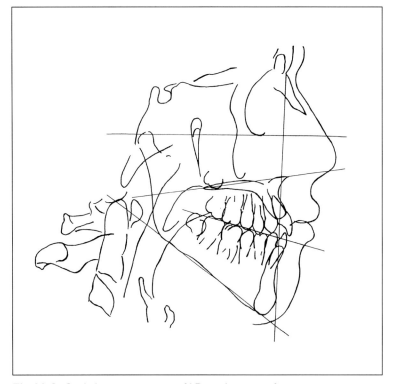

Fig 10-2 Cephalometric tracing of J.D. at the time of retention.

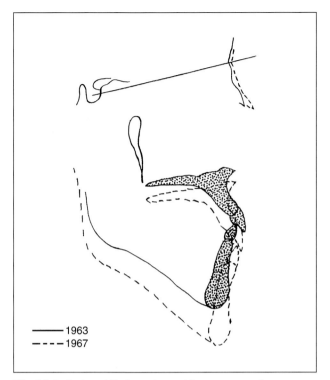

Fig 10-3 Patient J.D. Superimposition at start of treatment (1963) and at time of retention (1967) (superimposition on the S-N plane, registering on the anterior surface of sella).

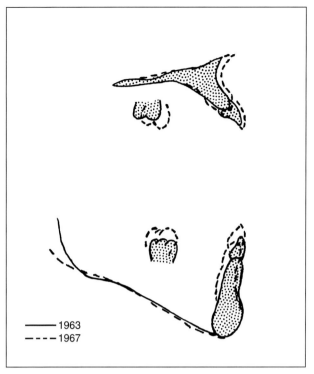

Fig 10-4 Superimpositions of J.D. in 1963 and 1967, indicating eruption of maxillary and mandibular molars incident to treatment.

Superimposition of progress lateral cephalometric radiographs (Fig 10-3) indicated that considerable mandibular growth had occurred during treatment. There was proportionately more increment in lower anterior facial height than posterior facial height and posterior oral cavity height. The mandibular plane had maintained its steepness. Mandibular growth and treatment procedures seemed to have positioned the chin more downward and forward, increasing lower anterior facial height.

The premaxilla was still tipped up anteriorly, while the posterior aspect of the palate was tipped down. In evaluating treatment of a slight maxillary retrusion in light of contemporary knowledge, it appears that headgear therapy should not have been undertaken. Unfortunately, the cervical appliance aided in excessively erupting the maxillary molars (Fig 10-4), resulting in the maxillary incisors being positioned above the occlusal plane.

Fifteen years after dismissal from retention, the maxillary retrusion was still evident; with an

excellent anteroposterior relationship of the chin to the forehead, midface concavity became more evident. A Class I molar relationship and an acceptable posterior occlusion still existed (Fig 10-5), but now the incisors were either edge-to-edge or in a slight open bite relationship. The centric cephalometric radiograph (Fig 10-5) showed that the palate was still observed to tip cranially, progressing anteriorly to the premaxillary area. The maxillary retrusion was measurable, and lower anterior facial height was excessive. Posterior oral cavity and ramal height had increased, but not commensurate with lower anterior facial height. The maxillary incisors were somewhat proclined and the functional occlusal plane now approximated the incisal edges of both the maxillary and mandibular incisors. The two-step occlusion was no longer evident. In the 15-year postretention period, there had been considerable eruption and mesial positioning of the maxillary molar as well as considerable eruption of the maxillary incisors (Fig 10-6), resulting in both the posterior and anterior dentition

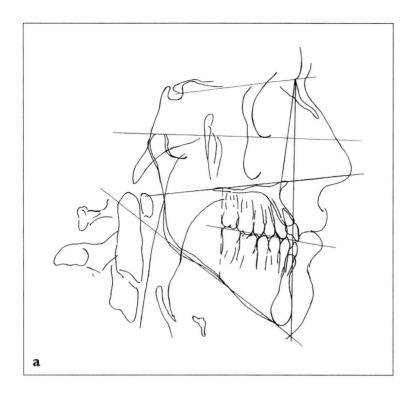

a

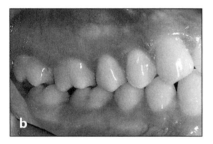

b

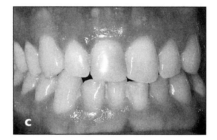

c

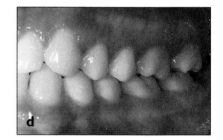

d

Fig 10-5 Patient J.D. *(a to d)* Tracing of lateral cephalometric radiograph and photographs of occlusion in 1981.

being positioned along the occlusal plane. The mandibular molars had erupted, but the increase in lower anterior facial height had kept improving the vertical position of the incisors so that now the incisal edges were closer to the level of the functional occlusal plane and there was a physiologic correction of the two-step occlusion.

Superimposition of progressive radiographs (Fig 10-7) indicated that considerable mandibular growth had occurred from the time of dismissal to the 15-year postretention cephalogram. Maxillary anteroposterior growth had been much less than mandibular growth, and the palate had dropped more in the back than in the premaxillary region—a difference in anterior and posterior vertical nasomaxillary growth.

With the appreciable mandibular growth the chin had positioned noticeably vertically, as well as anteriorly. All in all, appreciable mandibular growth had resulted in proportionately more vertical than horizontal positioning of the chin. Anteriorly, an open bite was evident when the posterior teeth were in occlusion. This represents a case where, subsequent to orthodontic correction and growth, a patient who had started with a deep overbite progressed to an open bite occlusion (Fig 10-8).

It certainly would have been advantageous if, somehow, such an undesired outcome could have been prevented—an instance where an ounce of prevention would truly be worth a pound of cure.

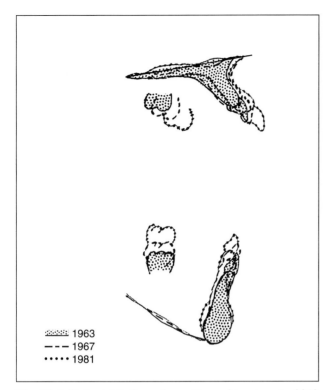

Fig 10-6 Patient J.D. Superimposition of tracings in 1963 (start), 1967 (retention), and 1981, indicating eruption and positional changes in molar and incisors.

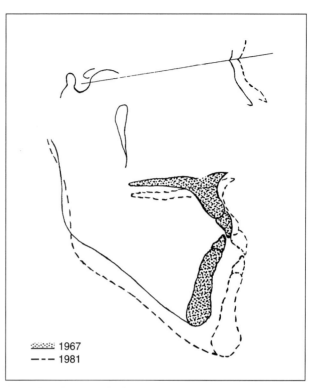

Fig 10-7 Patient J.D. Superimposition depicting direction and extent of growth from retention to 1981 records.

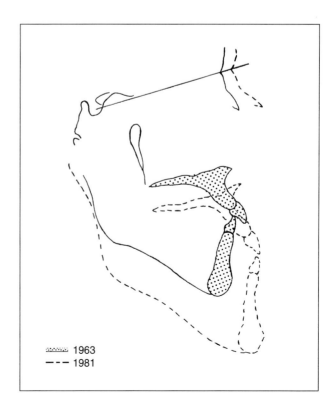

Fig 10-8 Patient J.D. Superimposition of 1981 on 1963 tracings indicates progression from deep bite to anterior open bite.

Characteristics of a Skeletal Open Bite

If something is to be prevented, there must be some insight into what exactly is being prevented before decisions can be made as to how, when, and where preventive measures are to be initiated, especially in such a loosely defined category as skeletal open bite. Perhaps clues will be found in a description of salient characteristics reported in a 1964 open bite study[1] that defined many dentofacial skeletal relationships, seemingly expressed as vertical problems and exhibiting persistent open bite malocclusions at later age levels.

Although the study had been undertaken on individuals past the early growing years, subsequent to eruption of the permanent dentition, characteristics of the skeletal open bite were defined that may be distinguishable at early ages and that may be pertinent to the early treatment of this tendency. First, there were many more open bites evident at an early age than observed at a later age,[2] indicating that the age gradient is an important factor in open bite malocclusions. Therefore, it was hypothesized that environmental factors leading to open bite may be operative at early age levels. These could include such habits as thumb and finger sucking, mouth breathing incident to enlarged adenoid tissue and/or nasal turbinates and a concomitant lower mandibular posture, or fronted tongue posture incident to enlarged tonsillar tissue. Open bite could even be correlated with yet inadequate growth of the jaws to accommodate the disproportionately large size of the more early-maturing tongue that must posture forward for accommodation within the oral cavity. However, the study found that many of the pertinent skeletal relationships that manifested themselves as a persistent open bite at later age levels were vertical problems. It is logical to assume that many early-developing open bites were precursors of the so-called "skeletal" open bite diagnosed at later age levels. In that study, the skeletal-dental configuration of 25 subjects with open bites in the permanent dentition was compared with a group of 30 subjects with normal occlusions. Following are some of the more

pertinent differences in dentoskeletal relationships. Excessive lower anterior facial height tended to coexist with a comparatively shorter posterior facial height. Additionally, a steeper mandibular plane and a significantly more open gonial angle were evident, as well as some retrusion of both the nasomaxillary complex and the chin relative to the cranium (Fig 10-9). Surprisingly, the open bite patients exhibited markedly supraerupted maxillary molars and incisors; this was sometimes evident in the mandibular molar and incisor dentition as well, although on a more individual basis. The significance of the findings of supraerupted molars cannot be overemphasized, since the over-erupted molars can effectively retroposition the mandible and thereby increase lower anterior facial height; excessive eruption could be instrumental in creating and perpetuating an open bite. At that time, a statement was made that skeletal open bites are grossly evident at later age levels and certainly must have been developing during earlier growth periods.

Early Causative Factors Contributing to Development of Open Bite

To a degree, the aforementioned observation could be substantiated by several studies undertaken at the Eastman Dental Center that have demonstrated that certain adverse functional activities can cause varying degrees of deformation of the jaws consistent with the undesirable features of an anterior open bite. For example, in one study[3] 34 strong thumb suckers were studied using cephalometric radiographs and cineradiographic recordings. It was found that the posterior height of the nasomaxillary complex in the thumb-sucking subjects was greater than that found in the control sample (Fig 10-10). Additionally, in the thumb suckers, the mandible frequently exhibited evidence of deformation in that the body seemed to be bent more in a downward and backward direction relative to the ramus. The architectural deformation of both the maxilla and the mandible were recognizably directed toward expressing

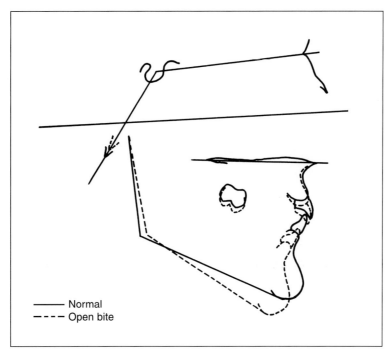

Fig 10-9 Composite indicating differences in skeletal open bite sample compared with control sample.

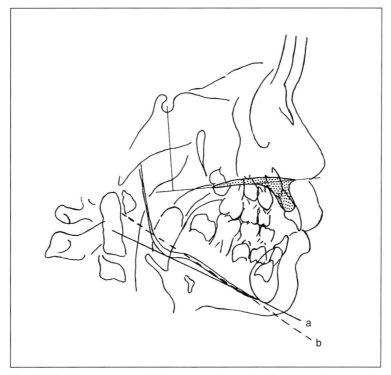

Fig 10-10 Tracing of a cephalometric radiograph taken on a thumb-sucking patient. Downward tip of the posterior aspect of the hard palate seems to predetermine an increased posterior nasomaxillary height. The dashed line (b) passing through the greatest concavity anterior to gonion—rather than the more conventional mandibular plane (a)—indicates a greater bending of the body of the mandible relative to the ramus.

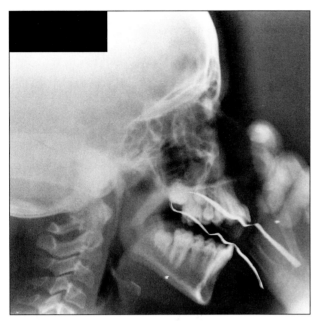

Fig 10-11 Lateral cephalometric headplate of a patient in the posture of thumb sucking. Disarticulation of the occlusion and other dentoskeletal relationships is evident.

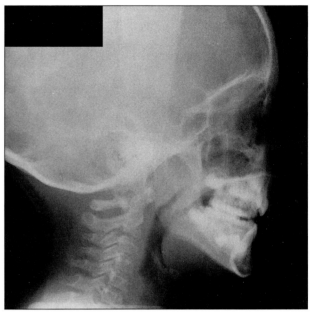

Fig 10-12 Cephalometric radiograph of a mouth-breathing youngster incident to enlarged adenoid tissue in the nasopharynx. Skeletal configurations and relationships, as well as mouth-breathing characteristics, can be noted.

increased anterior lower facial height and an open bite. Added to this, increased maxillary molar eruption due to the more-than-usual disarticulation (Fig 10-11) of the dentition can increase posterior dentoalveolar height, causing the mandible to assume a more open posture. This mandibular posture, in combination with inhibition of maxillary incisor eruption and proclination of the mandibular incisors incident to the digit-sucking process, can cause an anterior open bite and conceivably be the forerunner of a later skeletal open bite.

In other studies at Eastman, adverse alterations of the skeletal jaws were also noted in subjects with potential mouth-breathing habits incident to enlarged adenoids and/or enlarged nasal turbinates. In one study,[4] 33 subjects with enlarged adenoids were compared with a comparable sample of youngsters with minimal dimension to their adenoid mass; in another study,[5] 30 subjects having turbinate masses occupying more than 70% of the nasal cavities (as measured on frontal cephalometric radiographs) and no evidence of enlarged adenoids were

compared with control subjects exhibiting less than 60% turbinate obstruction. Findings relative to the skeletal morphology of the face and the relationships of the jaws were similar in both studies. Both groups of subjects had (1) a significant degree of maxillary retrusion, (2) some degree of counterclockwise rotation of the hard palate as indicated by an increase in posterior nasomaxillary height, (3) some degree of clockwise rotation of the mandible resulting in increased retrognathism and increased lower anterior facial height, and (4) a clinically observable bending of the body of the mandible relative to the ramus in the antegonial regions (Fig 10-12). One can readily recognize that some of these skeletal configurations and postural relationships of the jaws are somewhat similar to those observed in the strong thumb suckers. Evidently some similar functional factors must be operative in these two adverse and different functional problems that lead to similar results. In one instance, mouth breathing is a functional rest posture causing a disarticulation of the mandible associated with a parting of the lips. In

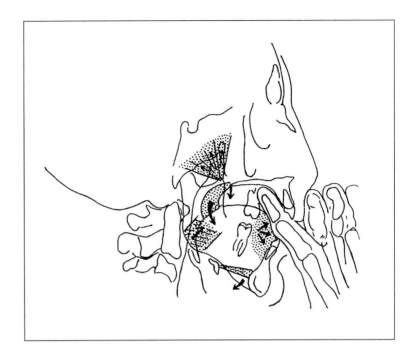

Fig 10-13 Depiction of muscle influences (stippled areas) in shaping the architecture of the jaws in a strong, longtime thumb sucker, ie, bringing the posterior aspect of the hard palate downward and mandibular bending anterior to the gonial region.

essence, this rest posture of the mandible can facilitate further eruption of the posterior teeth, causing increment in lower anterior facial height. Strong and prolonged thumb sucking, likewise, necessitates a disarticulation of the mandible to permit placement of the digit into the oral cavity, allowing the molars to erupt excessively and cause increment in lower anterior facial height. In all probability, some similar muscular influences are operative either in the establishment of postural changes of the jaws or actively functioning to alter skeletal configuration. In mouth breathing, in addition to parting of the lips, the tongue is postured downward and forward to permit passage of air through the oral cavity. Muscular interconnections between the soft palate, tongue, and pharynx cause a downward and somewhat forward influence on the posterior border of the hard palate, which, with time and growth, explains the increment in posterior nasomaxillary height. In the more open posture of the mandible during rest, the suprahyoid muscles attached to the body and symphysis of the mandible are pulling downward and backward while the muscles associated with the ramus are maintaining a postural stabilization.

This may explain the bending of the mandibular body relative to the ramus, as well as the increment in lower anterior facial height that is positionally maintained with molar eruption.

Similar muscular influences bring about the skeletal deformation noted in the thumb-sucking group, with the difference being that strong periodic muscular forces are being exerted during digit sucking, rather than the continual resting postural forces operating during mouth breathing. It was noted cineradiographically that, during strong thumb sucking, the tongue was pressing forcibly against the thumb and the lingual surfaces of the mandibular incisors (Fig 10-13). Not only was this creating a proclination of the mandibular incisors, but the tongue, via the glossopalatine muscle, was pulling the soft palate downward and forward. This, of course, maintained an airway for nasal respiration, but likewise pulled in a downward and forward direction on the posterior border of the hard palate—a forceful muscular activity that could reasonably explain the increased posterior height of the nasomaxillary complex. The ramal muscles (such as the temporal, masseter, and internal pterygoid) stabilize the mandible, pre-

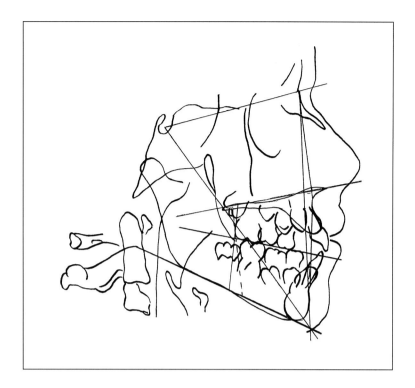

Fig 10-14 Cephalometric tracing of F.R. taken at the initial visit in 1963, evidencing certain characteristics of a developing skeletal open bite.

venting excessive pressure on the intruded thumb and, of course, keep the mandible disarticulated, permitting the suprahyoids to place downward and backward forces on the body and symphysis, and it probably explains the bending of the body relative to the ramus—mandibular skeletal deformation similar to that noted in the mouth breathers. Two different habits, one outcome. In essence, excessive vertical development in the posterior region of the maxilla and/or excessive eruption of the molars combined with the configuration and postural changes of the mandible, contribute to the development of excessive lower anterior facial height and an inadequate overbite or open bite.

It is the interplay of posterior vertical facial development relative to anterior vertical facial growth that appears to be significantly responsible for the development of vertically related malocclusions such as skeletal open bite. Once this concept is accepted, then the desirability of removing its precipitating factor(s) must be acknowledged. Furthermore, if the configuration and position of the skeletal jaws can be adversely affected with continued growth, correc-

tion or control should be undertaken as early as possible. If treatment is undertaken before and during active growth periods, ie, the period of transitional dentition, it may be possible to prevent further maldevelopment.

Early Open Bite Treatment

It is at the time that vertical jaw and alveolar growth are strongly active that treatment should be initiated to mechanically prevent the expression of full vertical development in the posterior region of the occlusion. By so doing, mandibular posture can be prevented from opening excessively in the anterior dentoalveolar region while continued expression of vertical development in that region may maintain an acceptable overbite.

Patient F.R. is an example of being able to minimize posterior dentoalveolar growth and preclude the development of an open bite incident to treatment and growth. The patient presented during the early transitional dentition with a retrognathic, convex facial pattern. Significantly, the palatal plane was observed to incline

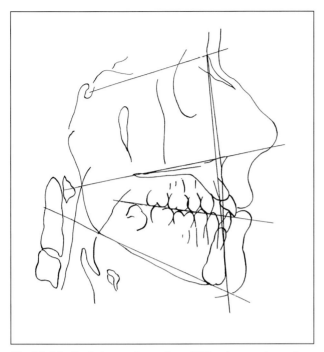

Fig 10-15 Cephalometric tracing of F.R. taken at time of retention in 1968.

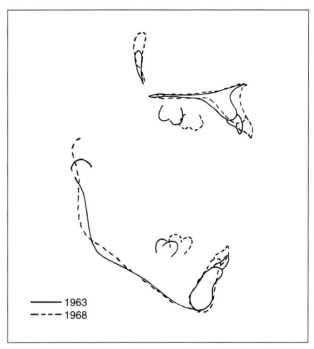

——— 1963
- - - - 1968

Fig 10-16 Superimposition of tracings of F.R. from 1963 and 1968, indicating growth and dentoalveolar changes incident to growth and treatment.

cranially, in progressing from the posterior nasal spine to the anterior nasal spine (Fig 10-14), causing the premaxilla to tip up, a noticeable characteristic of some skeletal open bite problems. As the posterior of the hard palate was somewhat tipped down, there was some decrease in posterior oral cavity height. The ramus seemed comparatively short, and some steepness to the mandibular plane was noted.

Dentally, a Class I molar relationship was noted, with proclined maxillary and mandibular incisors, along with a small anterior open bite. Both maxillary and mandibular incisors were positioned considerably forward of the jaw profile (A-Po) line. It was decided to extract maxillary first premolars to permit retraction of the maxillary incisors and reduce the high degree of facial convexity and to extract mandibular second premolars to minimize retraction of mandibular incisors while achieving dental alignment and orthodontic correction. A Nance holding arch was placed on the maxillary first molars to serve as anchorage and to minimize eruption of those teeth. Incident to treatment (Fig 10-15), SNA had been reduced noticeably with a retroposi-

tioning of point A relative to nasion. More significantly, the maxillary first molars had been prevented from erupting excessively, even after removal of the holding arch during appliance therapy. Some mesial positioning of those teeth was also noted, incident to growth and orthodontic therapy. The maxillary incisors were erupted and retropositioned commensurate with the extent of eruption of the maxillary molars (Fig 10-16). In the mandibular arch, there was further eruption as well as mesial movement of the molars and considerable eruption of the incisors. In retrospect, it might have been advisable to use a maxillary bite block or a mandibular lingual arch to minimize mandibular molar eruption. Subsequent to treatment, the anterior open bite was closed, with approximately 15% to 20% overlap. The Class I molar relationship was maintained, and occlusal interdigitation and alignment were considered retainable.

During the period of orthodontic therapy, considerable growth had taken place which, as might be expected, was much more evident in the mandible than in the maxilla. The mandible grew downward and forward (Fig 10-17). There

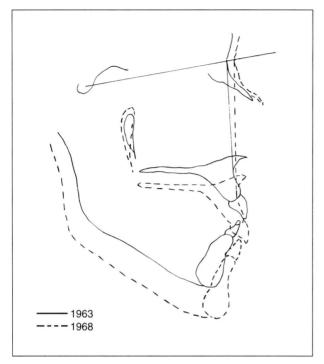

Fig 10-17 Superimposition (F.R.) of 1963 and 1968 tracings, indicating jaw relationships incident to growth and treatment.

— 1963
---- 1968

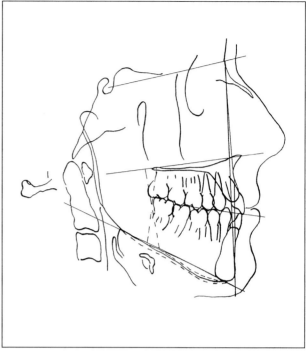

Fig 10-18 Tracing of lateral cephalometric radiograph of F.R. taken in 1979.

seemed to be slightly more posterior than anterior lower facial height development. As a consequence, in addition to minimizing maxillary molar eruption, it was possible to close the anterior open bite. Because of the retropositioning and uprighting of the anterior teeth, as well as growth, there was considerable improvement in facial convexity and skeletal relationships.

In analyzing the case 11 years postretention (Fig 10-18), it became evident that there was good maintenance of overbite correction. Growth had continued to occur in both jaws. The maxilla had continued to grow anteroposteriorly, with point A coming downward and forward (Fig 10-19); commensurate with this growth, the full dentition had likewise been positioned occlusally and forward (Fig 10-20), and the maxillary incisor edge had approximated the level of the posterior occlusal plane. During this period the third molars had likewise

erupted and were in full occlusal contact. Concomitantly, good anteroposterior and some vertical growth of the mandible had taken place, positioning the mandibular dentition more mesially as well. The chin had moved slightly more anteriorly than vertically. The functional occlusal plane was observed to pass through the tip of the mandibular incisor. The overbite had decreased, but not to the extent of an open bite. Again, there was similarly slight eruption of both molars and incisors to maintain occlusal plane levels. Growth in ramal and lower posterior oral cavity height had occurred, and, although the premaxilla was still tipped cranially, control of the posterior vertical height permitted maintenance of the bite closure years after treatment (Fig 10-21). Mandibular anterior malalignment was noted during the postretention years, but the slight overbite had been maintained (Fig 10-22).

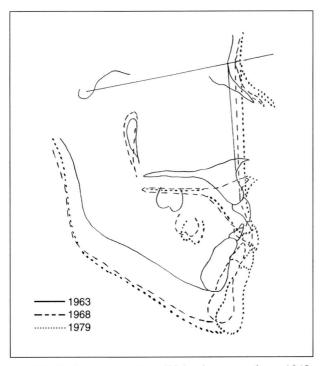

Fig 10-19 Superimposition (F.R.) of tracings from 1963, 1968, and 1979 on the S-N plane registering on sella, indicating growth and changes of the maxilla and mandible.

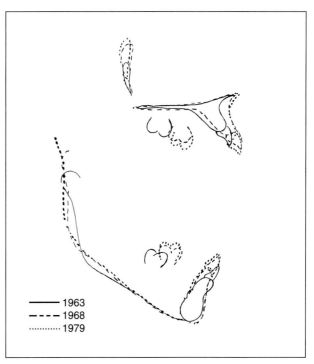

Fig 10-20 Patient F.R. Dentoalveolar changes incident to growth and treatment.

Fig 10-21 Superimposition of beginning and final cephalometric tracings of F.R. An anterior open bite did not develop.

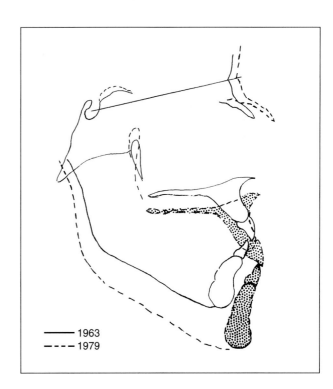

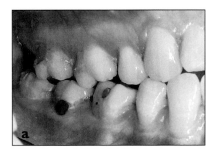 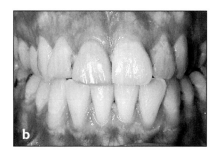 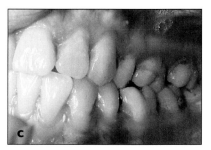

Fig 10-22 Patient F.R. *(a to c)* Final records of occlusion recorded in 1979.

Principles of treatment

Prevent increment in posterior oral cavity height

The ounce of prevention that the orthodontist must exert is to either prevent eruption of the molars or, if possible, to facilitate depression of these teeth.

The significance of supraerupted molars in skeletal open bite cases, younger and older, cannot be overemphasized, because over-erupted molars can effectively lower and reposition the chin, thereby increasing lower anterior facial height. The ensuing increase in posterior dentoalveolar height incident to the postural opening of the mandible can result in excessive lower anterior facial height and an open bite malocclusion. We are not referring to inadequate anterior dentoalveolar eruption, but to a more-than-desired posterior dentoalveolar eruption. This can be well demonstrated by a small study conducted in the orthodontic department at Eastman Dental Center. Six orthodontic students had photographs of their anterior dentition taken with their teeth in occlusion and with graduated thicknesses of soft mouthguard wafers placed bilaterally between the most posterior molars. Photographs and lateral cephalometric radiographs were taken at 1 mm gradients from 0 to 5 mm.

Figures 10-23 and 10-24 show the occlusion and the analogous cephalometric radiograph tracings with the teeth in occlusion, with 1 mm of bilateral wafer thickness, and with a 3-mm thickness of soft wafers. Increment in anterior open bite is clearly evident, and the extent of anterior opening is disclosed. Cephalometric tracings (Fig 10-25) distinctly reveal the extent of opening of the mandibular symphysis and the definitive increase in lower anterior facial height. Clearly, small degrees of eruption of the posterior teeth will result in a much greater opening of the anterior occlusion as well as posture the symphysis downward. Orthodontic therapy must be directed toward preventing counterclockwise rotation of the nasomaxillary complex and maxillary dentition while augmenting the counterclockwise rotation of the mandible and its dentition. Fixed holding appliances have been shown to be useful adjuncts in preventing eruption of molars. The mandibular lingual arch that has been adjusted away from the lingual surfaces of the mandibular incisors prevents eruption of the mandibular molars and at the same time permits eruption and uprighting of the mandibular incisors. Likewise, transpalatal holding arches and Nances are helpful adjuncts in preventing eruption of maxillary molars and permitting retroclination and eruption of the anterior teeth.

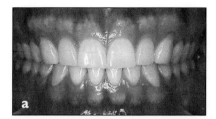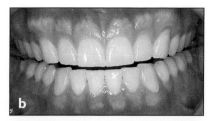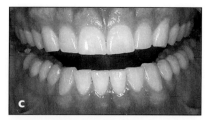

Fig 10-23 Intraoral view of P.D.'s anterior occlusion *(a)* with the teeth in occlusion, *(b)* with a 1-mm-thick wafer between the most posterior molars, and *(c)* with a 3-mm-thick wafer between the most posterior molars. Note the anterior opening of the bite.

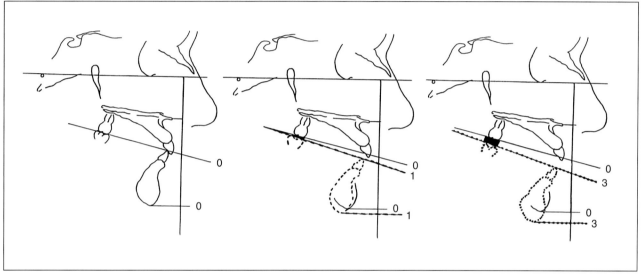

Fig 10-24 Tracings of lateral cephalometric radiographs of P.D. with the teeth *(left)* in occlusion, *(center)* biting on a 1-mm wafer, and *(right)* biting on a 3-mm wafer.

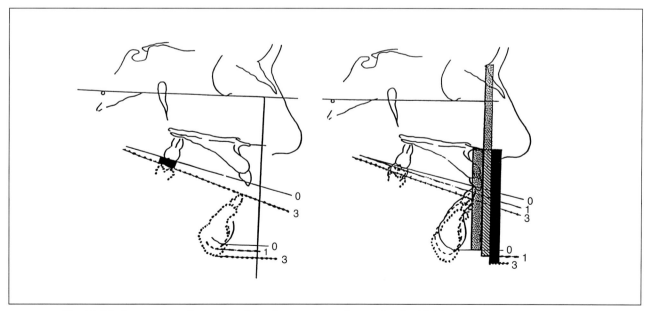

Fig 10-25 Superimposed tracings of the three tracings depicted in Fig 10-24 showing the extent of lower anterior facial height incident to wafer placement: teeth in occlusion (stippled bar), 1-mm wafer thickness (striped bar), and 3-mm wafer thickness (black bar).

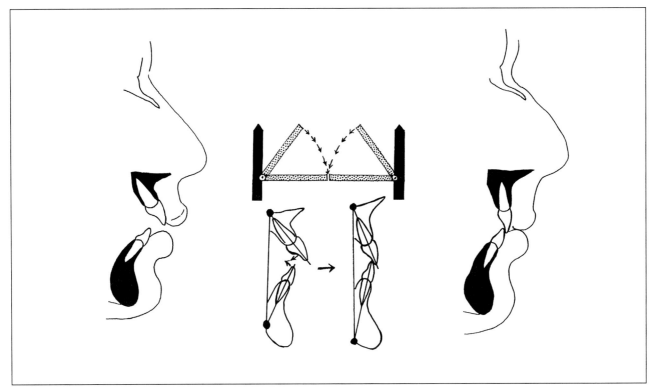

Fig 10-26 Illustration of the drawbridge principle in anterior open bite closure by lingual tipping of maxillary and mandibular incisors.

Close the drawbridge

Retroclination of the maxillary and mandibular incisors is particularly important since it fulfills the "closing the drawbridge" principle (Fig 10-26). When a drawbridge opens, the two sections tip away from each other (proclining maxillary and mandibular incisors); when it closes, the two halves tip or hinge toward each other (retroclining anteriors), approximating or overlapping to effectively close the bridge (or the open bite).

Bite-block depression

At young ages, occlusal bite blocks may be helpful in preventing eruption of posterior teeth. A study[6] was undertaken at the Eastman Dental Center, using 45-degree oblique films to evaluate the effects of posterior bite blocks on the occlusion. In the adult (Fig 10-27), when the bite block exceeded the freeway space by a considerable dimension, intrusion of the opposing posterior teeth was noted. In growing individuals, although it did not cause a discernible intrusion of the posterior teeth, it did serve to prevent eruption of these teeth (Fig 10-28). As an additional benefit, the bite block was instrumental in uprighting mesially tipped posterior teeth by applying pressure to the distal of the molars. In growing individuals, occlusal onlays on palatal developers and holding arches, as well as on removable bite blocks themselves—when they do not overly exceed the freeway space—have effectively inhibited molar eruption. This inhibition, whether it be maxillary, mandibular, or both, likewise prevents an opening rotation of the mandible and mandibular arch. In growing individuals, the posterior occlusal bite block has been helpful in maintaining the existing anterior vertical dimension and in precluding increase in lower anterior facial height. Today the adjunct of occlusal posterior

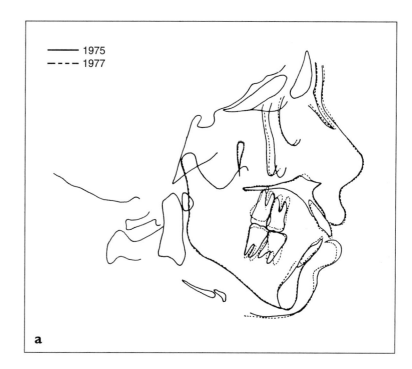

Fig 10-27 Patient M. R. *(a, b)* Cephalometric tracings and *(c to e)* photographs of maxillary bite block in situ, indicating depression of posterior teeth during bite-block therapy on an adult.

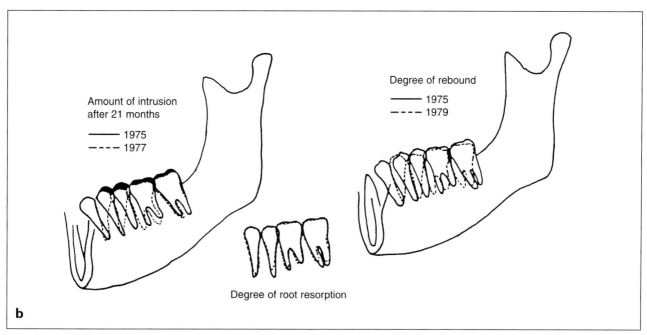

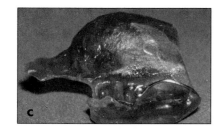
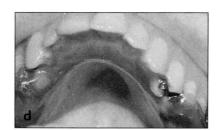
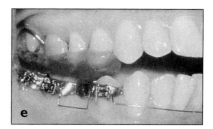

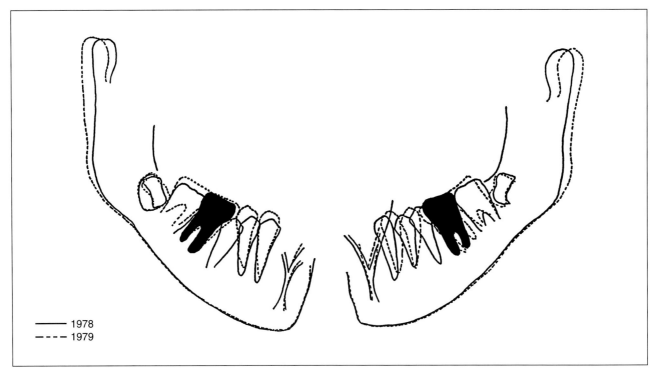

1978
---- 1979

Fig 10-28 Tracings of a growing individual undergoing bite-block therapy, demonstrating prevention of continued eruption of posterior teeth.

bite block is frequently used in those patients whose facial growth tends to be vertically directed, indicating the possibility of an open bite (Fig 10-29). Reference is made to those patients having limited lower posterior facial height, excessive upper posterior facial height, excessively erupted molars, or excessive antegonial bending of the mandible. In these cases, it is especially important to prevent any downward and backward retropositioning of the mandibular symphysis. The posterior occlusal bite block is fabricated to index the occlusal surface of the posterior teeth of one arch and its action is directed toward the occlusal surface of the molars of the opposing arch, using the orofacial muscles and occlusal forces to create pressures on those teeth in an effort to preclude eruption and, if possible, achieve some depression of those teeth. The addition of occlusal onlays is

particularly desirable in children with vertical developmental patterns where the extrusion of posterior teeth would serve to therapeutic disadvantage.

Control of posterior vertical development

In many instances it is desirable to depress molars as part of therapy to reduce lower anterior facial height. In the growing child, especially the youngster whose palate dips down posteriorly and has increased posterior nasomaxillary height (inadequate vertical ramal growth), it is even more advantageous to control the vertical development of the posterior area of the maxillary complex. It has been found that a high-pull or vertical-pull headgear can effectively depress maxillary molars and maintain vertical control of the posterior aspect of the palate. A cephalo-

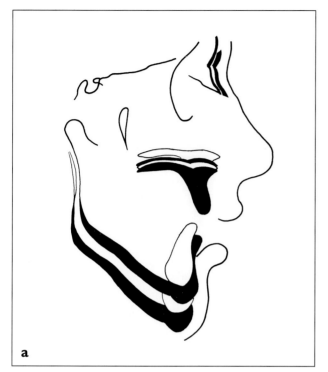 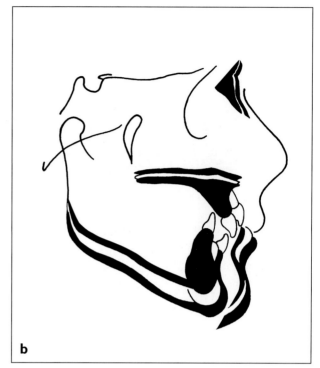

Fig 10-29 Superimposed cephalometric radiographic tracings of an individual with a facial growth pattern that seems predominantly vertical *(a)*. In contrast, *b* depicts a growing individual in whom the vertical positioning of the chin is not excessive in comparison with its anterior positioning.

metric radiographic study was conducted at Eastman Dental Center to evaluate the effects of high-pull headgear therapy[7] (in conjunction with full appliances) on 10 children being treated during active stages of growth in the transitional dentition. All the youngsters had successful resolution of an open bite malocclusion to an acceptable overbite relationship incident to the orthodontic procedures. It was determined that the high-pull headgear and orthodontic appliances had held vertical dentoalveolar development in the maxillary molar region to a minimum; in some instances, depression of these teeth was noted. The maxillary molars and their alveolar processes seemed to be retarded in vertical development and, more importantly, the high-pull therapy seemed to inhibit further counterclockwise rotation of the palate, thus restraining further vertical (down-

ward) movement, with growth, of the posterior palate while the anterior aspect of the palate was permitted to move downward with continued anterior maxillary growth. During this period, the maxillary anterior dentition and its related alveolar process continued to develop and erupt away from the level of the palate. It is interpreted that the extraoral appliance was able to exert an orthopedic influence on the nasomaxillary complex; the tipping of the palate indicated that, with growth, a clockwise rotation of the maxillary complex had ensued, which eventually aided in anterior bite closure. It is worthy to note that precautions should be taken to concomitantly prevent mandibular molar eruption, either with a maxillary bite block or a mandibular lingual arch, to permit the mandible to rotate upward and forward to achieve contact of the mandibular molar with the maxillary

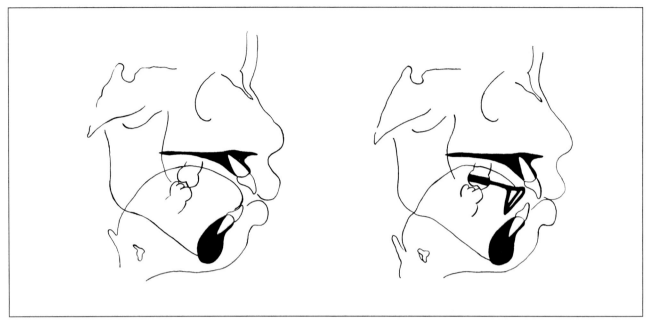

Fig 10-30 Tracing of a thumb-sucking child before and after placement of a crib to stop the habit. Note that the crib approximates the cingulum area of the mandibular incisors to act as a barrier to thumb placement.

molar, which is being positioned at a higher level. Counterclockwise rotation of the mandible is helpful in anterior bite closure; continued mandibular molar eruption reduces the extent of this rotation and increases the difficulty in bite closure.

It should be noted that these open bites—more usually related to deformation and malrelationships in the back of the oral cavity—are unlike those caused by excessive tongue dimension or fronted tongue posture such as that necessitated by tonsillar overgrowth. The tongue, because of dimension, posture, or position, can preclude or impede eruption of individual teeth or segments of the dentition. Very frequently the tongue fronting, and even passive digit sucking where the thumb does not extend beyond the anterior alveolar process, can result in an anterior open bite by reducing eruption of the incisors. This should be considered an ante-

rior dentoalveolar open bite and not the type of posterior jaw deformation commonly noted in a skeletal open bite. In the former instances, where inadequate development of the anterior dentoalveolar process is evident, treatment to permit continued eruption of the anterior teeth is indicated. Mechanical appliances can be placed to discourage sucking habits (Fig 10-30); tonsils can be removed to permit a retroposturing of the tongue (Fig 10-31); one can even await favorable growth changes to permit a disproportionately large tongue to be contained within the confines of the skeletal jaws (Fig 10-32). It should be re-emphasized that these are instances where inadequate anterior dentoalveolar development can be evident.

Thus, of prime import in the early treatment of so-called "vertical growth," or open-bite tendencies, is the necessity of reducing, preventing, or at least minimizing vertical dentoalveolar

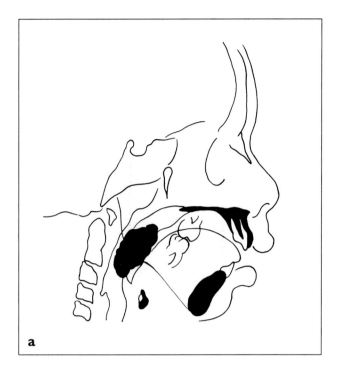

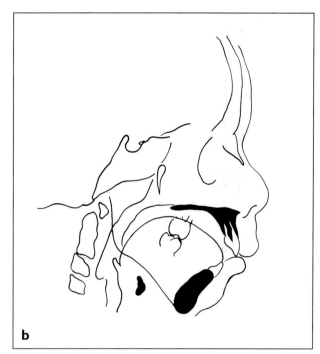

Fig 10-31 Progressive cephalometric radiograph tracings of an individual with enlarged tonsils before *(a)* and after *(b)* a tonsillectomy and adenoidectomy. The composite superimposition *(c)* indicates a change in tongue posture and noticeable eruption of the maxillary incisor teeth.

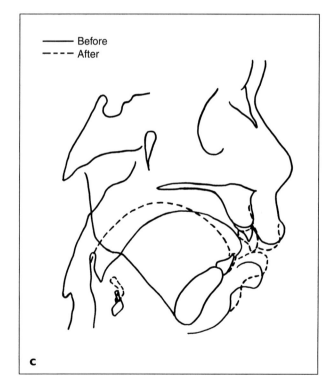

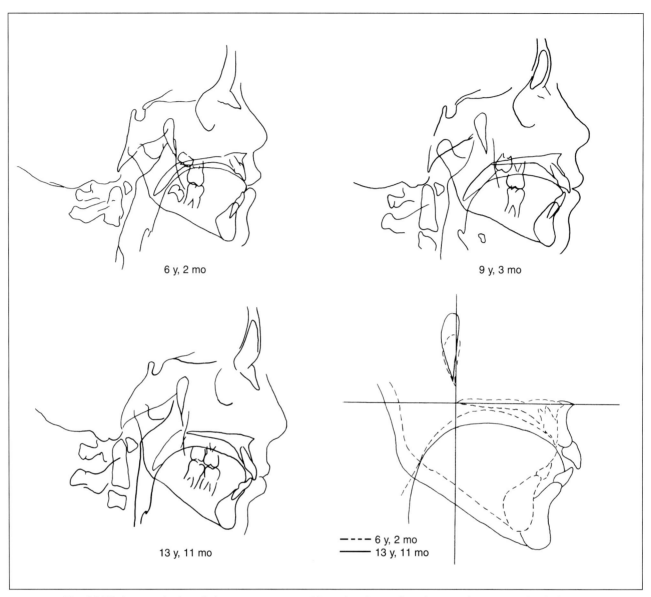

6 y, 2 mo

9 y, 3 mo

13 y, 11 mo

- - - - 6 y, 2 mo
───── 13 y, 11 mo

Fig 10-32 Longitudinal cephalometric tracings of lateral radiographs taken on the same individual over an approximate 7-year span; no orthodontic treatment was undertaken. The composite indicates growth changes, changes in tongue posture, and anterior bite closure.

development and molar eruption in the posterior region of the dentition, which is, in other words, an attempt to prevent a disproportionate increase in lower anterior facial height. Controlling vertical increment in the posterior region of the dentition may preclude an undesirable repositioning of the mandibular symphysis farther from the palate. In these instances an ounce of prevention may be the most effective cure.

In treating at early ages, the orthodontist can reasonably become a "re-director" of growth patterns rather than solely a worrier of tooth position. In these instances, the orthodontist is truly a "face former" as well as a "tooth mover"; a mover and a repositioner of jaws. It seems that the orthodontist's greatest influence may reside in controlling the vertical relationship of the molars and, thereby, the vertical and anteroposterior position of the chin. In a way, the orthodontist can play a role in posturing and molding the foundation for the teeth, rather than solely redistributing the teeth along the foundation. The orthodontist will have to become more knowledgeable and will have to learn to encourage growth, redirect growth, work with it and against it, rather than solely around it. To accomplish this, the orthodontist, will, of necessity, treat younger and younger people in order to influence the greatest amount of growth that it is feasible to influence.

References

1. Subtelny JD, Sakuda M. Open-bite: Diagnosis and treatment. Am J Orthod 1964;50:337–358.
2. Worms FW, Meskin LH, Isaacson RJ. Open-bite. Am J Orthod 1971;59:589.
3. Polson AP. A Cephalometric and Cineradiographic Study of the Influence of Thumbsucking on Oral Facial Skeletal Configuration [thesis]. Rochester, NY: Univ of Rochester, 1979.
4. Cancelli F. The Effects of Adenoid Tissue on the Morphology of the Mandible and the Palate [senior research]. Rochester, NY: Eastman Dental Center, 1980.
5. Etengoff R. Nasal Airway Obstruction and Its Effects on Maxillary Growth [senior research]. Rochester, NY: Eastman Dental Center, 1980.
6. Buck R. A Study of the Treatment Effects of the Posterior Occlusal Bite Block [senior research]. Rochester, NY: Eastman Dental Center, 1979.
7. McHugh F. A Cephalometric Study of Maxillary Molar Tooth Movement [research study]. Rochester, NY: Eastman Dental Center, 1972.

Part IV

Skeletal Dysmorphology
Jaw Malocclusions

Chapter 11

Maxillary Skeletal Jaw Dysmorphology: Cleft Lip and Palate

The question could rightfully be asked, "Why include a discussion of cleft lip and palate treatment when the incidence is so much lower than the more common, more readily recognized malocclusions?" In response it can be pointed out that, each year since the initiation of the orthodontic curriculum at Eastman Dental Center, the following observation has been made: If I (Subtelny) were told that I must restrict myself to one type of malocclusion with which to teach orthodontics, I would choose the entity cleft lip and palate for a multitude of reasons. Orthodontics is concerned with form, function, and change with time. Cleft lip and palate is an aberration in form of the maxilla and the overlying soft tissue, particularly the form of the lip and the nose. Cleft palate is not only an alteration in the form of the skeletal maxillary complex, but it also involves a misplacement and disarrangement of the parts of the maxilla; as a consequence, it definitely affects the maxillary dentition in context and in placement. Orthodontic students must know and understand the skeletal configuration as well as misconfiguration of the forms of the jaws.

A cleft lip is not only a disfiguration affecting the appearance of the face but also a disruption of the musculature of the upper lip; thus it affects the function of lip structures. The lip, in its contiguous relationship to the dentition, can have an effect on the position of the teeth. A cleft lip has a disruption in lip musculature and, as such, can have a developmental effect on the spatial relationship of the parts of the cleft maxilla, with a detrimental effect on tooth positions. Correction of the cleft lip has been shown to cause an alteration in the function and the influence of the lip on the underlying skeletal architecture as well as the dentition. Orthodontic students must understand muscle function and its influence on form. The study of cleft lip and palate enables the student to understand muscle function, as well as malfunction, and to see its influence on the occlusion incident to its influence on form.

It is readily acknowledged that growth of the facial structures is important to orthodontics. Growth represents change with time. Cleft lip and palate offers an excellent opportunity not only to see changes with time, but to understand growth in dysmorphic types of relationships and to understand muscular influences on growth. Knowledge of dysmorphic growth leads to a better understanding of the more normal growth of the well-formed craniofacial complex. Malrelated and misplaced parts grow aberrantly and can lead to differences of facial structural relationships, and with it, placement of the dentition. The orthodontic student can better understand not only the influence of growth on form and function but conversely, can understand the influence of form and function on growth. Growth is acknowledged and discussed, but a need exists to have a better understanding of growth to comprehensively conduct therapeutic procedures on orthodontic patients.

Additionally, the cleft lip and palate entity has representation of every type of malocclusion known to affect noncleft individuals. It has its share of Class II and Class III malocclusions. It has its share of vertical problems such as deep bite and open bites, crossbites of all types, malaligned and drastically rotated as well as malpositioned teeth; and it has its share of malocclusions that lie primarily in discordant skeletal parts with aberrant growth patterns.

One other observation can be made pertinent to the present discussion. It seems that the incidence of craniofacial dysmorphology is on the increase, indicating that in coming years there will probably be a growing number of these patients needing care and rehabilitation. Paul Fogh-Anderson,[1] a Danish plastic surgeon, has conducted extensive studies on the etiology and incidence of cleft lip and/or palate. In his 1939 doctoral dissertation he indicated that the incidence was approximately 1 in 760 births.[1] In 1968 he reported that the incidence had dramatically increased to 1 out of every 500 live births in Denmark.[2] Whether this represents a genetic progression or the influence of environmental factors on development is yet to be ascertained, but it represents an increment in incidence.

It should be recognized that all individuals during the formative embryonic stages, prior to 3 months of postconception development, manifest clefts of the lip and palate. During approximately 5 to 7 weeks postconception, closure of the lip and primary palate, which is basically the premaxillary region that includes the four maxillary incisors, occurs. This closure occurs bilaterally during normal embryological development. This is not meant to be a discourse on embryology, but it seems important to mention that all developing individuals manifest a bilateral cleft of the lip and primary palate (premaxilla) prior to the union of these parts to create what will eventually be the normal architecture of the lip and alveolar process. Later in embryological development, approximately 7 to 10 weeks postconception, the two palatal shelves unite with the nasal septum to form a complete palate. Developmentally, it can now be visualized as a more normal palate and, subsequently, a more normal maxillary jaw incident to union with the primary palate and the processes of the maxillary region. Clefts of the lip and palate occur in all developing individuals during the embryological stage and it is subsequent to that stage 3 months postconception that an intact nasomaxillary complex is finally recognized as normal morphology. Something occurs during embryological development that dictates the eventual dysmorphology of a cleft lip and/or palate.

Descriptive Anatomy of Clefts

Differences in timing explain the variety of forms observed within the entity of cleft lip and palate. Pruzansky's[3] statement, "All clefts are not alike," is very true because much heterogeneity is to be found in cleftness. In essence, one can say that variation is the name of the game. Differences in developmental time sequences will dictate differences in location and extensiveness of clefts of the lip and/or palate. Prior to lip closure, the embryo exhibits clefts on each side of the eventual philtrum area of the upper lip. If there is no closure on either side, then a bilateral cleft of the lip will be manifested at birth. At times, however, one side will close and the other will not; the outcome will be a unilateral cleft of the lip, right or left. Here again variation can be noted in that there may be partial closure (incomplete cleft) or there may be nearly full closure. If there is no closure whatsoever, then the cleft will extend from the vermilion border of the upper lip into the nares (complete cleft) (Fig 11-1). An incomplete (partial) cleft can be as minimal as a simple notch in the lower border of the upper lip vermilion, with some manifestation in the premaxillary alveolar region. Partial clefts can occur unilaterally or bilaterally, and within each of these types, individual variations can be found.

In dealing with cleft dysmorphology, one also learns to "never judge a book by its cover." Because of the time difference in embryological development, individuals may be born with a cleft of the lip but not of the palate. On the

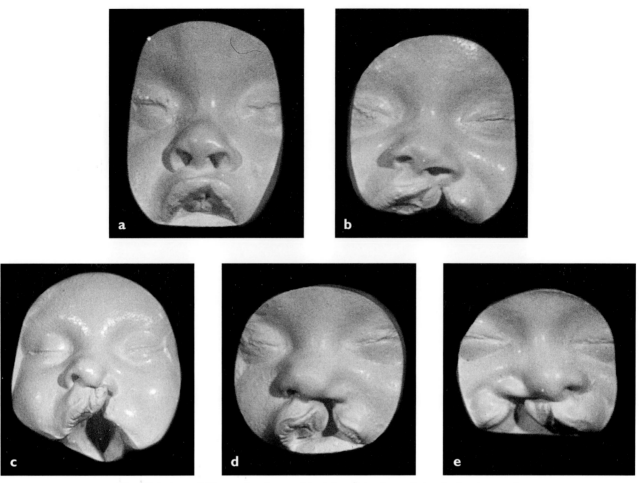

Fig 11-1 *(a to e)* Casts of patients with clefts of the lip; variation is clearly noted.

other hand, people may not have a lip cleft but, with the later time sequence in embryological development, may manifest a palatal cleft of varying degrees posterior to the premaxilla. Again, variation (Fig 11-2) is the name of the game when classifying clefts of the palate. If one of the palatal shelves unites with the nasal septum, then it is a unilateral cleft of the palate and could be either right or left. A complete unilateral cleft of the lip and palate is manifested as a cleft through the lip and the premaxillary region, and a palatal cleft extending into the nasal cavity on one side. In a unilateral cleft of the palate, there is an opening into the nasal cavity on the side of the cleft. This in itself could be complete or partial and, when it is in-

complete, the cleft will usually be anatomically manifested posteriorly to varying degrees, from the nasopalatine foramen toward the uvula. Thus, it may be a unilateral cleft of the entire hard palate, of portions of the more posterior aspect of the hard palate, or solely of the soft palate. If neither of the palatal shelves unites with the nasal septum, a bilateral cleft palate is manifested, in which case there is a palatal opening into both nasal cavities. In a complete bilateral cleft, there is usually a bilateral cleft of the lip and alveolar process as well as the palate on both sides of the nasal septum; the premaxilla and nasal septum are united and quite observable from the palatal perspective. As with clefts of the lip, clefts of the palate can be uni-

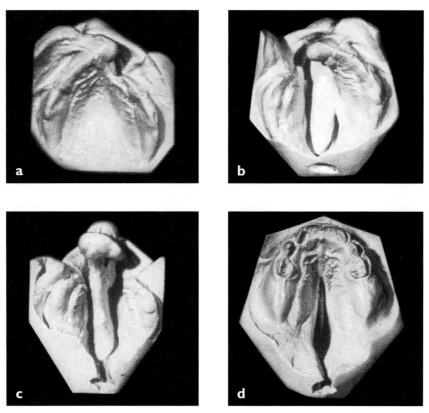

Fig 11-2 *(a to d)* Casts of patients with clefts of the palate. Variation is again clearly evident. (From Bardach J and Morris HL. *Multidisciplinary Management of Cleft Lip and Palate*, 1990. Reprinted with permission from Saunders.)

lateral or bilateral, but vary in extent and configuration; clefts of the palate alone with the lips and alveolar processes intact (posterior clefts) may also be seen. Once again, variation is the name of the game.

Clefts: What and How

When one looks at the congenital cleft, one begins to wonder whether the cleft represents an insufficiency of tissue or whether the parts of the lip and palate were simply displaced, resulting in an opening. Several studies have been undertaken on cleft youngsters: cast studies[4,5] and radiographic studies.[6] Measurements were taken to determine whether the open palatal cleft rep-

resented a deficiency (lack of tissue) or was simply an opening between adequately developed tissues that have somehow been displaced. Frontal laminagraphic sections (Fig 11-3) of the maxillary complex at the level of the most inferior point of the zygomaticomaxillary junction were obtained on 127 cleft palate children 3 years of age and younger and 50 noncleft children. These laminagraphic sections afforded a clear view of the nasal cavities, the palatal structures, and the outer aspects of the maxilla itself. Palatal dimensions (Fig 11-4) were taken on each individual to determine palatal shelf width, providing some indication whether there was a deficiency of tissue. The distance between the lateral borders of the nasal cavity provided information whether there was displacement of the

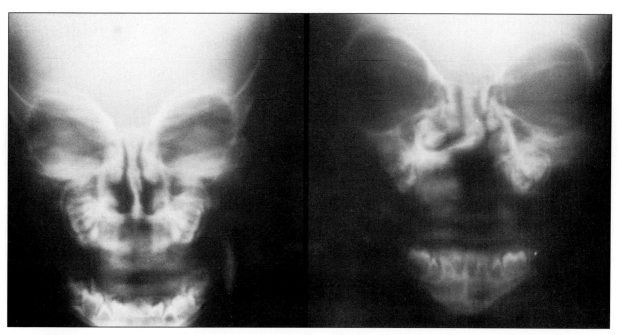

Fig 11-3 Laminagraphic sections of a noncleft individual *(left)* and of an individual with a unilateral cleft of the lip and palate *(right)*, clearly depicting differences in anatomy and relationship of parts in the nasal cavities and the maxillae.

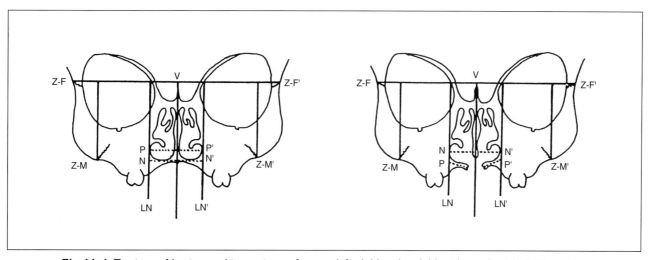

Fig 11-4 Tracings of laminagraphic sections of a noncleft child and a child with a palatal cleft illustrating measurements taken to evaluate deficiency and/or displacement of palatal tissue.

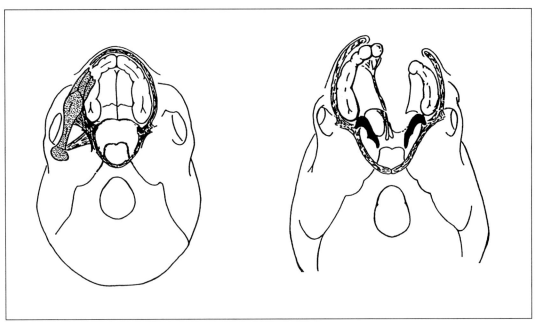

Fig 11-5 Artistic depiction of the ring of orobuccopharyngeal musculature encircling the nasomaxillary complex in noncleft individual (partial mandible stippled) *(left)* and unilateral cleft lip–and–palate individual *(right).*

parts of the skeletal jaw away from the cleft. It was ascertained that deficiency and/or displacement could be present. Again, variation could occur within individual cleft patients as well as within the cleft types themselves, albeit there was some degree of deficiency in all cleft types. In some instances much deficiency of tissue was evident; in others, only minimal deficiency. In some instances lateral displacement of the maxillary bones was evident and in others it was not so evident; again, this seemed to vary between individuals as well as within cleft types. The unilateral cleft palate subjects showed the least evidence of displacement as well as deficiency, and as before, it manifested to varying degrees from individual to individual. The differences are not pertinent to the present discussion except to acknowledge the presence of displacement and to project a hypothesis as to how displacement of the maxillary bones can occur at the prenatal level. Deficient tissue can be more readily understood on a congenital basis, but to explain the displacement of the parts of the maxilla is

more complex. It must be recognized that muscles in the head and neck are developing and functioning during embryonic and fetal life. Tongue muscles and cervical muscles have been shown to be capable of function at early developmental ages. Regional stimulation has been observed to cause tongue and lip movements as well as flexure movements in the cervical region.[7-9] There is a ring of orobuccopharyngeal musculature (Fig 11-5) that encircles the maxillary complex from the lips right around to the pterygomandibular raphe and is continuous with the superior constrictor muscle of the pharynx, which courses back to become part of the pharyngeal complex. This ring of muscle encompassing the maxilla is loosely analogous to a rubber band encircling a rolled-up scroll of paper.

A cleft of the lip represents a disruption in the continuity of the muscular ring in the anterior part of the maxillary region (Fig 11-5). If it is unilateral, it is on one side alone; if it is bilateral, it is on both sides of the premaxillary region.

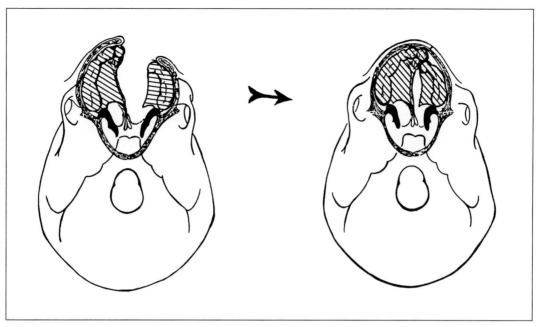

Fig 11-6 Artistic depiction of the reconstruction of the muscular ring (orobuccopharyngeal musculature) following cleft lip surgical repair. (From Bardach J and Morris HL. *Multidisciplinary Management of Cleft Lip and Palate*, 1990. Reprinted with permission from Saunders.)

Usually co-existent with complete clefts of the lip are complete clefts of the alveolar process in the premaxillary region (either unilateral or bilateral) and a complete cleft of the palate including the soft palate musculature. Of importance, cleft lip is a disruption in the orobuccopharyngeal muscular ring. A comparatively large tongue can exert pressures on the cleft bony segments, opening the avenue for displacement of the cleft parts of the maxillary complex. The tongue can push the premaxillary element anteriorly and the posterior jaw segments laterally. In the complete unilateral and bilateral cleft, the circumoral musculature during prenatal development does not have the continuity to counteract the tongue forces, so the cleft musculature itself creates adverse, outwardly directed forces on the cleft bony segments. The cleft disruption of the lip musculature precludes the possibility of their normal molding influence on the maxillary segments; unequal and asymmetric forces are exerted on the maxillary cleft structures, tending to pull the bony segments in a lateral direction.

It is hypothesized that the inequality of these muscle forces during prenatal development is the mechanism whereby the displacement of the maxillary bony segments occurs, resulting in the increased width of the nasal cavities.

Muscle and Muscle Molding

One of the first procedures in rehabilitating a cleft lip and palate is directed toward an obvious and immediate need to improve facial esthetics by surgically closing the cleft lip. This is most frequently done in the early months of postnatal life, usually before 3 months of age. A surgical repair of the cleft lip consists of reconstructing lip architecture and attempting to realign the muscle fibers on each side of the cleft. In other words, the cleft lip is closed for esthetic purposes but additionally serves to reinitiate the continuity of the muscular ring that encompasses the maxilla and underlies the lip epithelium (Fig 11-6). The reconstructed lip muscula-

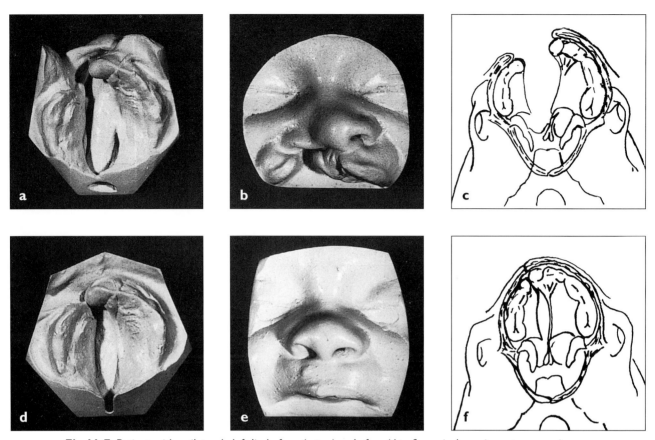

Fig 11-7 Patient with unilateral cleft lip before *(a to c)* and after *(d to f)* surgical repair; note approximation of the cleft alveolar segments. (From Bardach J and Morris HL. *Multidisciplinary Management of Cleft Lip and Palate,* 1990. Reprinted with permission from Saunders.)

ture initiates or creates compressive forces on the displaced maxillary bony segments. Varying responses can be noted in the spatial relationship of the underlying nasomaxillary parts and the alveolar segments incident to the molding affect of the reconstituted lip musculature. In some instances, the lip pressures may cause an approximation of the cleft alveolar segments within a short time, resulting in an acceptable maxillary arch contour (Fig 11-7). Sometimes the lip forces overly displace one or both of the maxillary segments medially and the premaxillary segment posteriorly, causing a constricted and distorted arch (Fig 11-8). The spatial relationships of the parts of the cleft maxillary jaw, prior to lip reconstruction, can be a strong factor in maxillary arch configuration following surgical lip repair.

In the newborn child, the maxillary bony segment displacement is usually most extensively expressed in the region of the eventual deciduous canine as well as a forward positional distortion of the premaxillary segment. This seems logical since the forward aspect of the cleft lip and alveolar process most usually occurs between the lateral incisor and canine. In some instances the reconstructed lip will mold and posteriorly position the anteriorly extended aspect of the premaxilla and reposition the smaller buccal segment medially, more in the canine region than in the tuberosity region, to a point of coaptation and good arch configuration. In other instances the smaller buccal segment can be displaced to the point of approximating the palatal process of the larger segment and even be overlapped by the premaxillary alveolar gum

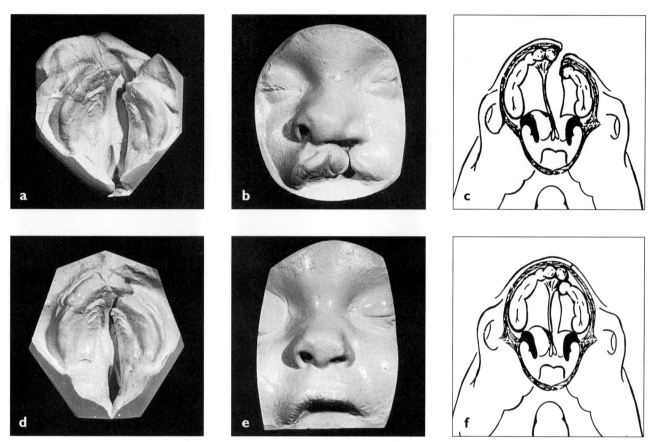

Fig 11-8 Plaster casts of an individual with a unilateral cleft of the lip and palate before *(a to c)* and after *(d to f)* surgical lip repair, illustrating constriction of the maxillary alveolar arch, premaxillary overlap of the smaller buccal segment, and narrowing of the palatal cleft. (From Bardach J and Morris HL. *Multidisciplinary Management of Cleft Lip and Palate,* 1990. Reprinted with permission from Saunders.)

pad, so that the eventual eruption of the deciduous canine will place it behind the deciduous incisors on that side. It has been shown that this molding effect is not restricted to the alveolar gum pad regions, but involves movement of the maxillary jaw segments as well, with a rearrangement of the nasomaxillary architecture (maxillary jaw segments) (Fig 11-9). This is a precursor to the dental arch distortion and a constricted malocclusion following eruption of the deciduous teeth. Pruzansky and Aduss[10] have shown that this molding movement of the posterior maxillary jaw segments will take place until the inferior nasal turbinate makes contact with the nasal septum. Concomitantly, a significant reduction in the width of the palatal cleft can occur, because it is a maxillary jaw movement and not solely an alveolar arch distortion

and reconfiguration. It is actually an opposite alteration of the prenatal bony jaw segment displacement. The muscle forces sometimes move the smaller jaw segments into a lingual relationship with the corresponding mandibular segment, narrowing the maxillary arch predominantly in the anterior or canine region and resulting in a crossbite. The usual smooth curve of the maxillary arch observed in noncleft individuals can be distorted into an inverted V, resulting in the greatest extent of crossbite being manifested in the canine region. As before, variation is the rule as to the varying degrees of reaction to the constricting effects of the reconstructed lip musculature.

Several studies have been undertaken to determine the incidence of constriction of maxillary segments in cleft lip and palate indi-

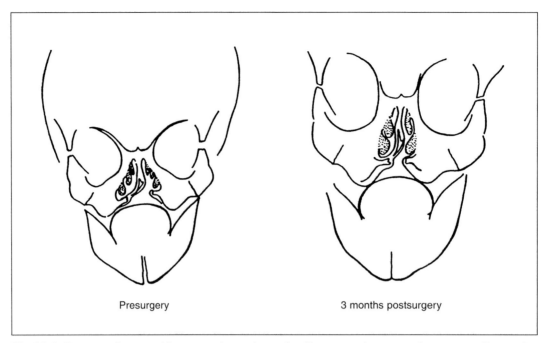

Presurgery

3 months postsurgery

Fig 11-9 Tracings of oriented laminagraphic radiographs, illustrating changes in the nasomaxillary architecture incident to growth and lip reconstruction in a unilateral cleft lip–and–palate individual.

viduals. The present discussion will center around the unilateral cleft, the most prevalent of the complete clefts, rather than the bilateral cleft of the lip and palate. In a documented study[11] conducted on longitudinal material obtained on unilateral cleft lip and palate children from infancy onward, it was determined that approximately 40% of the children exhibited collapse of the maxillary arch. Variation in the extent of collapse was evaluated by the number of dental crossbites; in some of the patients only the deciduous canine was in crossbite. This, of course, is in concord with the observation that there is greater medial distortion of the anterior aspect of the cleft jaw segment than is noted in the posterior buccal segment. It is important to emphasize again that the muscle action of the reconstructed lip can distort and constrict the maxillary alveolar arch and thereby create a potential malocclusion that can occur prior to the palatal surgery. It is also important to stress that the greatest effect of constriction is seen in the area of the cleft lip

repair in the more anterior regions of the mouth. With age and growth, the continued influence of the reconstructed lip musculature, superimposed upon the constrictive influences of scar tissue incident to palatal surgery, may cause a more pronounced crossbite to develop as the deciduous dentition erupts. Correction of the palatal cleft itself is usually undertaken at an appreciably later age than that of lip repair, usually 12 to 18 months of age. At any rate, lip and palatal closure usually occur before eruption of the complete deciduous dentition and incident to the constrictive muscle influences on the nasomaxillary complex. By that time, partial or even total crossbites will usually be seen on the side of the palatal cleft. It is emphasized that this occurs to varying degrees and, by documentation, only in approximately 50% of the young cleft lip and palate population. It is re-emphasized that crossbites are most usually incident to movements of the bony segments under constrictive muscle influences following surgical reconstruction.

Early Orthodontic Treatment in the Complete Cleft—Presurgical and/or Postsurgical?

In years past, different centers have reported attempts to obviate the development of a constricted deciduous arch by instituting what is called *presurgical oral orthopedic treatment*. It is not the purpose of this presentation to discuss such procedures per se, except to mention that not all centers are in accord with undertaking such procedures unless there are specific reasons to do so prior to reconstruction of the lip. In essence, these procedures require a series of molding and retentive appliances that gradually guide and mold the bony segments and alveolar processes into improved relationships, theoretically preventing the constriction of the bony parts. Many centers do not favor such a procedure, rationalizing that the malpositioned jaw parts can be altered to achieve proper correction after eruption of the deciduous dentition.

At this point, it seems desirable to propound mechanisms of orthodontic correction rather than variance in philosophies of timing and procedures. It is important to express the fact that, prior to birth, the segmental or geometric relationships of the parts of the cleft jaw are hypothetically created by the tongue and circumoral musculature within and external to the maxilla itself. After reconstruction of the cleft lip musculature, constrictive forces are created on the maxilla that can mold and move jaw segments so that, when the deciduous teeth erupt, they may be in varying degrees of malposition, most frequently crossbite. Considerable misconfiguration of the dentoalveolar complex may also occur in the posterior jaw segments, causing aberrant positioning of the cleft parts of the maxilla and misalignment of the erupting deciduous teeth in a malpositioned and misconfigured arch form. It is subsequent to the eruption of the deciduous dentition that the author recommends orthodontic treatment of the cleft lip and palate child.

During the deciduous dentition period, orthodontic therapy in the cleft lip and palate patient must be directed toward counteracting the adverse muscular influences that produced the maxillary constriction. Postoperative lip forces constrict the maxillary arch and, more pertinently, the supporting bone. As a consequence, orthodontic forces must be exerted toward moving the maxillary arch segments into a more acceptable position and normal arch configuration, expanding the maxillary occlusion to achieve both. Whereas there is substantial evidence that lip and tongue forces operative before birth move the cleft segments into malposition, there is also documented evidence that the reconstructed lip forces can again position the cleft maxillary segments into adverse geometric relationships. There is likewise substantial evidence that orthodontic forces applied in children with clefts of the lip and palate can move the unfused bony maxillary segments. Whereas treatment of the noncleft child involves the movement of individual teeth as well as tooth segments, orthodontic movement in a cleft individual can involve orthopedic as well as actual movement of jaw parts that contain the teeth.

This, of course, is contingent on an osseous binding not occurring in the bony palatal cleft incident to the surgical transposition of periosteal tissue, which can result in deposition of bone. If no bony connection is present in the alveolar and palatal bony cleft, then orthodontic treatment of the cleft lip and palate individual can result in an orthopedic effect (jaw segment movement) as well as an orthodontic effect (tooth movement). In actuality, orthopedic movement of the cleft jaw segments may be the more desired and the needed movement at early age levels. If the muscle forces of the reconstructed lip exert compressive forces on the jaw parts and move the bony segments out of alignment, orthopedic-orthodontic forces must counteract these forces and return the cleft jaw segments into position. Laminagraphic radiographs have substantially documented the observation that properly directed orthodontic forces do, in fact, move unfused bony maxillary segments[12] in young children with repaired clefts of the lip and palate. Substantial radiographic evidence has demonstrated an increase in width between the lateral borders of the nasal cavities following the application of orthopedic-orthodontic forces, more so in the anterior (canine)

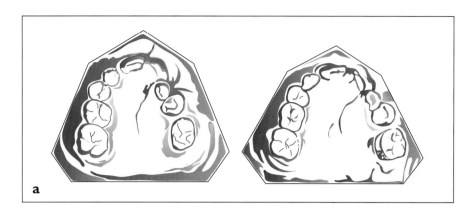

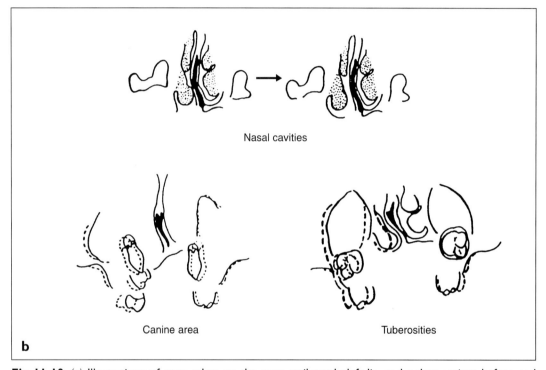

Nasal cavities

Canine area   Tuberosities

Fig 11-10 *(a)* Illustrations of casts taken on the same unilateral cleft lip–and–palate patient before and after orthodontic-orthopedic expansion. *(b)* Frontal laminagraphic radiograph tracings of selected areas taken at the same record times indicate increase in nasal cavity width. Dashed line depicts changes in unerupted canine crown positions and position of unerupted permanent molars after segmental movement.

region than in the tuberosity (molar) region; likewise, distances between the crowns of developing, unerupted permanent canines—well encased in the maxillary bones—have shown measurable increments (Fig 11-10). Notably, the inferior turbinates on the cleft side were at times observed to be moved away from previous contact with the nasal septum, increasing nasal airway space—further substantiation of orthopedic

movement of the cleft bony jaw segments, rather than the restricted movement of teeth.

As previously mentioned, a preference exists in some institutions to use molding plates (presurgical oral orthopedics) to reposition the cleft maxillary jaw segments prior to lip surgery and eruption of the teeth to align the alveolar gum pads into a more acceptable alveolar arch alignment. Unless there is an express need to undertake surgical lip closure, the author prefers to await full eruption of the deciduous dentition to position the cleft jaw segments. First, the mandibular deciduous dental arch is a clear guide as to the positioning of the cleft maxillary segments. The maxillary dentition can now be properly placed into its relationship with an existent, fully erupted mandibular deciduous dentition. It must be understood that the jaw segments are being moved and not the teeth. The maxillary deciduous teeth are holding mechanisms for the maxillary appliance to cause the repositioning of the jaw segments, containing them until the maxillary dentition is moved into good alignment with the mandibular dentition. When teeth are not present, considerable guesswork is involved in molding the maxillary alveolar arch segments into an acceptable relationship with the mandibular jaw.

Second, there are no specific clinical measures of alveolar arch deficiency in the cleft maxilla as to extent and location; it is subject to clinical judgment. If deficiencies are present in the cleft region of the maxillary alveolar processes, it is difficult to determine exactly where the gum pads must be positioned and in what geographic relationship they should be to each other. If it is not known how much of the cleft is due to tissue deficiency, there is no way of knowing where to place the open ends of the alveolar arch processes around that cleft. The presence of mandibular teeth readily enables one to determine where to place the maxillary teeth into an acceptable relationship with the mandibular arch. Furthermore, at very young ages, there is little probability of determining the extent or direction of mandibular growth in a short time interval. In presurgical oral orthopedics, there is no indication what the maxillomandibular relationship will be at the time of eruption of the deciduous dentition. In practice, an alveolar gum pad configuration is established and surmised to eventually be in an acceptable relationship with the conceptualized position of the mandibular dental arch at the time of eruption of the deciduous dentition. Spatial relationships of the maxilla are hypothesized without clear knowledge of what the rearranged maxillary segments will be relative to the mandible incident to growth.

Functional-Developmental Reasons for Early Orthodontic Treatment in Deciduous Dentition

According to the author's preference, orthodontics in the cleft lip and cleft palate child involving the early movement of jaw segments could, and preferably should, be undertaken after eruption of the deciduous dentition. Various expansion appliances such as the Arnold expander, the W-expander, or the palatal developer can readily reposition the cleft maxillary bony segments. It is important to remember that, at early age levels, permanent teeth are unerupted and developing in the maxillary cleft segments. As a consequence, early movement utilizing the deciduous dentition to reposition the maxillary jaw segments into a better buccolingual relationship can facilitate an improved spatial position for the eventual eruption of the succedaneous teeth, and better align them with their mandibular counterparts, reducing the potential for a buccolingual crossbite.

Many other reasons can be presented to initiate early orthopedic movement in the deciduous dentition rather than awaiting the eruption of a greater number of permanent teeth. A more desirable arrangement of the cleft parts of the maxilla can create a more harmonious maxillary bony architecture for the position, support, and function of the overlying cheek and reconstructed lip musculature. The circumoral musculature not only overlies the jaw structure, but is attached to it as well. When the supporting maxillary segments are optimally positioned, lip posture, continued lip development, and improved lip function may result. If nothing else, the improved foundation for the reconstructed upper lip may substantially improve the lip's appearance. Movement of the jaw segments can create a better oral environment for tongue posture and for tongue placement during speech and deglutition. When maxillary segments are excessively constricted and in a crossbite relationship, the tongue tends to assume a lower posture.

Creating a more normalized framework for the roof of the oral cavity enhances the probability of improved tongue activity during such

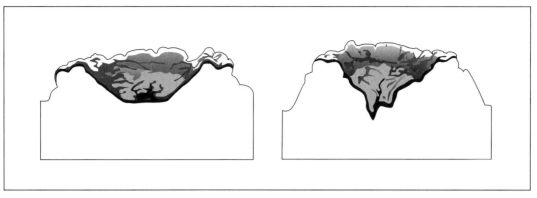

Fig 11-11 Cross-section of dental casts cut through the region of the first molars. *(left)* A noncleft-palate individual. *(right)* A cleft-palate individual with distortion and constriction of the maxillary palate clearly evident.

functional activities as speech, mastication, and deglutition. Abnormal scaffolding can cause, strengthen, and perpetuate compensatory adjustments of the tongue during these functions dictated by distorted and constricted oral cavity vault architecture (Fig 11-11) and malformed dental arches. When the palatal architecture is more acceptably arranged, it may be possible to minimize or even preclude the development of the misarticulations common to cleft lip and palate children. Articulatory speech skills are acquired and become increasingly more developed during early age levels, chronologically between 2 and 4 years of age, increasing the desirability of improved oral architecture at those ages. It has been stated that mature speech patterns are normally attained by 7 years of age, strongly suggesting that oral architecture reconstruction be achieved early—if possible during the deciduous dentition stages of dental development. During speech maturation, a distorted and constricted maxillary arch creates an undesirable oral environment for tongue placement during rest and function. Distorted proprioceptive cues are maintained and undesirably reinforced. Proper repositioning of the parts might give more room and create more appropriate cues to the tongue during both speech and deglutition; improved speech articulation patterns might be able to be maintained during the progressive maturational development of speech.

Overlap or close alveolar arch approximation might preclude the growth of the alveolar processes in the region of the cleft. Overlap might hinder eruption of teeth and maxillary alveolar arch development. Reduction of anterior dental and alveolar structure may hinder articulatory patterns by not providing proper proprioceptive clues for tongue-tip placement during rapid speech. Establishment of a more acceptable spatial relationship of the maxillary segments may enhance development of the maxillary alveolar processes, especially in the anterior areas of alveolar overlap, malposition, and containment. When one alveolar segment—usually the premaxillary segment—has been found to overlap and buttress against an adjacent alveolar segment, an impediment to alveolar growth and tooth eruption exists. Correction of the overlap, by repositioning the alveolar segments facilitates eruption of the contained teeth and, with that eruption, aids alveolar bone development. The contained alveolar process has been observed to develop vertically as well as anteroposteriorly concomitant with tooth eruption. Many times this alone has helped improve lip posture incident to added support and enhanced facial appearance.

It must be remembered that full eruption of the deciduous dentition has been preceded for considerable time by the surgical closure of the cleft lip and palate. Most usually the palatal cleft has been surgically corrected prior to the 18th

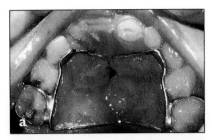 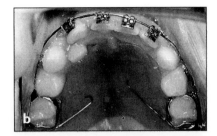

Fig 11-12 *(a, b)* A fixed maxillary lingual retainer in a young child with a repaired cleft of the lip and palate, orthodontically expanded in the deciduous dentition stage of development. Side by side: an acrylic palatal retainer needed to obdurate a palatal opening. This can be used, if desired, in conjunction with a fixed palatal lingual retainer, but must overlie the fixed retainer.

month of life and very frequently by 1 year, typically undertaken at such early ages to facilitate the development of proper speech patterns. In essence, orthopedic movement of the maxillary jaw segments counteracts the compressive forces of the overlying reconstructed lip musculature as well as the constrictive forces incident to any cicatricious tissue that may have developed following surgical closure of the palatal cleft. The orthodontic forces must overcome the strong compressive muscular forces of the buccopharyngeal ring and the constrictive forces incident to healing of the soft tissues overlying the palatal cleft, so orthopedic movements must be guided in proper directions and amounts in order to achieve desired jaw relationships as well as maxillary dentoalveolar arch alignment. These natural forces are continuous and maintain a degree of compressive strength; therefore, retentive appliances must be adequate to counteract these strong constrictive forces for extensive periods of time after proper jaw alignment. It has been noted that, whereas it might take considerable time to align the jaw segments, if proper retention is not utilized, the forces will undo the correction and cause a reversion toward the original arch malalignment very rapidly. Retention must be almost immediate. It's been observed that, although the orthodontic-orthopedic correction may take several months to achieve, it could be lost within 24 hours, so that retention planning becomes critical. A well-adapted, cemented maxillary lingual arch, properly designed and constructed (Fig 11-12) and inserted as soon as feasible following appliance removal (within an hour or two), can hold the maxillary alveolar segments at the desired geometric positions. It has the further advantage of minimizing material bulk in the palatal region, permitting the tongue to achieve and maintain a natural, higher posture in the oral cavity.

At times an opening of the palatal cleft may become evident following orthodontic movement in regions where there has been no surgical union, creating a potential speech problem. In many instances prior to palatal surgery in a unilateral cleft, the smaller jaw segment may approximate the palatal tissue of the larger segment in the anterior of the hard palate, or in a bilateral cleft with the premaxilla or the nasal septum on either side. In such cases, where coaptation of the tissue is evident, the surgeon will not undermine extensive tissue to achieve a surgical closure, maintaining a soft tissue surface contact closure. It is important to acknowledge that this tissue was not surgically united and the reopening of the palatal cleft anteriorly is a result of bony segmental repositioning. If an opening in the palate exists, then removable palatal coverage (Fig 11-12) would be indicated because of a need to obturate that opening. This can be done in addition to, and after placement of, the fixed lingual appliance. Removable

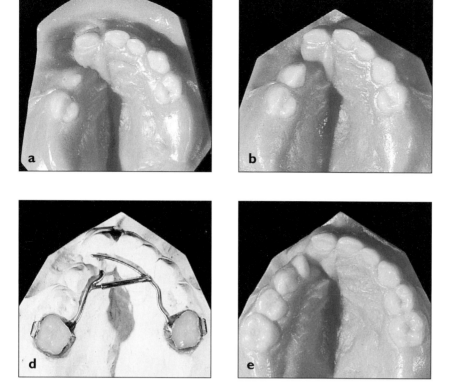

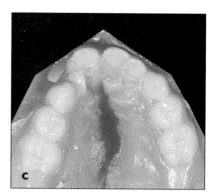

Fig 11-13 Patient G.S. *(a to c)* A unilateral cleft lip–and–palate individual with three progressive models showing dentoalveolar changes into the full deciduous dentition. *(d)* Maxillary casts of this patient with an Arnold expander in place (without coil) and *(e)* maxillary dentoalveolar arch after segmental expansion. The deciduous lateral incisor in the buccal segment and adjacent to the cleft is maintained in place to maintain bone.

palatal coverage alone is not recommended; loss or improper usage most probably would necessitate retreatment because of the rapid loss of what had been achieved through orthodontic expansion. Palatal coverage in conjunction with fixed retention can be used to preclude leakage of liquid or air through the opening into the nasal cavity and possibly through the anterior nares, which creates a social problem during eating as well as a nasal emission problem during speech. A speech problem would occur incident to loss of oral air pressure during the articulation of certain sounds. Nasality occurs, not from inadequate velopharyngeal (soft palate–pharynx) function, but from air leakage and a loss of oral air pressure incident to an opening in the palate. Of necessity, retention in early treatment stages must stay in place to preclude rapid relapse until succeeding periods of orthodontic correction are undertaken. This treatment might not occur until the transitional dentition period, after eruption of the permanent first molars and the maxillary incisors. As a consequence, this retention might be in place for a period of 3, 4, 5 years, or possibly longer, depending on eruption of maxillary permanent teeth albeit long before the full eruption of the permanent dentition.

As a rule, treatment in the deciduous dentition (Fig 11-13) must not necessarily be concerned with alignment of individual teeth as much as with jaw segment and alveolar arch alignment (Fig 11-14). Deciduous teeth will be lost, having lost root progressively from root tip toward the crown. However, full maintenance of the deciduous dentition as long as possible may be important, especially in the region of the cleft because, as long as root structure is present then surrounding alveolar bone is also present. Furthermore, maintaining alveolar bone in the cleft region for as long as possible helps to continue counteracting the ever-present constrictive forces of the reconstructed lip musculature; it also assures maintenance of the maxillary alveolar arch alignment for as long as possible, especially important during the times of eruption of the succeeding permanent teeth.

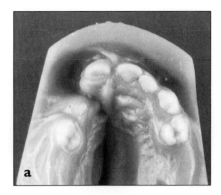
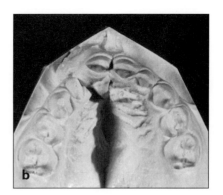
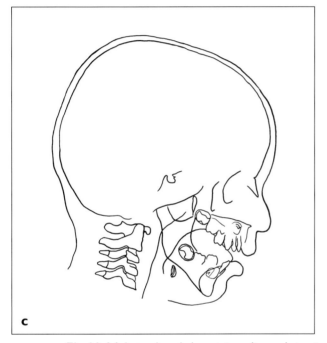
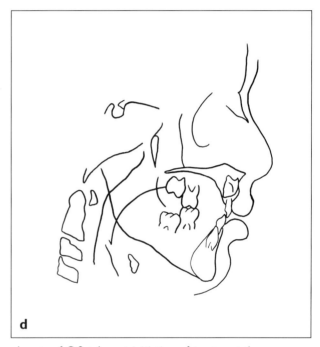

Fig 11-14 Lateral cephalometric radiograph tracings and casts of G.S. taken at initiation of treatment *(a, c)* and at the time of completion of initial segmental arch expansion *(b, d)*.

Orthodontic Therapy in the (Cleft) Transitional Dentition Stage of Development

A second phase of orthodontic treatment in cleft lip and cleft palate individuals usually occurs after eruption of the permanent molars and the permanent anterior dentition (Fig 11-15). Orthopedic bony segment movement can still be undertaken, if necessary, to reposition the parts of the cleft maxillary jaw provided no bony union has occurred in any region of the cleft.

Bone grafts placed in the alveolar cleft, as has sometimes happened, would preclude any further orthopedic movement because of direct continuity of bone across a previously open area. Sometimes an inadvertent transposition of periosteal tissue across the cleft occurs, causing a bony union between the two sides of the cleft and precluding orthopedic movement. This would occur when an extensive vomer flap has been done.[13] With no bony union, orthopedic repositioning of the jaw parts can still be undertaken and, again, should be done prior to concentrating on individual tooth movement. Once jaw segments are positioned as advantageously

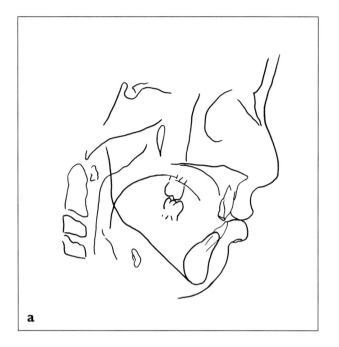

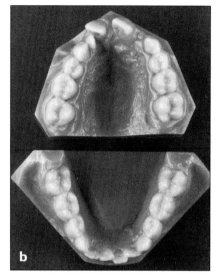

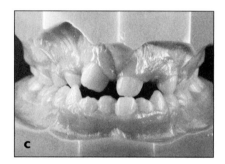

Fig 11-15 Patient G.S. *(a to c)* Tracing of lateral cephalometric radiograph and dental casts revealing malposition of incisors and recurrence of crossbites of the right deciduous canine and permanent central incisor regions incident to mandibular growth, indicating a need for a second phase of orthodontic treatment.

as possible, the second phase of cleft lip and palate treatment can be undertaken, involving more conventional orthodontic tooth movement and the placement of individual teeth into proper relationships.

Most frequently the maxillary anteriors, specifically those that border the alveolar cleft, will erupt in undesirable positions, many times with severe rotations and poor axial inclinations. Longitudinal lateral and frontal cephalometric radiographs[14] taken of unilateral cleft lip and palate subjects have shown that incisors bordering the cleft frequently erupt toward the cleft in a downward and backward direction, becoming more retroclined than normal. With continued eruption, these teeth tended to become more retropositioned with progressively increased tipping toward the cleft. Maxillary canines adjacent

to the cleft were significantly erupted less vertically than normal, indicating less vertical dentoalveolar development approximating the cleft. It can be surmised that any deficiency of bony tissue and the spatial relationships of the premaxillary segment relative to the posterior segment bordering the cleft, both before and after surgical correction, can highly influence the extent and path of eruption, as well as the erupted position of the teeth adjacent to the cleft. This further emphasizes the significance of early treatment to advantageously position the tooth-containing jaw segments. Incisors adjacent to the cleft might be inclined lingually rather than labially; they might be severely rotated with this lingual positioning; they might erupt almost horizontally into the cleft region rather than vertically toward the mandibular anterior dentition.

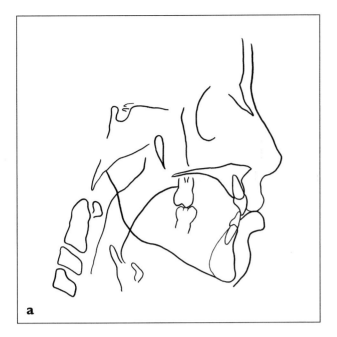

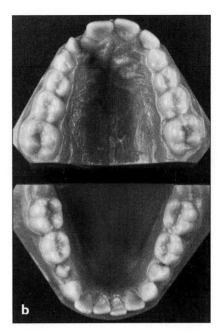

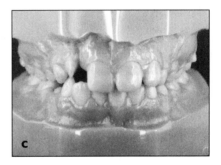

Fig 11-16 *(a to c)* Tracing of lateral radiograph and dental casts of G.S., after some additional segmental expansion and alignment of the erupted maxillary incisors. Note that the maxillary dental midline does not coincide with the mandibular dental midline.

In extreme situations they have erupted horizontally toward the lip; they have even been seen to erupt toward the nasal cavity rather than the oral cavity. Facial and dental midlines are severely disparate. Anterior teeth, particularly those bordering the cleft, are not only unesthetic but also may create functional problems in the anterior part of the dentition.

The malpositioning of the maxillary anterior teeth necessitates the initiation of orthodontic treatment at relatively early ages, preferably during or just subsequent to their eruption and most times long before complete root formation (Fig 11-16). Obviously these teeth must be moved for esthetic reasons if not for functional reasons. Individuals with a repaired cleft of the lip and palate many times have attention called to their lips and related facial structures almost solely incident to a surgical repair. Malpositioned maxillary incisors compound the esthetic problem so that added attention is called to the cleft problem. Psychosocial reasons alone dictate the advisability of initiating correction of the position of these teeth. It has also been observed by the author that orthodontic correction prior to the completion of root development can dictate better results. It has been the author's observation that, when severely rotated teeth are corrected prior to apical closure of the root, results are more stable in that the relapse tendency of the rotation seems to be less than customarily observed after full root development. This has been observed in noncleft individuals as well. Further, according to Rygh's[15] findings, it has been determined that there is considerably less root resorption in the incisors if they are moved prior to apical closure rather than after full development of root structure. It seems, therefore, that much less root resorption might be anticipated if these teeth are moved out of severely abnormal positions into better relationships prior to complete root development. Additionally, proper positioning of the incisors can be of value in the maturational process of the speech articulatory system. Many of the sounds in the English language require tongue-tip movements and proper environmental contacts for good articulation. When teeth are badly out of place, improper cues for tongue-tip contact can occur, so patterns of misarticulation can develop and be undesirably strengthened with time. Other reasons for early treatment of the anterior dentition also become apparent. Maxillary incisors can be moved out of crossbite which, in itself, may prevent abnormal mandibular shifting movements in order to achieve full occlusion. More advantageous masticatory patterns can ensue as early as possible from proper positioning of the dentition. The author is a strong advocate of initiating movement of the anterior teeth in these individuals as early in age as feasible.

Caution must be exercised in moving anterior teeth for purposes of dental midline alignment. Many times lateral incisors are observed to be in the bony segment distal to the cleft rather than in the premaxilla itself. These teeth cannot be moved out of bone in order to position them in proper contact with the central incisors. Teeth approximating the cleft margins on both sides of the cleft will have very little bone overlying that side of the root, so they cannot be moved laterally into the cleft area because they will be moved out of bone and cannot be maintained. Even though the soft tissue covering may be observed overlying the cleft, it cannot be concluded that the bone underlying that soft tissue is continuous and not a bony cleft. If there is a cleft of the bony alveolar process, the teeth cannot be moved to achieve contact relationships. Likewise, if bony clefts exist it may not be possible to move the maxillary incisors into a desirable relationship with the mandibular midline. The mandibular midline must be the major consideration provided, of course, there is no mandibular shift. Although the maxillary dentition must be placed as advantageously as pos-

sible to achieve a satisfactory occlusion with the mandibular dentition, midline relationships might be observably disparate and to some extent must be accepted. The only way that this can be overcome is by the placement of an alveolar bone graft at an early age, which will give bony continuity and provide for tooth movement. Many times this is done after eruption of the central incisors and prior to the eruption of the permanent canine, which is adjacent to the cleft margin. It is frequently recommended that an alveolar bone graft be undertaken in this region when the root of the unerupted canine is approximately one-half to two-thirds formed.[16] It has subsequently been observed that, in many of these cases, the permanent canine erupts into the bony graft itself and can be placed into position. Many times this is also done prior to full root development and eruption of the lateral incisors approximating the cleft, since it, too, might need bone in order to be properly placed. If a bone graft is to be undertaken in the maxillary alveolar region, it is usually done at this time rather than at much earlier periods. It must be remembered that, once a bone graft has been placed and bony continuity is established, orthopedic movement of the bony segments is no longer feasible. Consideration must also be given to the fact that once a bone graft is done in the maxillary alveolar region, maxillary growth is slightly retarded compared with cleft lip and palate patients in whom a bone graft has not been done.[17] Of course in cleft cases, grafted or not, some retardation of nasomaxillary growth has been observed to occur when compared with noncleft individuals. Although orthopedic segmental movement cannot be done in the cleft lip and cleft palate individual after a bone graft, it is feasible to move teeth into the graft in order to achieve better midline relationships. Another consideration is that the orthodontist has the privilege of additional time before the decision to undertake a bone graft must be made; teeth in the region of the cleft have been observed to develop and erupt somewhat later than those not adjacent to the cleft. Thus, chronologic age is not the criterion for the timing of an alveolar graft; the decision should be based on stages of root development and the possibility of tooth eruption into the graft region.

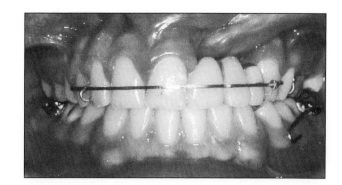

Fig 11-17 Maxillary Hawley retainer processed with a prosthetic replacement for a missing tooth at the site of the alveolar cleft.

Orthodontics during the transitional dentition stage of development in the cleft lip and palate patient usually involves extensive alignment of the anterior dentition. Incisors originally markedly malpositioned, poorly inclined, often severely rotated, and sometimes malconfigured must be adequately positioned. Movements that must be achieved are best accomplished with brackets and archwires and require significant root control position—all to be done with strong consideration of dental arch form and desired relationships in occlusion. If deciduous teeth are still present, they can be incorporated into the orthodontic mechanics for their anchorage values, but one must be aware that applied orthodontic forces will usually accelerate deciduous root loss. Again, care must continually be taken not to move any portion of a permanent tooth root through thin bone bordering the cleft, into the open bony cleft itself. The open alveolar cleft—if nongrafted—still imposes recognizable limitations on tooth position. After alignment of the anterior dentition, a period of retention must again be undertaken. If no bone graft has been placed in the alveolar region, then bony discontinuity of the nasomaxillary complex still exists. As a consequence, retention must be placed rapidly and withstand the compressive forces of the overlying repaired lip musculature as well as the constrictive forces of cicatricious tissue in the region of the palatal cleft

repair. Thus, the palatal aspect of retention is still very important, much as during the deciduous dentition period, but additionally, retention must contend with the anterior maxillary dentition where there has been much movement and correction of positions (such as rotations) of the incisors. The author usually prefers a well-fitting maxillary Hawley with a rectangular anterior wire, well adapted to the labial surfaces of the anterior teeth, with adequate acrylic built up incisally on the lingual surfaces of the maxillary dentition to not only withstand the compressive lip forces but to preclude rotation and inclination relapse of the anterior teeth. When there is a missing tooth or teeth in the cleft regions, a prosthetic replacement can be incorporated into the retainer for esthetic purposes as well as maintenance of the open area in the dental arch (Fig 11-17). The retainer must fit very well to withstand the ever-present forces of relapse and, again, must be placed within a very short time (hours—not days) in order to minimize relapse movement of the dentition as well as possible movement of the bony segments themselves. The compressive lip forces are ever present and must continually be withstood. This further emphasizes the desirability of an alveolar bone graft during or following the transitional dentition period of treatment. As previously stated, prior to the time of permanent canine eruption and preferably when the root of the

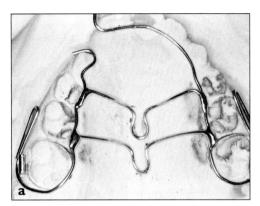 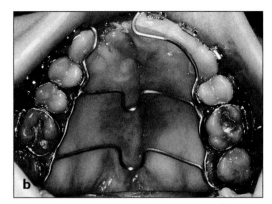

Fig 11-18 *(a)* Removable retentive bone graft appliance with palatal loops that can be activated to create tension forces on the bone graft. *(b)* Fixed retentive bone graft appliance cemented onto the maxillary dental arch via the first molar bands. Loops can be activated to create tension forces.

unerupted canine on the side of the cleft is approximately one half to two thirds formed. If a bone graft has been done and good bony continuity exists (stabilizing the cleft maxillary jaw parts) then greater resistance to the compressive lip forces are operative, permitting somewhat greater latitude in the construction and placement of the retentive appliance.

After achieving the most ideal alignment of the anterior teeth, either a prolonged, continuous period of retention must be undertaken or an alveolar bone graft should be surgically placed to preclude rapid collapse of the bony expansion achieved and to preclude relapse tendencies of the dentition that has been moved into place. If retention is the decision of choice, missing or unerupted anterior teeth can be included on the retainer for esthetic as well as retention value. Placement of anterior prosthetic dental units helps to insure retention wear on the part of the patient because of the added esthetics in the maxillary anterior region. Again, the retainers should cover any palatal opening to preclude loss of liquid into the nasal cavity or loss of intraoral air pressure during speech.

If a bone graft is done in the alveolar cleft, additive retention values are achieved incident to the stabilization of the bony segments as well as added support to the retainer, particularly in the alveolar crest region. When a bone graft is placed—usually harvested from the iliac crest—

all care is taken to completely encompass the graft with a palatal mucoperiosteal flap and a gingivolabial flap anteriorly to ensure maintenance of the graft. The harvested spongy bone is introduced at the level of the floor of the nose and placed in the alveolar area to alveolar crest level, occupying considerable volume. When the decision is made to undertake a bone graft, the use of a retentive, but potentially tension-producing, "bone grafting" appliance is strongly recommended, so that the orthodontic correction done so far will not be minimized or lost during the period before and almost immediately after the surgical procedure. If not done, strong and continuous muscular forces and tissue healing forces incident to the surgery will permit rapid segmental relapse, as well as the more conventionally understood movement of individual teeth. This appliance can be removable or fixed (cemented) (Fig 11-18), but must be carefully constructed to allow surgical access, be adequately retentive, and allow for the creation of tension forces in the bone graft area at the proper time after surgery. Chierici[18] has shown that tension forces, lightly placed on a bone graft, will help maintain that graft and new bone will form in the grafted area, much akin to periodontal tension forces causing new bone development. After a period of healing, the appliance can be removed and teeth can be orthodontically moved into the grafted area;

unerupted teeth such as canines can erupt into the grafted area and their periodontal fibers can maintain the viability of bone in the grafted area. If the need exists, osseointegrated implants can be placed in the grafted bone area. An alveolar bone graft may not be recommended or even feasible in some cases, but where applicable, it can greatly aid in the stabilization of the cleft bony segments and improve the integrity of the maxillary arch, permit eruption and placement of teeth within the arch, and many times eliminate the need for prosthetic adjuncts.[19-21] In addition, of course, are the esthetic benefits to be accrued in supporting the upper lip, both in the nasal floor area and in the dentoalveolar area.

Maxillary Retrusion and Orthopedics—All Stages of Dental Development

One other factor needs to be strongly considered in early orthodontic treatment processes (pre-adult dentition) in the cleft lip and palate individual—reduced nasomaxillary growth. During the many stages of craniofacial growth and more particularly during the later stages of growth, retrusion of the nasomaxillary complex—the midface—may become increasingly more obvious incident to the reduced expression of skeletal growth in that area. The mandibular region—the lower face—may continue to grow and, with a perceptible degree of retardation of maxillary growth, disharmony in facial appearance may develop, along with a developing anterior crossbite. In such cases, it becomes increasingly important to institute treatment measures directed toward improving the facial profile and facial appearance (Figs 11-19a to 11-19j), and to enhance the forward development of the midfacial region (Fig 11-20).

As has been mentioned in the previous discussion on early treatment of skeletal maxillary retrusion, the orthopedic face mask has proven useful in stimulating forward maxillary skeletal development. Clinically, very encouraging results have been attained in developing bone in the midfacial area. Also as previously mentioned, it

has been found desirable to advance the maxillary incisor apices prior to initiating face-mask use. Advancement of the incisor root tips has been observed to develop bone in the anterior maxillary region below the anterior nasal floor. This position of the incisor root tips has also seemed to be of help in nasomaxillary development when forward-directed forces were placed on the maxillary complex via the face mask.

It has also been observed, and corroborated by several research studies, that the extent of maxillary development was highly dependent on the individual stage of maturation.[22-24] Patients who had not reached their peak of pubertal growth, and when a good deal of facial growth could still be anticipated, exhibited the greater amounts of anteroposterior skeletal maxillary development and thereby improvement in facial profile relationships. Face-mask therapy, when needed, could be undertaken at any age. It has been successfully used to advantage from the time of the complete deciduous dentition (prior to eruption of the permanent first molars and permanent incisors) through succeeding stages of maturation. Propitiously if at all possible, this orthopedic therapy should be initiated at least by the time of the beginning of the adolescent growth spurt, since the greatest changes in the forward development of the nasomaxillary complex occurs during the early stages.

If an early bone graft has been placed in the bony cleft area, it has been observed that some degree of retardation could be anticipated in nasomaxillary growth, which could result in gradually progressive retrusion of the midfacial region. As mentioned, this is frequently done prior to full development of the unerupted maxillary canine root, and sometimes prior to the eruption of the permanent maxillary lateral incisor adjacent to the cleft. Any retardation of maxillary growth due to the surgical placement of the bone graft can be overcome with a face mask. Forces are used to enhance development of the maxillary complex and to maintain the maxillary dental arch in its proper relationship anterior to the mandibular dental arch. Recognition must be given to the fact that all correction in the anteroposterior dental relationship is not solely due to forward development of the maxillary region. It has been shown that much

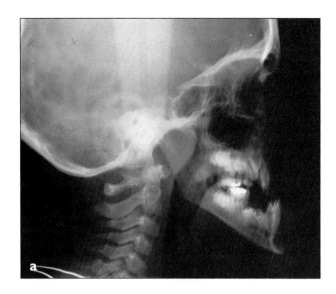

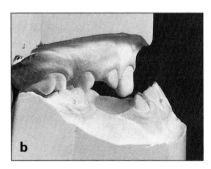

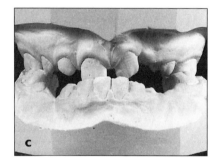

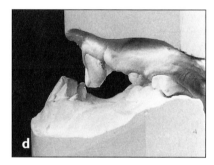

Fig 11-19 *(a to d)* Lateral cephalometric radiograph and dental casts of a young individual with a repaired unilateral cleft lip and palate showing severe maxillary retrusion and resultant malocclusion.

of the facial profile improvement results from the chin becoming positioned more downward and less forward of the maxilla than could be normally anticipated. In cases studied, a greater-than-normal increase in anterior lower facial height was noted. This change in the chin position seemed to result from increment in molar eruption, especially maxillary molar eruption. With the anteroposterior nasomaxillary ad-

vancement and with the more vertical positioning of the chin, the overall effect is some increase in facial convexity and an observable improvement in facial appearance. This also makes it clinically obvious that the direction of mandibular growth can be very important in the correction of facial disfigurement in cleft lip and palate patients. In treating cleft lip and palate, the orthodontist cannot totally concentrate on

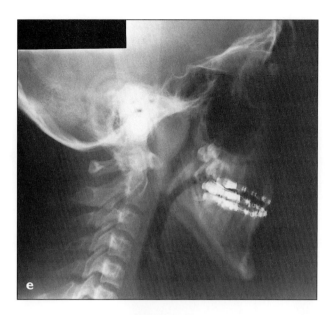

Fig 11-19 *(e to h)* Lateral radiograph and dental casts indicating the orthopedic and orthodontic correction of the maxillary retrusion and resultant dental relations.

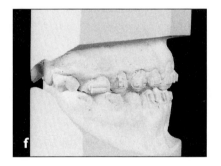
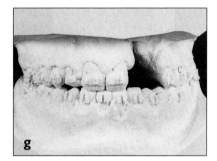
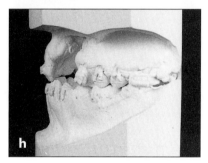

maxillary growth and its anteroposterior position, but must equally consider mandibular growth and its positional relationship. It is again recommended that this sort of therapy be initiated at early age levels when the orthodontist can take advantage of the greatest degree of potential maxillary growth. It must be recognized that after any stage of orthodontic and/or orthopedic treatment, face mask or otherwise,

retention mechanisms must be placed as well as carefully planned; most often in cleft lip and palate patients, retention will be prolonged indefinitely, if not for a lifetime (Fig 11-21). Retention is an adjunct to orthodontic treatment of cleft lip and palate individuals at all ages and stages of development (Fig 11-22).

In cleft lip and palate patients, orthodontic treatment does not end with completed early

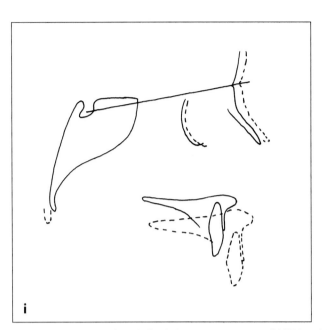

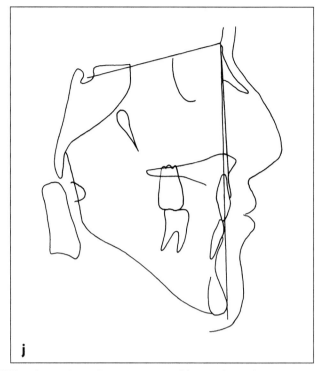

Fig 11-19 *(i, j)* Cephalometric tracings of 1974 and 1979 radiographs, indicating extent of forward maxillary development, and tracing of 1979 radiograph showing jaw profile relationships and resultant soft tissue facial profile.

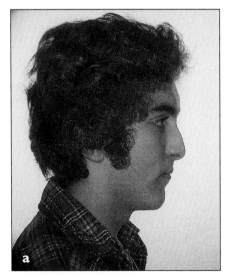

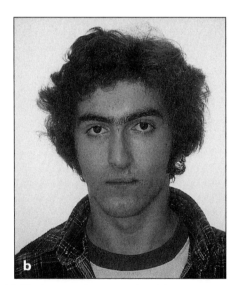

Fig 11-20 *(a, b)* Photographs of patient in Fig 11-19 showing changes in facial features incident to orthodontic procedures.

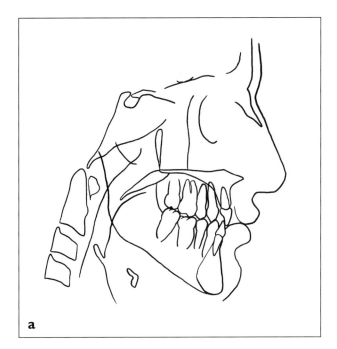

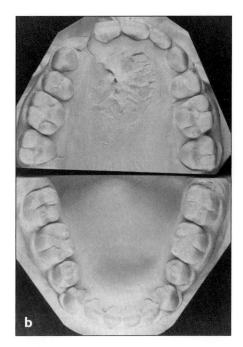

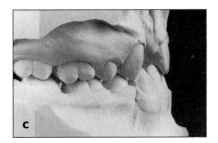

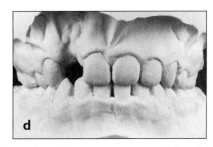

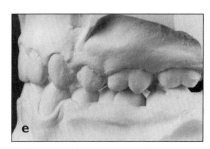

Fig 11-21 Patient G.S. *(a to e)* Lateral cephalometric tracing and dental casts at the time of completion of orthodontic treatment. At this time, full-time retention was mandated and a retainer with a prosthetic tooth was placed.

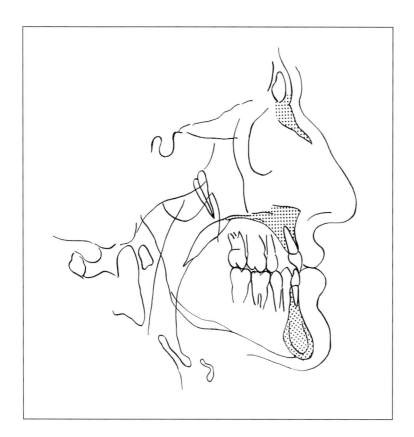

Fig 11-22 Cephalometric lateral tracing of patient G.S. at 32 years of age.

stages, but of necessity must continue, stage by stage, into and beyond the time of the complete adult dentition, including the reduced stages of craniofacial growth (Fig 11-23). Treatment will still be necessary at the time of adult dentition and, at times, require the adjunctive help of orthognathic surgery or nasomaxillary skeletal advancement by means of distraction osteogenesis (as illustrated in Figs 11-24 and 11-25), but those aspects are beyond the purview of this treatise. Suffice it to say orthodontic care for the individual with a cleft lip and palate continues throughout the lifetime of that individual. Orthodontics at all ages and stages of development plays a valuable role in attempts to achieve as near an ideal result as possible in the complete rehabilitation of an individual with the skeletal dysmorphology of cleft lip and palate. It necessitates a thorough knowledge of the anatomy and functional physiology of the congenitally affected structures, supplemented with a knowledge of changes with time and growth and how those changes relate to facial appearance and occlusion.

Fig 11-23 *(a to f)* Records taken of G.S. at 48 years of age, indicating results and long-term stability. This was truly a long-term follow-up of a patient from young childhood (2 years) to full adulthood (48 years).

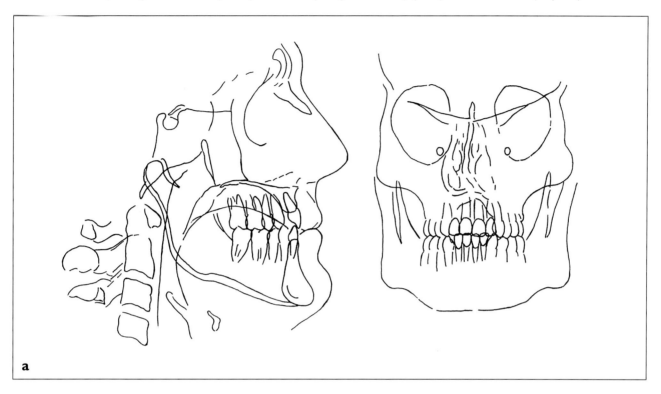

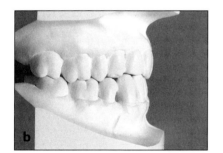
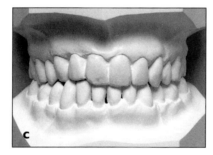
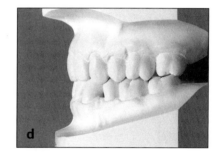

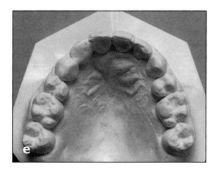
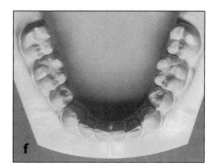

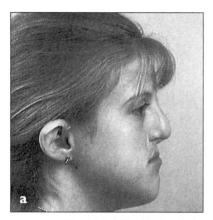 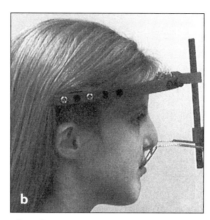 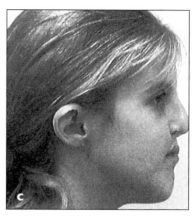

Fig 11-24 Profile facial photographs of a patient with a surgically repaired bilateral cleft and palate who underwent maxillary distraction osteogenesis to improve facial appearance. The patient was missing her premaxilla and all of her maxillary incisors. The photographs were taken predistraction *(a)*, with the rigid external distraction device in place *(b)*, and after distraction *(c)*. (Courtesy of Dr A. Figueroa and Dr J. Polley, University of Illinois at Chicago.)

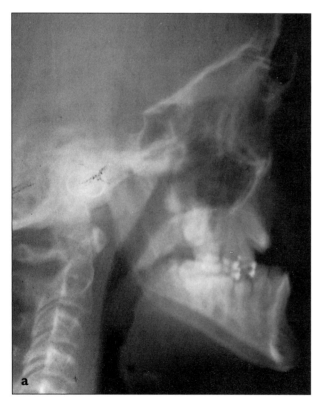 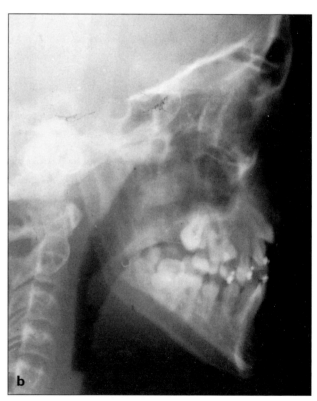

Fig 11-25 *(a, b)* Radiographs taken before and 3 months after distraction.

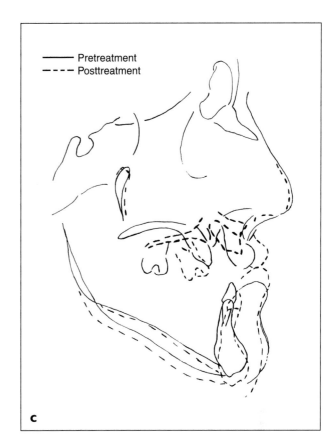

Fig 11-25 *(c)* Superimposed tracings revealing skeletal and soft tissue profile changes incident to the distraction procedure.

References

1. Fogh-Anderson P (ed). Inheritance of Hare Lip and Cleft Palate. Copenhagen, 1942.
2. Fogh-Anderson P. Increasing incidence of facial clefts, genetically or nongenetically determined? In: Longacre JJ (ed). Craniofacial Anomalies: Pathogenesis and Repair. Philadelphia: Lippincott, 1968.
3. Pruzansky S. Description, classification and analysis of unoperated cleft lips and palate. Am J Orthod 1953; 39:590.
4. Peyton WT. The dimensions and growth of the palate in the normal infant and in the infant with gross maldevelopment of the upper lip and palate. Arch Surg 1931; 22:704.
5. Peyton WT. Dimensions and growth of the palate in infants with gross maldevelopment of the upper lip and palate: Further investigations. Am J Dis Child 1934; 47:1265.
6. Coupe TB, Subtelny JD. Cleft palate-deficiency or displacement of tissue. Plast Reconstr Surg 1960;26:600.
7. Humphrey T. The relation between human fetal mouth opening reflexes and closure of the palate. Am J Anat 1969;125:317–344.
8. Humphrey T. Reflex activity in the oral and facial area of the human fetus. In: Bosma JF (ed). Second Symposium on Oral Sensation and Perception. Springfield, IL: Charles C. Thomas, 1970:195–233.
9. Humphrey T. Development of oral and facial motor mechanisms in human fetuses and their relation to craniofacial growth. J Dent Res 1971;50:1428–1441.
10. Pruzansky S, Aduss H. Arch form and the deciduous occlusion in complete unilateral clefts. Cleft Palate J 1964;1:411.
11. Pruzansky S, Aduss H. Prevalence of arch collapse and malocclusion in complete unilateral cleft clip and palate. Trans Eur Orthod Soc 1967;1–18.
12. Subtelny JD, Brodie AG. An analysis of orthodontic expansion in unilateral cleft lip and cleft palate patients. Am J Orthod 1954;40:686.
13. Prydso, Holm, Dahl, Fogh-Anderson P. Bone formation in palatal clefts subsequent to palato-vomer plasty. Scand J Plast Reconstr Surg 1974;8:73–78,197.
14. Ogidan O, Subtelny JD. Eruption of incisor teeth in cleft lip and palate. Cleft Palate J 1983;20:331–341.

15. Rygh P. Periodontal responses to orthodontic forces. In: McNamara JA Jr, Ribbens KA (eds). Malocclusion and the Periodontium, monograph 15, Craniofacial Growth Series. Ann Arbor, MI: Univ of Michigan, 1984:17–42.

16. Abyholm FE, Bergland O, Semb G. Secondary bone grafting of alveolar clefts: A surgical/orthodontic treatment enabling a non-prosthodontic rehabilitation in cleft lip and palate patients. Scand J Plast Reconstr Surg 1981;15:127–140.

17. Friede H, Johanson B. A follow-up study of cleft children treated with primary bone grafting, I: Orthodontic aspects. Scand J Plast Reconstr Surg 1974;8:88–103.

18. Chierici G. Experiments on the influence of oriented stress on bone formation replacing bone grafts. Cleft Palate J 1977;14:114–123.

19. Boyne PJ, Sands NR. Combined orthodontic-surgical management of residual palato-alveolar cleft defects. Am J Orthod 1976;70:20–37.

20. El Deeb M, Messer B, Lehnert MW, Hebda TW, Waite DE. Canine eruption into grafted bone in maxillary alveolar cleft defects. Cleft Palate J 1982;19:9–16.

21. Turvey TA, Vig K, Moriarty J, Hoke J. Delayed bone grafting in the cleft maxilla and palate: A retrospective multidisciplinary analysis. Am J Orthod 1984;86:244–256.

22. Simonsen R. The Effects of Facemask Therapy [senior research]. Rochester, NY: Eastman Dental Center, 1982.

23. Galletto L. Cephalometric Evaluation of Dentofacial Changes Incident to Facemask Therapy [senior research]. Rochester, NY: Eastman Dental Center, 1988.

24. Glauser J. Timing of Facemask Therapy Based on Skeletal Maturation [senior research]. Rochester, NY: Eastman Dental Center, 1995.

Chapter 12

Mandibular Skeletal Jaw Dysmorphology

Dysmorphologic development of the mandible, either congenital or acquired, invariably alters facial configuration, provided the variance is unilateral or develops bilaterally at different rates. Hemifacial microsomia, a dysmorphology of one side of the mandible, is the second most common congenital anomaly of the face, second to cleft lip and palate.[1,2] It occurs in approximately one out of 5,600 births.[3] Generally more males than females are affected (3:2)[4–6] and there seems to be a predilection for the right side.[7] At present there is no specific mechanism that has been proven as the definitive etiologic factor, that is, causative in hemifacial microsomia, but it is acknowledged that such mandibular dysmorphology has an undesirable affect on the occlusion. According to the adage, "As the jaws grow...," there is an accompanying effect on the position of the dentition.

Asymmetric mandibular development is the earliest manifestation of hemifacial microsomia; the mandible is usually shorter, retrusive, and narrowed on the affected side. This disparity may become more pronounced with time since growth on the unaffected side will outpace that of the affected side. There are wide spectrums of differences in the extent of mandibular malformation in individual cases, but with hemifacial microsomia, usually some deviation from the av-

erage can be noted in the nasomaxillary complex on the affected side, which may be reflected in reduced bony height and width, as well as in the height of the dentoalveolar process.[7,8] Because of the vertically shortened maxilla and mandibular ramus, diminished dentoalveolar height results in the occlusal plane being tilted cranially on the affected side. The chin is deviated toward the affected side and some degree of deformation of the external ear is usually found to be associated with this deformity.[9] There is a great degree of heterogeneity among hemifacial microsomia patients. The ramus itself may range from complete agenesis to identifiable—but grossly malformed—structures such as condyles and coronoid processes, to simply a decrease in dimension.[10,11] Pertinent to this discussion and of eventual pertinence to treatment, there is also some degree—quite variable—of muscular underdevelopment.[12] Severe underdevelopment of bone seems to be associated with severe underdevelopment of the muscles of mastication,[13] although not in direct correlation. The diminution in muscle development actually provides the rationale for introducing early orthodontic-orthopedic forces in the treatment of these individuals but it may not be feasible to do so until a sufficient number of teeth—at minimum deciduous—has erupted.

Treatment of Hemifacial Microsomia

Surgery: Costochondral rib grafts—cartilage and bone

Unquestionably, surgery is often a consideration and sometimes a necessity in the care of these individuals, depending on the severity of the mandibular deformity—particularly in the ramal region. In the past, for example, if there was a severe deficiency of ramal tissue and absence of a condyle, some surgeons would advocate early placement of a costochondral rib graft in an attempt to replace the absent temporomandibular joint (TMJ) and the absent or deficient ramus,[14–18] hoping the graft would provide growth potential via the cartilage as well as a replacement of deficient bony tissue. It was hoped that, in children, the grafted side would approach normality and the face would grow to achieve reasonable symmetry and appearance. Placement of these grafts was recommended at early ages for psychosocial reasons, as well as to replace the facial tissues for growth purposes. Follow-up studies over several years yielded varied and sometimes confusing results.[19,20] Costochondral grafts were generally found to grow, but varied greatly in the rate, amount, and direction when compared with the nonaffected side. Again, variation was the name of the game! In some cases, the grafted side grew less than the nonaffected side; in other cases the grafted side kept pace with the unaffected side, while in still other cases undesired greater growth was demonstrated on the grafted side, actually leading to a unilateral Class III malocclusion. This has raised speculation whether reported differences in soft tissue matrices, such as muscular tissues, might not be a factor in the variables noted. It has been found[21] that there is a reduction in the volume of some of the masticatory muscles on the affected side of those individuals with marked mandibular dysmorphology, but there is also marked variability from individual to individual. However, there seems to be general agreement that there is a relationship between the neuromuscular functional activity of some of the mandibular muscles and the extent of mandibular dysmorphology in hemifacial microsomia patients.[22–24]

Strongly suggesting benefits to self-image, it is generally recommended that this type of graft surgery be performed at age 5 or 6, with the realization that further surgery may be needed in adolescence. Consideration is also given to the fact that vertical nasomaxillary growth is being progressively affected incident to the mandibular dysmorphology, assuming the maxilla to be normal in all developmental aspects at birth but being kept from fully growing vertically because of the vertical, structural hypoplasticity of the affected mandible. In fact, this may not be true because concordant defects can likewise be found in the zygomatic and even the orbital region in some of these patients at birth. Studies of hemifacial microsomia individuals have shown that vertical asymmetry and the disparity between the two sides does not unflaggingly increase with time.[25] In some longitudinal studies it has been shown[26] that growth on the affected side corresponded to the growth on the other side; in this regard the degree of disparity did not change with age. Growth can occur in both rami on a parallel basis, indicating that facial asymmetry in hemifacial microsomia is not necessarily a progressive deformity.[27]

In a study[28] documenting vertical midfacial growth after surgical placement of a costochondral graft in an affected ramus, it was found that some patients exhibited symmetric growth of the rami and, when teeth were orthodontically erupted into the surgically created open bite, a long-term successful outcome ensued. The occlusal plane leveled from side to side incident to vertical alveolar and midfacial growth. Comparing the occlusal cant to the cant of the nasal cavity floor revealed that alveolar increment was "more significant than midfacial growth"; in other words, vertical maxillary alveolar growth was greater than vertical nasomaxillary growth. Some cases were considered unsuccessful: those individuals exhibited more severe cants to the occlusal plane. This seemed to be related to the severity of the overall deformity. The authors concluded, "Success depends on maintenance of the open bite and regulation of tooth eruption to produce vertical mid-facial and dentoalveolar growth."

Orthodontic care—Hemifacial microsomia

Hard tissue grafts, such as costochondral grafts, are sometimes placed when there is severe deficiency of ramal and condylar tissue; it is recommended that such a graft be placed early, approximately 5 or 6 years of age. The purpose, of course, is to increase the size of the underdeveloped and dysmorphic ramus and concomitantly to preclude what is presumed to be a secondary deformation of the nasomaxillary complex on that side.[29] It should be pointed out that such dysmorphic mandibles will usually grow—with or without placement of surgical grafts. It was pointed out in the case of M.M. (chapter 6) that, surprisingly, a discernible ramus and condyle did develop where radiographic records at birth had revealed severe deficiency of ramal tissue—only a gonial region and a semblance of a coronoid process were evident. Also surprisingly, it grew to an appreciable dimension albeit definitely smaller than the unaffected side. Our philosophy is to try to stimulate whatever growth potential exists in the existent tissue, to do this orthodontically and orthopedically, and to undertake surgical intervention when and if necessary. Orthodontic procedures are instituted as early as possible after eruption of the deciduous dentition and when the necessary cooperation is achievable, realizing that eventually maxillary deformity will be expressed as well as the more evident mandibular dysmorphology. Furthermore, much of the maxillary deformity is expressed in the vertical plane and eventually in a reduction in the maxillary dentoalveolar height on the dysmorphic ramal side.

The main objective of our orthodontic-orthopedic approach in these cases is to stimulate vertical development of the ramus and both the maxillary and mandibular dentoalveolar vertical dimensions on the dysmorphic side at as early an age as is feasible. This is accomplished by progressively repositioning the mandible toward a more symmetric relationship with the more acceptably structured maxillary jaw, causing an open interocclusal space and increasing dentoalveolar heights on the dysmorphic side by erupting posterior teeth toward each other. It is rationalized that vertical repositioning of the mandible will stretch muscle, and the ensuing tensile forces will stimulate the formation of new bone, much akin to an exostosis improving vertical skeletal dimensions. Bringing the posterior dentition into occlusion should help maintain the new mandibular position, improve facial symmetry, and, it is hoped, camouflage the congenital dysmorphology. As has been mentioned in chapter 7, this is accomplished with unilateral bite blocks on the nonaffected side. Change in the postural position of the mandible, in changing spatial relationships to musculature, causes alteration in force distribution and may result in bone apposition and lengthening on the affected side. In the relatively few hemifacial microsomia patients who have been available for orthodontic treatment, favorable increments in length and vertical height were noted; however, increase in width, which also is necessary for good facial appearance was not adequately achieved. This shortcoming is also characteristic of surgical undertakings. Of course, surgical augmentation will often be helpful, but not always necessary, being highly dependent on the extent of the congenital deformity. Surgical procedures can be undertaken at any stage when deemed desirable, but it may not be recommended to undertake these procedures too early in rapidly growing individuals and to await more advantageous timing. It is our philosophy that orthodontic-orthopedic therapies should be implemented as early in the growing ages as is feasible and that surgery be delayed until later stages of growth. Before undertaking a discussion of a more contemporary procedure (distraction osteogenesis), which is pertinent to these congenital dysmorphic cases, it seems advisable to present cases related to past experiences.

Case presentations

Patient A.S. A male child born with hemifacial microsomia was referred for orthodontic evaluation at 7 years of age (1985) (Fig 12-1). CT scans of the head obtained at that time (Fig 12-2) revealed the following. Images of the osseous structures showed absence of the right external auditory canal, with a small right base of the skull associated with asymmetry of the facial bones and mandible. The right zygomatic

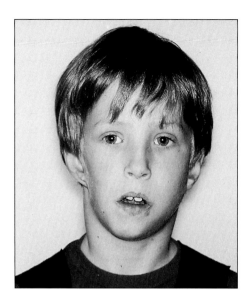

Fig 12-1 Frontal photograph of A.S., who has congenital mandibular right hemifacial microsomia. Note the facial asymmetry with chin deviation to the right and inadequate width, as well as lower face vertical shortness on the right.

arch had not completely developed. The malar bone on the right side was small. The right maxilla was maldeveloped compared with the normal left. The entire right mandible was poorly developed, having incomplete formation of the condylar head and neck, body of the mandible, and coronoid process. There was a definitive shift of the mandible to the right. Orthodontic evaluation indicated Class I molar relationships on both sides, but there was a Class II canine relationship on the affected side. There was a distinct midline discrepancy, with the mandibular dentition toward the right, as well as a limited mouth opening of only 25 mm. Additionally, there was a severe cant of the posterior occlusal plane, the right side being more cranial. There was no history of TMJ sounds or pain. Upon palpation, the left masseter muscle felt stronger and broader than the right; the temporal muscles felt approximately equal in size and synergistic in function, although there was severe deviation of the mandible toward the right on opening.

His lateral cephalometric radiograph (Fig 12-3) revealed a marked retrognathic, convex facial pattern, despite the fact that maxillary retrusion was likewise skeletally discernible, with an NA-FH of 80.5 degrees (mean 88.1 degrees). There

was marked steepness of the mandibular plane, more on the right side—the congenitally dysmorphic side. The frontal radiograph (Fig 12-4) revealed severe deformity of the right mandible, with skeletal deficiency in the ramal and gonial regions (both vertically and laterally) and a severe chin deviation to the right. There was an obvious tilt of the nasal floor (roof of the mouth) cranialward on the right in concordance with the cant of the posterior occlusal plane.

At this early stage of treatment, it was decided to initiate cervical headgear therapy to expand, erupt, and rotate the molars. Concomitantly, a mandibular unilateral (left) bite block would be used to open the vertical, stretch the muscles, and develop the right vertical dentoalveolar dimensions. After correction of the maxillary molars, we would then shift to maxillary unilateral (left) bite block for similar reasons. Later it was decided to periodically use a functional appliance (Harvold-type) to help correct the skeletal chin position and to aid in mandibular body, ramal, and dentoalveolar development. At the proper time, full orthodontic appliances were to be utilized with both orthodontic and orthopedic forces until surgical therapy, if and when indicated, would be performed.

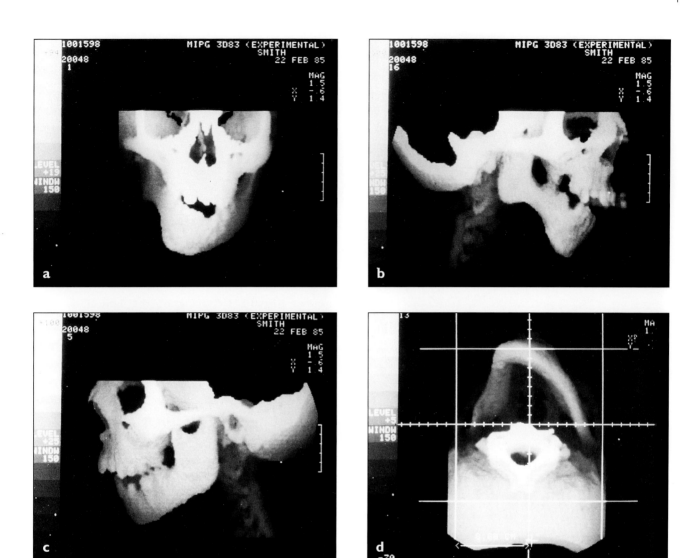

Fig 12-2 Computed tomography scans of A.S. showing mandibular right hemifacial microsomia. *(a)* Frontal scan indicating the similarity of the facial skeleton to the overlying features seen in the facial photograph. *(b)* Scan of the right side; note the short ramal height of the right mandible as well as the severe antegonial bending of the body of the right mandible—the side with hemifacial microsomia. *(c)* Scan of the left mandible, which is not congenitally skeletally deformed. Differences are apparent. *(d)* Scan of the inferior view of the mandibular jaw. The body length shortness and skeletal deformity are apparent when compared to the more normal left side.

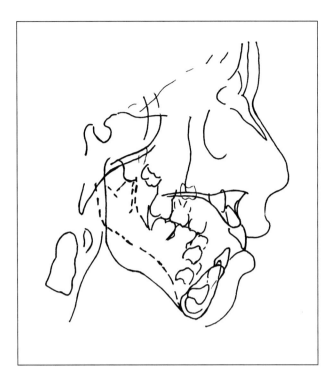

Fig 12-3 Tracing of the lateral cephalometric radiograph taken of A.S. at the time of orthodontic evaluation. The deformity and inadequacy of the right mandible is outlined by the dashed line.

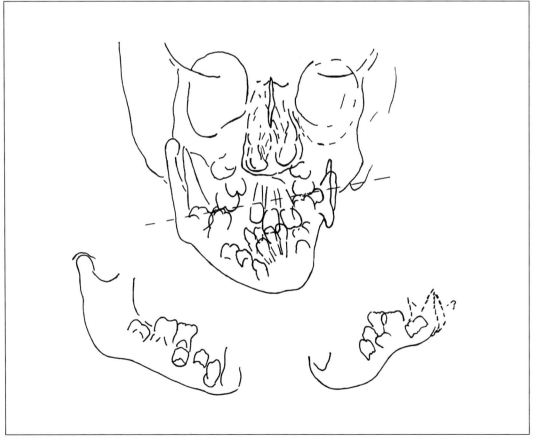

Fig 12-4 Tracings of the frontal and the right and left oblique cephalometric radiographs of A.S. Note the skeletal deformity and ramal shortness as well as inadequacy of the right mandible.

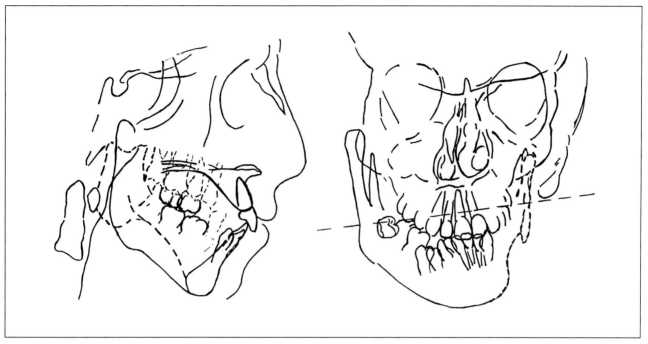

Fig 12-5 Tracing of the lateral and frontal cephalometric radiographs of A.S. at 12 years of age, after a period of orthodontic therapy. Changes incident to growth and, to some extent, incident to stimulation via orthodontic therapy are noted in comparison to the earlier records.

This therapy was pursued with some degree of improvement over a period of years. Progressive evaluation of records (Fig 12-5) revealed that growth and some favorable change had occurred. There was additional vertical mandibular growth on the right, as well as development in width. There was improvement in the cant of the posterior plane. Ramal height had increased on both sides but increment in severe antegonial notching on the affected side was obvious. The increase in ramal height seemed to be relegated to the gonial region, the coronoid process, and the condylar area—all presumably due to muscle and connective tissue pull. Dentoalveolar improvement could probably be ascribed to orthodontic forces. At this point, it was decided to initiate surgical procedures for jaw reconstruction, and the patient was readied for surgery. Surgery was planned in two stages:

Stage I
• Extraction of mandibular third molars
• Maxillary Le Fort I osteotomy and correction of the maxillary cant; rigid internal fixation

• Bilateral ramal osteotomies of the mandible (extraorally); rotation of the mandible to the left and autologous graft of the right ramus; rigid internal fixation

Orthodontic therapy was resumed several weeks postoperatively.

Stage II (approximately 1 year following stage I)
• Facial contour revision—right mandibular ramus, if desired
• Genioplasty, if needed
• Rhinoseptoplasty, if desired

As proposed in the first stage, two-jaw surgery was performed with considerable improvement in skeletal, dental, and soft tissue facial relationships as visualized on cephalometric radiographs (Fig 12-6). Postsurgically, there was an apparent widening of the nasomaxillary complex, increase in right ramal height, and an apparent increment in width at the ramal and gonial level. What was apparent on the lateral and frontal cephalograms was an inability to remove

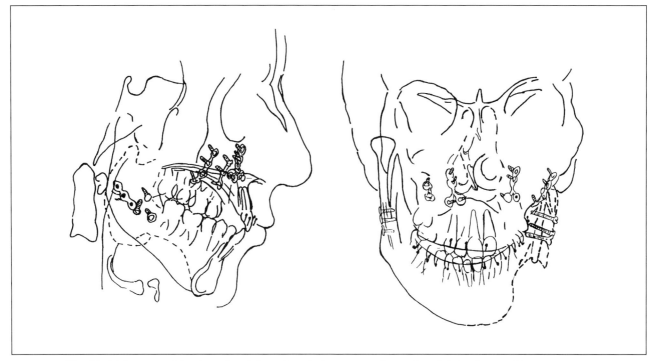

Fig 12-6 Tracings of the lateral and frontal cephalometric radiographs of A.S. taken at 14 years of age after two-jaw surgery was performed to improve dentofacial skeletal relationships. The rigid surgical fixation was readily discernible on the radiographs.

the severe antegonial notching. Considerable improvement was noted in dental relationships, including the midline (albeit not full correction) and in vertical dentoalveolar relationships, leading to immediate improvement in the cant of the posterior occlusal plane. Facial photographs indicated notable improvement in frontal facial appearance; however, profile retrognathism persisted. Surgery was performed in early December 1992 and orthodontic treatment was reinitiated in April 1993 after many delays. Follow-up orthodontic treatment again involved periodic bite-block therapy to improve and preserve vertical relationships and to improve and refine dental relationships. The patient was subsequently placed into retention (Fig 12-7).

Of particular pertinence to this discussion are the mandibular changes, more specifically in the ramal regions of this individual incident to growth and therapy. Superimposition of longitudinal oblique radiographs gives some indication of the changes. On the unaffected (left) side, it was possible to superimpose on the lower bor-

der of the mandible from the gonial region anteriorly and on the symphyseal region to obtain two different visualizations. On the dysmorphic side, it was almost impossible to satisfactorily superimpose for interpretation, but superimposing (best fit) on the anterior of the mandibular lower border registering on the symphyseal region permitted some insight into the changes. On the affected side, there was increment in the ramal region vertically and posteriorly, from the apparent coronoid process to the gonial region. This occurred during periods of bite block and activator wear, as well as in orthodontic therapy. Considerable change occurred, particularly in the rather elongated and acute gonial region, as previously observed on the frontal headplates. Increase in ramal height and width was likewise noted on the unaffected side, although the gonial region remained with similar contour and obtuseness; on this side, increase in condylar height was clearly observed. Some time after surgery, new records revealed considerable change in the dysmorphic right side of the

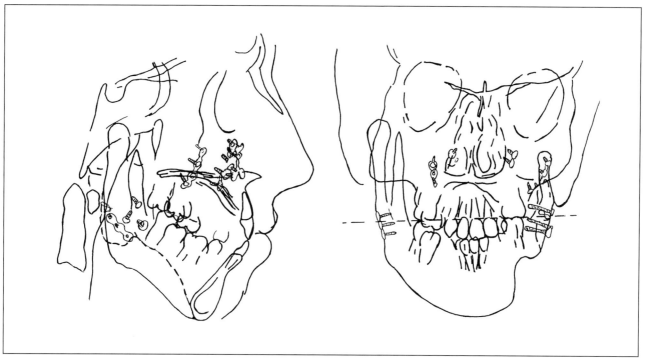

Fig 12-7 Tracings of the lateral and frontal cephalometric radiographs taken at the age of 17 years, following postsurgical orthodontic therapy and the placement of retention appliances.

mandible. Surgical reconstruction had added dimension vertically as well as posteriorly to the right ramus. Bone seemed evident anterior to gonion, making that region broader and flatter, with a strange configuration and acuteness to the antegonial notch; the fixation screws were quite evident. Increment in right ramal width was clearly evident on the frontal cephalograph, with an appearance simulating an onlay graft. Changes were also observed in the antegonial region. Reconstruction and repositioning of the nasomaxillary structures, the left mandibular ramus, and the dentition (including the cant of the occlusal plane) were noted (Figs 12-6 and 12-7). Part of the nonaffected left ramus seemed to be positioned posteriorly and had a bony indentation on its posterior border, posterior and superior to the gonial region (probably related to the surgical attempt to improve facial symmetry). Increased condylar, coronoid, and posterior dentoalveolar heights were likewise noted.

When the final oblique radiographs were evaluated in 1996, little change could be noted on the mandible's nonaffected side; there was almost no further increment in condylar height relative to the gonial region. The condyle, however, was angulated and positioned more posteriorly relative to the posterior surface of the ramus, while the posterior bony indentation above the gonial region seemed smoother and less pronounced. However, the affected (right) ramus and mandibular body were more altered in configuration (Fig 12-8). It was difficult to determine whether this was configurative or positional. There was more severe and acute antegonial notching in addition to considerable remodeling of the ramal and gonial region, probably due to altering functional forces during growth as well as orthodontic and orthopedic influences. Incident to these changes were visible tendencies toward a return to some of the undesirable features of the cant of the occlusal plane. The foregoing is evidence that, even with morphologic changes through surgery, there will be changes—some desirable and some undesirable—resulting from continued growth and the

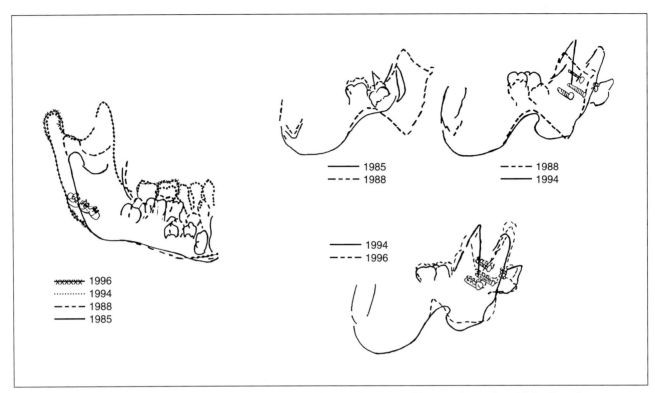

Fig 12-8 Superimposed tracings of the left and right cephalometric oblique radiographs of A.S. taken during the 11-year period of orthodontic treatment and growth. Differences of the left mandible, morphologically more normal, and the right mandible, the congenitally dysmorphic side, are apparent.

various functional, muscular influences, influences that the orthodontist must try to control as early as possible to achieve the most desirable results in such skeletal dysmorphology.

Patient B.B. This patient's deformity was not as extensive at birth as was the previous patient's; as before, no surgical procedures involving the facial skeleton were undertaken. The patient was treated orthodontically with an orthopedic approach and the understanding that the parents had no desire for a surgical undertaking.

B.B. was born in 1978 with left facial microsomia. CT scans of the head were taken in 1985, with the following findings: hypodevelopment of the left temporal bone and left pinna, with no evidence of an external auditory canal. The middle ear cavity was poorly developed, if present at all. The inner ear structures (cochlea and vestibule) appeared to be present but were probably malformed. The internal auditory canal

was also present but appeared to be directed anteriorly compared with the right side. The left portion of the mandible was less developed than the right. The condyle and TMJ were less developed than their right counterparts and there was absence of the left zygomatic process of the temporal bone.

All in all, there was hypoplasia of the left temporal bone, the left mandible, and the left temporomandibular joint area. Subsequent TMJ scans and MRIs confirmed the hemifacial microsomia of the left mandible and temporal bone, revealing a small condyle, a small, or "pseudo" disc, an incomplete zygomatic arch, a poorly developed middle ear, and absence of the external auditory canal on the left side.

Tc99m-labeled MDP was administered intravenously to evaluate cellular activity in the condylar region compared with that found in the fourth lumbar vertebra (L4). The right-sided ratio was approximately 1.4 relative to L4, which is

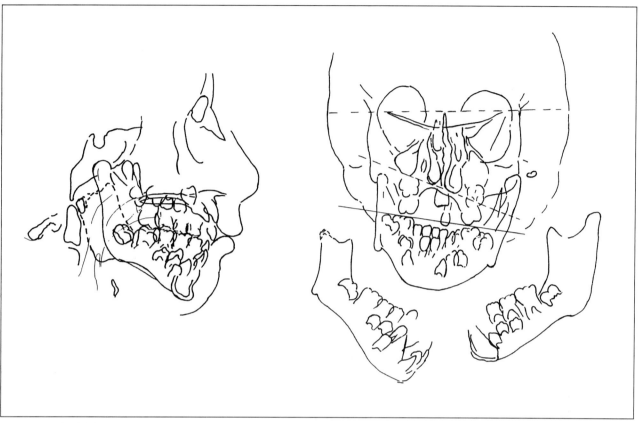

Fig 12-9 Tracings of the lateral, frontal, and right and left mandibular oblique cephalometric radiographs taken of B.B. at 7 years of age, showing congenital left hemifacial microsomia. Note the skeletal facial asymmetry affected by the maxilla and mandible. The vertical shortness of the left mandibular ramus and the concomitant reduced dimension of the condyle are likewise to be noted.

within normal limits for the patient's age, but the left-sided ratio was markedly reduced at 1.1 relative to L4, indicating severely limited growth potential of the left condyle. The patient had undergone several periods of surgical reconstruction of the left external ear with cartilage implants and soft tissue repositioning and was referred for orthodontic evaluation in 1985. At that time, the first CAT scans and conventional orthodontic records were taken (Fig 12-9). The oblique radiographs revealed a much-reduced left ramus and condyle; the frontal radiograph clearly disclosed skeletal facial asymmetry with obvious left-sided deficiency vertically and laterally. This was not only evident relative to the mandible, but to the maxilla as well, with severe cants of the nasal floor (nasal cavity shortness on the left side) and the occlusal plane, being more cranially positioned on the left.

The patient was in the early transitional stage of dental development; the permanent incisors had not yet erupted, but treatment was initiated shortly after records were taken and analyzed. A maxillary unilateral (right) bite block was implemented to disarticulate the dentition, to preclude eruption of the right posterior teeth, and to permit eruption and vertical positioning of the posterior teeth on the left (affected) side (Fig 12-10). It was hoped to achieve, if possible, added vertical growth on the hemifacial side of the face. A year later, the bite block was replaced with a functional appliance in an attempt to shift the lower midline into a more desirable position and encourage anteroposterior and vertical growth of the left mandible (Fig 12-11). This was replaced the following year with a combination Herbst appliance and palatal expander, again, in an effort to

[251]

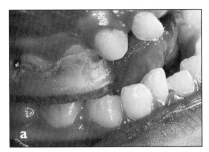
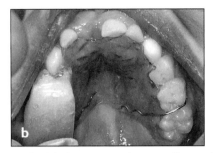
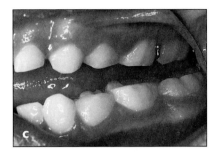

Fig 12-10 *(a to c)* Intraoral views of B.B.'s dentition with a maxillary right unilateral bite block in place. When the mandibular posterior teeth are in contact with the unilateral bite block, the left dentition is disarticulated, allowing dental eruption on the dysmorphic left side.

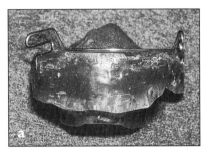
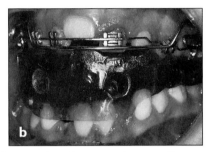

Fig 12-11 Patient B.B. *(a, b)* Views of the functional appliance used in an effort to align midlines and move the left mandible anteriorly, hoping for soft tissue tension to stimulate added growth of the left dysmorphic mandible.

enhance any potential growth on the affected side. Evaluating the records taken in 1989 (Fig 12-12), one will note that there has been generalized growth of the craniofacial complex; however, skeletal facial asymmetry is still marked. Of significance, growth of the affected ramus is definitive and positive—although of limited amount—and at least comparable to the nonaffected side; in addition, ramal shape and condylar configuration are somewhat more defined. Coexistent is greater steepness of the mandibular plane and increased antegonial notching on the affected side. The overall impression is that of improved skeletal facial asymmetry, although the lateral, or width, dimension is still a problem. The patient was still in the late transitional dentition stage, approximating the time of premolar eruption.

The following year, full appliance therapy was instituted, but with continuance of right unilateral bite block therapy to facilitate increment in the left maxillary posterior dentoalveolar complex by continued stepping down the archwire on that side. This therapeutic approach with full appliance therapy was continued until 1993 when the mandibular left posterior segment was erupted to increase vertical. At this time, because of developing arch length problems, it was decided to extract two mandibular central incisors in order to achieve anterior alignment and to compensate for the fact that the crestal aspects of these teeth were being crowded and moved out of the labial alveolar plate. The mandibular lateral incisors were moved orthodontically into the positions of the central incisors and the canines were moved into the positions of the laterals. As can be noted on the progress records (Fig 12-13), there is some semblance of improvement in the skeletal facial symmetry, albeit still a deficiency in width (lateral dimension) on the left. There seems to have been additional vertical growth

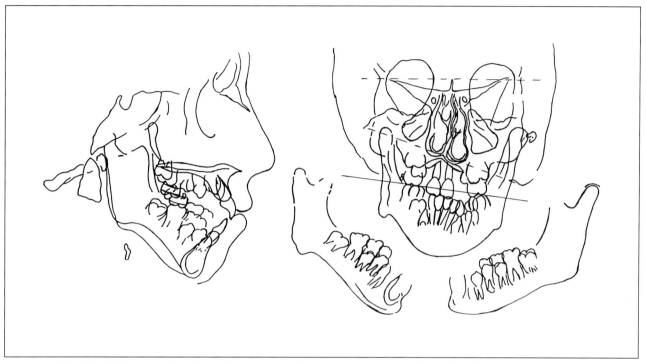

Fig 12-12 Tracings of the lateral, frontal, and oblique cephalometric radiographs of B.B. taken at 11 years of age after the periods of appliance therapy to stimulate growth and improve facial symmetry. A more defined structure in the condylar region of the left side can be noted.

of the ramus on that side, with elongation in the gonial region as well as possibly in the condylar region. On the oblique radiographs, ramal height increment is evident on both sides. There is some improvement in the cant of the occlusal plane and in the disparate vertical height within the nasal cavity; however, it must be acknowledged that head positioning is questionable, at best, with any hemifacial microsomia patient with ear and external auditory ear canal malformation. Comparative evaluations, therefore, are rather tenuous and must be interpreted with a high degree of caution. On the lateral cephalogram, steepness of the mandibular plane is obviously increased, antegonial notching is more pronounced, anterior teeth are more proclined, and an open bite has developed, now requiring further appliance therapy to correct axial inclinations and control lower anterior facial height.

As subsequent appliance therapy was continued, there was periodic utilization of a func-

tional activator until the placement of retainers. Retention consisted of a mandibular lingual splint for the two incisors and adjacent canines (serving as lateral incisors) and a fixed maxillary combined lingual–transpalatal arch to preclude eruption and constriction (Fig 12-14). Prolonged retention was anticipated. New records were taken in 1998 (Fig 12-15) when the patient was on his way to college. At that time, the oblique radiographs as well as the Panorex revealed a shortened but markedly defined left ramus with a condyle-like structure and a discernible coronoid process. There was marked antegonial notching, with minimal bony dimension, in the mandibular body anterior to the gonial region, inferior to the still open apices of the left third molar, and markedly close to the lower border of the mandible. Although there was measurable increment in the height of the left ramus, skeletal facial asymmetry was clearly existent. Again, the deficit in lateral dimensions was

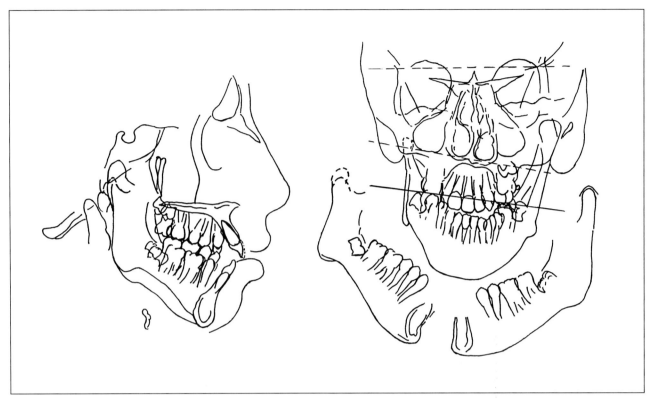

Fig 12-13 Tracings of the lateral, frontal, and oblique cephalometric radiographs taken of B.B. at 15 years of age. Some improvement, although not optimally sufficient, in skeletal facial symmetry and the vertical height of the left ramus can be noted.

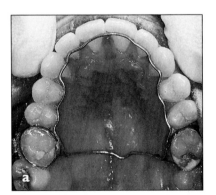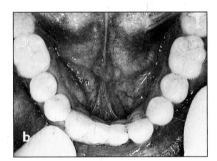

Fig 12-14 *(a, b)* Maxillary and mandibular intraoral views of the retention mechanism used for B.B.

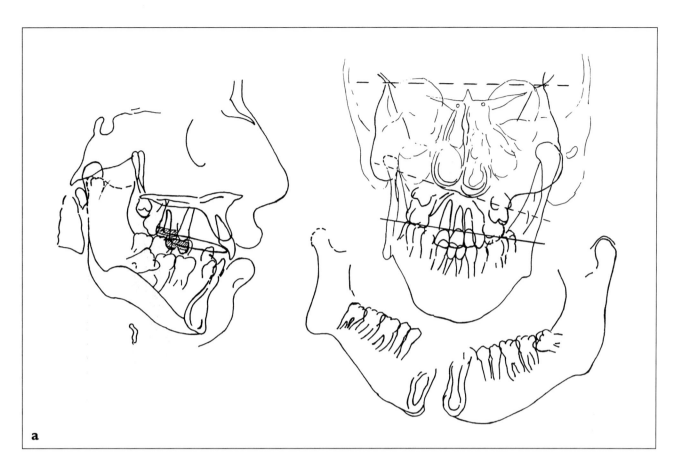

a

Fig 12-15 *(a, b)* Tracings of the lateral, frontal, and oblique cephalometric radiographs of B.B. at 20 years of age. The skeletal deficit still evident in the facial skeleton is due to inadequacy in width in the left ramal region.

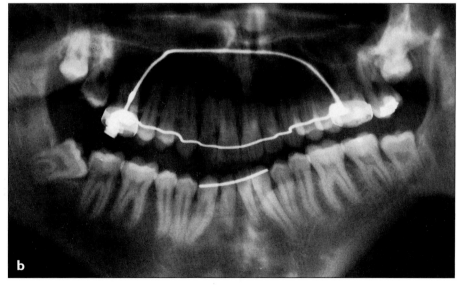

b

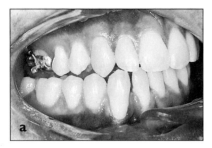 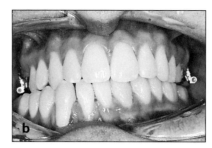 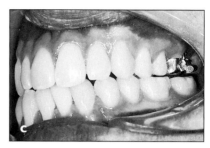

Fig 12-16 Intraoral views of B.B.'s occlusion upon completion of orthodontic treatment. Full-time retention was required and monitored periodically.

clearly evident. Nevertheless, visual facial appearance was somewhat improved, as was the occlusion and the appearance thereof (Fig 12-16). On the lateral cephalogram, differences in right and left mandibular configuration and dimensions were obvious, all of which resulted in two levels of posterior occlusion. Furthermore, dramatic steepness of the mandibular plane was obvious, but it was well camouflaged by the overlying soft tissues. All in all, a reasonable outcome to a somewhat severe congenital developmental problem and mandibular growth problem was achieved. The point to be made is that orthodontic-orthopedic continuous control seemed to enhance skeletal mandibular development; the additional bony growth—although an exostosis brought about (probably) by muscular influences—seems to have helped facial appearance as well as the occlusion. However, the still uncontrollable element is the lateral dimensions of the mandible and lower face.

Distraction osteogenesis

Contemporarily, distraction osteogenesis is recommended for the treatment of individuals born with hemifacial microsomia. Distraction osteogenesis has evolved from the realization that

tensile forces can be instrumental in developing new bone, provided there is controlled interaction with a blood supply and an eventual period of reorganization and consolidation. Many of the current distraction osteogenesis procedures are an outgrowth of the work of Ilizarov[30,31] and incorporate histologic sequences seen in the healing of bony fractures. The first phase in bone fracture healing is the stage of inflammation, with the formation of a hematoma around the bone fragments. This is followed by transformation into a blood clot, subsequent infiltration of capillaries and proliferating cellular elements, and replacement with granulation tissue. A soft callus develops incident to a fibroblastic conversion of the granulation tissue into fibrous tissue. In distraction osteogenesis, the requisite of initiating tensile forces on the soft callus by the distraction appliances is instituted using graduated, periodic forces, basically pulling the soft callus in opposite directions.

These tensile forces result in the newly forming tissue orienting in the line[32] of the presumably equal and opposite tension "pull" and the soft callus fibrous tissue aligning in the direction of distraction. Several days after the initiation of distraction, capillaries invade the fibrous tissue toward both bony segments as well as the created open area between the segments, supplying cells capable of becoming fibroblasts, chondroblasts, and osteoblasts.[33,34] Subsequently, osteoblasts lay down osteoid tissue on closely related collagen fibers, developing into bone spicules. Bony development is initiated at the walls of the two proximal segments and progresses toward the gap created by the distraction forces. The distraction space is continually kept open by the opposing tensile forces; osteogenesis in the residual opening continues throughout the period of distraction. After cessation of the distraction forces, there is gradual bone regeneration within the open area, and eventually there is a remodeling of the bone regenerate into more mature bone. In essence, growth stimulates new bone formation incident to tensile forces.

As previously stated, distraction osteogenesis has been successfully undertaken in the treatment of hemifacial microsomia where increase in unilateral mandibular bone length is needed. However, the patient with a complete absence of the ramus and condyle is presently not considered a candidate for this procedure. When the distraction procedure is feasible, an oblique subperiosteal coricotomy is usually made at the angle of the mandible on the lateral surface—many times from the retromolar area to behind the gonial angle. The cut is made through the cortex to the cancellous bone, but does not include the medial or internal cortical layer. Intraosseous stainless steel pins are inserted on both sides of the coricotomy and perpendicular to it to attain the desired vector of distraction, and joined by a softer distraction screw. Five to 7 days postcorticotomy, distraction forces are initiated by opening the screw 1 mm per day. Distraction is done only on the lateral aspect of the mandible in an effort to permit elongation of the mandible to simulate a normal pattern of growth in a tridimensional direction. When the distraction procedure starts, the bone elongation occurs mainly in the outer, or external, cortex and cancellous bone. At the end of the second week, it is conceptualized that the distraction forces actually fracture the lingual cortex. The distraction continues until the pro-

jected elongation of the hypoplastic mandible is achieved, usually 3 to 4 weeks. The screws are left in place until there is radiographic evidence of new cortical bone formation, usually 6 to 8 weeks following cessation of distraction, at which time the screws can be removed.

This process of new bone generated across a gap that is gradually widened by controlled procedures has introduced dramatic clinical implications for the lengthening of a shortened, deficient mandible, as noted in Figs 12-17a to 12-17k. In treating cases of unilateral hemifacial microsomia or bilateral micrognathia, mandibular length has been increased 12 to 28 mm—a remarkable change.[35,36] Where indicated, it has even been found that the condylar head could be appreciably enlarged and, with additional growth, could continue to increase in size. The distraction procedure has likewise been beneficial in the reconstruction of a new condyle, such as instances where there has been loss of a condyle incident to a tumor.[37]

A distinct advantage of osteogenesis distraction is that functional activities can be carried on during the distraction process. Conceptually, function is encouraged to maintain and even to accelerate growth on the distracted side. The sometimes overlooked factor is the ability of masticatory and facial muscle function before, during, and after osteogenesis distraction to enhance bony tissue development. Coincident with this is an apparent increment in soft tissue dimension that seems to lead to an improvement in facial symmetry and appearance. However, the one limitation yet to be overcome and which is apparent in the literature seems to be attaining sufficient dimension laterally; improvement occurs visually to some degree because of the soft tissue covering, but the desired improvement is still difficult to achieve, especially with the high possibility of lateral deficiency in the cranial base, as well as in the mandibular ramus and condyle. The authors have had very limited experience with osteogenesis distraction, but feel it to be of such great importance as a comparatively new procedure in the treatment of maxillary and mandibular skeletal deficiency to acknowledge its existence and potential significance.

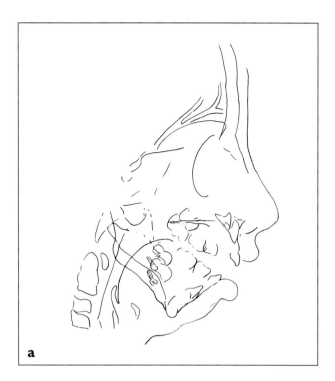

a

Fig 12-17 Patient R.T. *(a)* Lateral radiograph tracing of a 3-year-old patient born with congenital bilateral facial microsomia (complete left condylar and ramal hypoplasia and right condylar hypoplasia), taken (July 22, 1994) 1 week after both sides of the mandible were reconstructed with costochondral rib grafts.

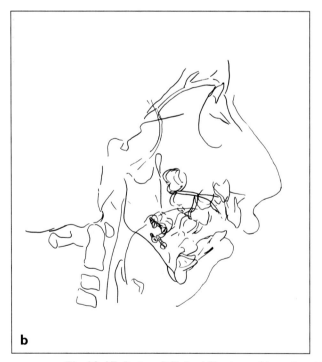

b

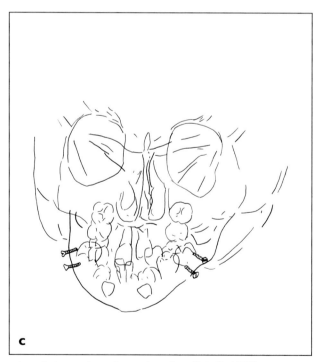

c

Fig 12-17 Patient R.T. *(b, c)* Tracings of lateral and frontal cephalometric radiographs taken (July 2, 1997) just before removal of screws after the costochondral rib grafts failed to achieve desired mandibular growth. A decision was made to initiate distraction osteogenesis procedures.

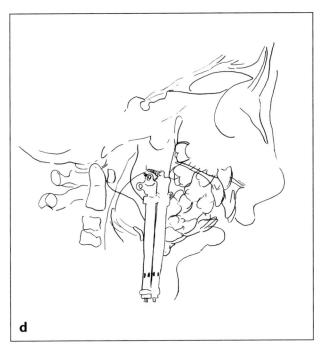
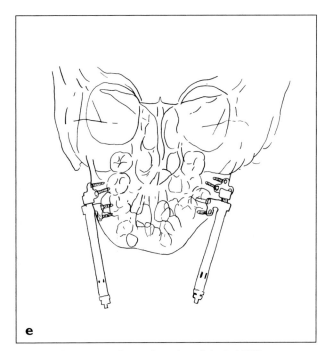

Fig 12-17 Patient R.T. *(d, e)* Tracings of lateral and frontal cephalometric radiographs taken (July 8, 1997) after placement of the distraction osteogenesis appliance.

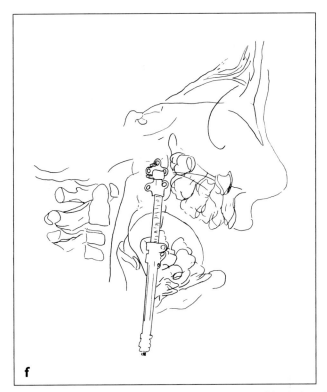
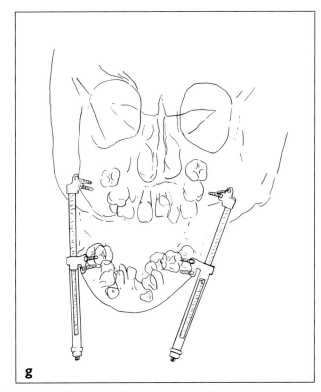

Fig 12-17 Patient R.T. *(f, g)* Tracings of lateral and frontal cephalometric radiographs taken (August 14, 1997) after completion of active distraction osteogenesis.

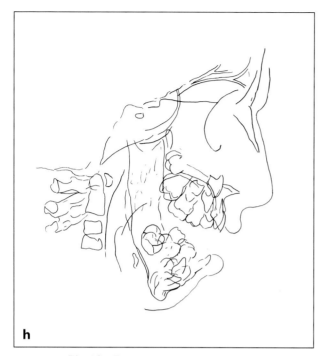

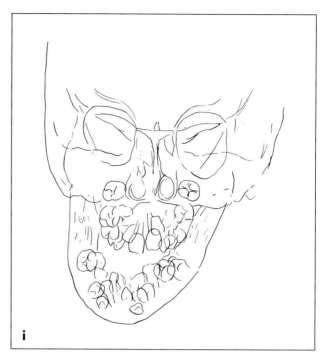

Fig 12-17 Patient R.T. *(h, i)* Tracings of lateral and frontal cephalometric radiographs taken (October 30, 1997) after removal of the distraction appliance. New bone has developed in both ramal regions, and the mandible now appears longer and somewhat straight on both sides, with a distinct vertical dimension.

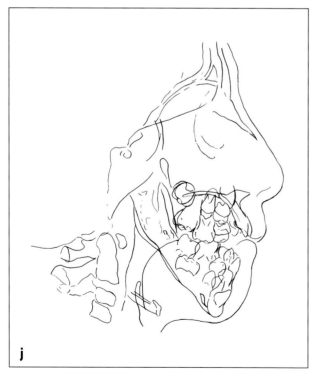

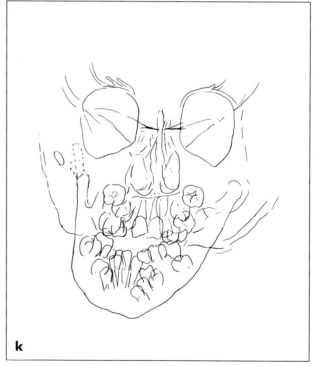

Fig 12-17 Patient R.T. *(j, k)* Tracings of the lateral and frontal cephalometric radiographs taken (March 16, 1999) approximately 15 months after completion of the distraction osteogenesis procedure. Both sides of the mandible still appear long, with short rami and open gonial angles. There has been considerable eruption of posterior teeth, and an anterior open bite with excessive lower anterior facial height is clearly evident. The patient will undergo orthodontic treatment.

References

1. Kaban LB, Mulliken JB, Murray JE. Three-dimensional approach to analysis and treatment of hemifacial microsomia. Cleft Palate J 1981;18:90–99.
2. Murray JE, Kaban LB, Mulliken JB. Analysis and treatment of hemifacial microsomia. Plast Reconstr Surg 1984;74:186–199.
3. Grabb WC. The first and second branchial arch syndrome. Plast Reconstr Surg 1965;36:485.
4. Gorlin RJ, et al. Oculoauriculovertebral dysplasia. In: Syndromes of the Head and Neck, ed 2. New York: McGraw-Hill, 1976:546–552.
5. Rollnick BR, Kaye CI. Hemifacial microsomia and variants: Pedigree data. Am J Med Genet 1983;15:233–253.
6. Smith DW. Facio-auriculo-vertebral spectrum. In: Recognizable Patterns of Human Malformation, ed 3. Philadelphia: Saunders, 1982:497–500.
7. Coccaro PJ, Becker MH, Converse JM. Clinical and radiographic variations in hemifacial microsomia. Birth Defects 1975;11:314–324.
8. Grayson BH. Analysis of craniofacial asymmetry by multiplane cephalometry. Am J Orthod 1983;84:217–224.
9. Figueroa AA, Pruzansky S. The external ear, mandible and other components of hemifacial microsomia. J Maxillofac Surg 1982;10:200–211.
10. Pruzansky S. Not all dwarfed mandibles are alike. Birth Defects 1969;5.
11. McCarthy JG. Craniofacial microsomia. In: Serafin O, Georgiade NG (eds). Pediatric Plastic Surgery. St. Louis: Mosby, 1984:499–517.
12. Kane AA, Lo LJ, Christensen GE, Vannier MW, Marsh JL. Relationship between bone and muscles of mastication in hemifacial microsomia. Plast Reconstr Surg 1997;99:990–999.
13. Fischer CE, et al. Quantitative assessment of muscular underdevelopment in hemifacial microsomia. [Transactions of the Eighth International Congress on Cleft Palate and Related Craniofacial Anomalies, 1997, Singapore].
14. Munro IR. One-stage reconstruction of the temporomandibular joint in hemifacial microsomia. Plast Reconstr Surg 1980;66:699–710.
15. Munro IR, Lauritzen CG. Classification and treatment of hemifacial microsomia. In: Caronni EP (ed). Craniofacial Surgery. Boston: Little, Brown, 1985:391–400.
16. Obwegeser HL. Correction of the skeletal anomalies of otomandibular dysostosis. J Craniomaxillofac Surg 1974;2:73–92.
17. Ware WH, Brown SL. Growth centre transplantation to replace mandibular condyles. J Craniomaxillofac Surg 1981;9:50–58.
18. Ware WH, Taylor RC. Cartilaginous growth centers transplanted to replace mandibular condyles in monkeys. J Oral Maxillofac Surg 1966;24:33–43.
19. Munro IR, Phillips JH, Griffin G. Growth after construction of the temporomandibular joint in children with hemifacial microsomia. Cleft Palate J 1989;26:303–311.
20. Mulliken IR, Ferraro NF, Vento AR. A retrospective analysis of growth of the constructed condyle-ramus in children with hemifacial microsomia. Cleft Palate J 1989;26:312–317.
21. Marsh JL, Baca D, Vannier MW. Facial musculoskeletal asymmetry in hemifacial microsomia. Cleft Palate J 1989;26:292–302.
22. Converse JM, Coccaro PJ, Becker M, Wood-Smith D. On hemifacial microsomia: The first and second branchial arch syndrome. Plast Reconstr Surg 1973;51:268–279.
23. Figueroa AA, Pruzansky S. The external ear, mandible and other components of hemifacial microsomia. J Craniomaxillofac Surg 1982;10:200–211.
24. Vargervik K, Miller AJ. Neuromuscular patterns in hemifacial microsomia. Am J Orthod 1984;86:33–42.
25. Rune B, Surnas KV, Selvik G, Jacobsson S. Roentgen stereometry with the aid of metallic implants in hemifacial microsomia. Am J Orthod 1983;84:231–247.
26. Polley JW, Figueroa AA, Liou EJ, Cohen M. Longitudinal analysis of mandibular asymmetry in hemifacial microsomia. Plast Reconstr Surg 1997;99:328–339.
27. Kearns G, Kaban LB, Padwa BL, et al. Progression of facial asymmetry in patients with hemifacial microsomia. J Oral Maxillofac Surg 1997;55(suppl 3):48.
28. Padwa BL, Mulliken JB, Maghen A, Kaban LB. Midfacial growth after costochondral graft construction of the mandibular ramus in hemifacial microsomia. J Oral Maxillofac Surg 1998;56:122–127.
29. Vargervick K. Sequence and Timing of Treatment Phases in Hemifacial Microsomia. New York: Alan R Liss, 1983.
30. Ilizarov GA. The tension-stress effect on the genesis and growth of tissues, I: The influence of stability of fixation and soft-tissue preservation. Clin Orthop 1989;238:249–281.
31. Ilizarov GA. The tension-stress effect on the genesis and growth of tissues, II: The influence of the rate and frequency of distraction. Clin Orthop 1989;239:263–285.
32. Delloye C, Delefortrie G, Coutelier L, Vincent A. Bone regenerate formation in cortical bone during distraction lengthening: An experimental study. Clin Orthop 1990;250:34–42.
33. Irianov YM. Spatial organization of a microcirculatory bed in distraction bone regenerates. Genij Orthopedii 1996;1:14–18.
34. Irianov YM. Scanning electron microscopy of distraction regenerate. Genij Orthopedii 1996;2-3:131–132.
35. Molina F, Ortiz-Monasterio F. Mandibular elongation and remodeling by distraction: A farewell to major osteotomies. Plast Reconstr Surg 1995;96:825–840; discussion 841–842.
36. Diner PA, Kollar E, Martinez H, Vasquez MP. Submerged intraoral device for mandibular lengthening. J Craniomaxillofac Surg 1997;25:116–123.
37. Stucki-McCormick SU. Reconstruction of the mandibular condyle using transport distraction osteogenesis. J Craniomaxillofac Surg 1997;8:48–52.

Part V

How Early and Why Early?

Chapter 13

Maturational Development and Facial Form Relative to Treatment Timing

Leonard S. Fishman, DDS

It is important for the clinician to be able to unveil the developmental uniqueness of an individual, especially at a young age, so that the timing and design of treatment modalities can be most advantageously facilitated. Correlation of information integrating a child's maturational age, facial form, and proposed treatment mechanics is essential if a successful treatment result is to be achieved. Chronologic age is not a reliable developmental yardstick, as it is not necessarily correlated with the maturational age of the patient.[1-3]

Treatment initiated during growing periods requires an understanding of the past and the predicted maturational profile of the patient and its influence on the developing facial form. Incremental skeletal and soft tissue changes in the face and their associated growth rates are closely correlated with an individual's patterns of maturational development.[4-6] Dental development, especially when related to tooth eruption, is poorly correlated with general and facial skeletal growth.[7,8]

The Concept and Evaluation of Maturational Age

The concept of maturation refers to the progress an individual makes toward the adult state. Since all individuals express their own

unique developmental time scale, it is important to have some means of identifying one's maturational profile. The orthodontist is mainly concerned with the childhood and adolescent periods of development.

The hand-wrist radiograph has long been a common tool for evaluation of skeletal age since the many bones in the wrist develop in an orderly, sequential manner throughout the entire growth period. Three common approaches have been used in the past to assess hand-wrist radiographs. The atlas system involves the matching of a hand-wrist radiograph with a standard series of chronologically oriented radiographic images. The patient's hand-wrist radiograph is matched with the most appropriate example in the atlas, and the conformity or discrepancy between the chronologic age of the patient and the chronologic age assigned to the standardized film is noted.[9,10] A second assessment variation involves matching features of many individual bones and then assigning point scores to the stages revealed.[11] Another method emphasizes alterations in bony shapes and establishes ratios between linear measurements of the long bones of the hand and wrist; the grading of the indicators and ratios is then calculated to determine the skeletal age.[12]

It is important not to interpret differences between chronologic and maturational age as abnormal. A particular evaluation may not be average but, as a consequence, is not necessarily abnormal. This is a common misconception relative to the interpretation of maturational age. Within the usual orthodontic population it is possible that a child may be associated with a significant developmental abnormality but such is rarely seen. For the most part, almost all orthodontic patients are normal in development. They may demonstrate wide variability between their maturational and chronologic ages, but they are still within the acceptable parameters considered normal in development. Some children are simply developing within a more advanced or more delayed time frame. Everyone expresses their own unique pattern of development.

At all developmental stages, the maxilla completes a larger percentage of its skeletal growth when compared with the mandible, resulting in significantly more later mandibular growth expressed during late adolescence. Although mandibular growth will sometimes lag slightly behind the general skeletal maturity of the body, it can be considered to be closely correlated. Growth curves representing incremental skeletal increases per unit of time of statural height and mandibular development are very similar.[13,14] By understanding the maturational and associated growth patterns being expressed, treatment and its timing can be more rationally coordinated for the patient.

System of Skeletal Maturation Assessment[14,17]

To properly identify the maturational age of an individual, it is essential that both maturational stage and maturational level be assessed. *Maturational stage* refers to the amount of progressive skeletal development that has occurred toward adulthood. The respective stages are designated by utilizing specific skeletal maturity indicators (SMIs) identified on hand-wrist radiographs. *Maturational level* refers to the rate of maturational development, whether it be advanced, average, or delayed relative to chronologic age. Individuals can demonstrate the same maturational stage (SMI) but vary relative to their maturation level. In these situations, individuals will exhibit differences in the lengths of

time between the maturational stages, in the percentages of total growth completed, and in the associated velocity of growth.

Maturation stages

Skeletal maturity indicators have been identified for both the childhood and adolescent periods of development.[15,16] The skeletal maturity indicators were selected on the basis of sequential stability of occurrence, relatively even chronologic distribution, and ease of identification on radiographs. The objective is to identify the most advanced maturational stage that exists on the individual hand-wrist radiograph.

As seen in Fig 13-1, the six late childhood indicators commonly associated with early orthodontic treatment (SMI F to K) involve stages of development of specific carpal bones, phalanges, and a metacarpal bone.

SMI F: appearance of scaphoid and/or trapezoid bones
SMI G: overlapping of trapezium and trapezoid bones
SMI H: fourth finger, distal phalanx; epiphysis as wide as diaphysis
SMI I: fourth finger, distal phalanx; epiphysis wider than diaphysis
SMI J: second finger, proximal phalanx; epiphysis as wide as diaphysis
SMI K: first metacarpal (thumb); epiphysis as wide as shaft

As seen in Fig 13-2, the adolescent skeletal maturity indicators (SMI 1 to 11) involve stages of development of specific phalanges, the adductor sesamoid of the thumb, and the radius bone.

SMI 1: third finger, proximal phalanx; width of epiphysis as wide as or wider than diaphysis
SMI 2: third finger, middle phalanx; width of epiphysis as wide as or wider than diaphysis
SMI 3: fifth (little) finger; width of epiphysis as wide as or wider than diaphysis
SMI 4: ossification of adductor sesamoid of thumb

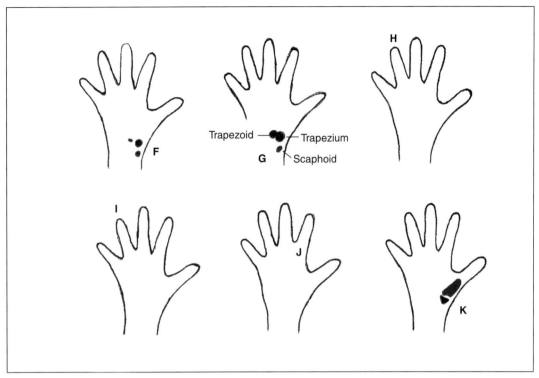

Fig 13-1 Childhood stages of maturation (SMI F to K).

SMI 5: third finger, distal phalanx; capping of both sides of epiphysis

SMI 6: third finger, middle phalanx; capping of both sides of epiphysis

SMI 7: fifth finger, middle phalanx; capping of both sides of epiphysis

SMI 8: third finger, distal phalanx; complete fusion

SMI 9: third finger, proximal phalanx; complete fusion

SMI 10: third finger, middle phalanx; complete fusion

SMI 11: radius; complete fusion (skeletal growth completed)

Figure 13-3 illustrates the approximate timing of these childhood and adolescent stages of maturation as related to an average developmental growth curve. Although small preadolescent growth spurts can occasionally occur, the late childhood period is usually one of relatively slow growth. The adolescent period of development can be arbitrarily divided into periods of accelerating growth (SMI 1 to 3), high growth rate including peak velocity of growth (SMI 4 to 7), and decelerating growth (SMI 8 to 11). It is particularly important to establish the relationship of each SMI to the relative steepness of the growth curve, as an increase in velocity is directly correlated with an additional increase in incremental facial growth.

Clinically, it is often advantageous to further distinguish additional stages of maturational development, particularly during the high velocity growth period and during late adolescence. Proper timing of headgear treatment and the decisions regarding timing of facial surgery are common examples of benefiting from their use. Initiating headgear treatment during a period of rapid growth will yield significantly better results as compared with using a headgear during a slower growth period. Surgery can be timed rel-

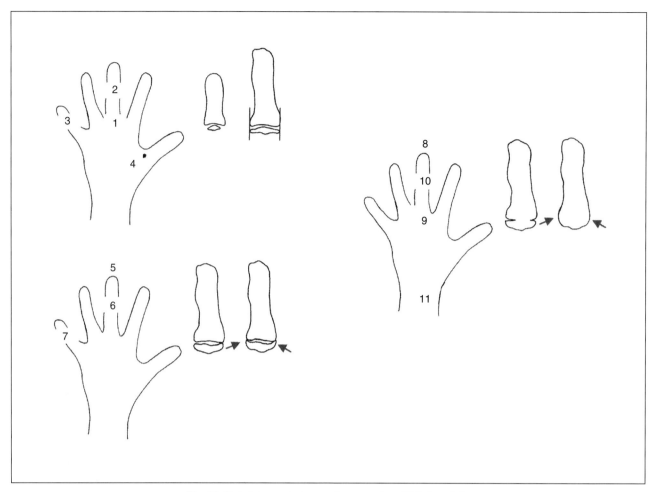

Fig 13-2 Adolescent stages of maturation (SMI 1 to 11).

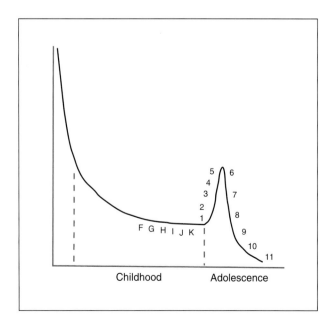

Fig 13-3 Relationship of late childhood and adolescent maturation stages to developmental growth curve.

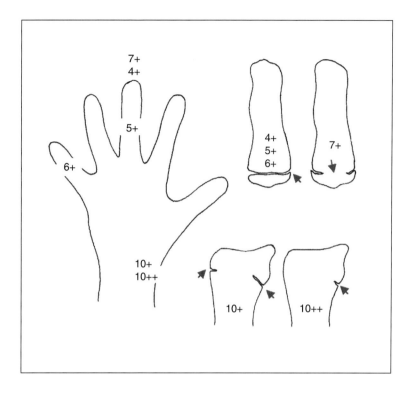

Fig 13-4 Intermediate stages of maturation.

ative to the patient's expected maturational development. As will be discussed later in this chapter, advanced maturers can possibly be considered for surgical intervention before growth is completed. Identifying intermediate stages of maturation during late adolescence helps to more definitively consider available options.

As seen in Fig 13-4, six intermediate SMIs that are easily identifiable have been established for this purpose.

SMI 4+: SMI 4 exists, but only medial (thumb side) side of third finger, distal phalanx is capped.

SMI 5+: SMI 5 exists, but only medial side of third finger, middle phalanx is capped.

SMI 6+: SMI 6 exists, but only medial side of fifth (little) finger, middle phalanx is capped.

SMI 7+: SMI 7 exists, but only central and medial side of third finger, distal phalanx is fused.

SMI 10+: SMI 10 exists, but only the central area of radius is fused.

SMI 10++: SMI 10+ exists, but only the central area and ulnar (distal) side of the radius are fused.

Maturation levels

Growing individuals demonstrate the same SMIs at widely varying chronologic ages. This is illustrated in Tables 13-1 and 13-2 where mean and ±1 standard deviation chronologic age values of the SMIs and maturation levels are listed for the late childhood period.

Level A, advanced maturers

Level B, average maturers who are closer to being advanced

Level C, average maturers who are closer to being delayed

Level D, delayed maturers

The female and male chronologic age values of the maturation stages and their associated maturational levels for the adolescent period of development are demonstrated in Tables 13-3 and 13-4.

It becomes evident why the level of maturation must be taken into consideration when maturational age is to be determined. As demonstrated in these tables, a wide range of chronologic age variation exists between advanced and delayed maturers even when they are at the same maturation stage. For example, as seen in Table 13-3, an advanced female adolescent who demonstrates a maturation stage of SMI 8 is approximately 12 years 3 months of age, while a delayed maturer who demonstrates the same SMI is 14 years 3 months of age. As seen in Table 13-4, a delayed male will terminate growth at approximately 18 years 8 months of age, while an advanced maturer will terminate growth almost 3 years earlier at approximately 15 years 10 months of age. Individuals who demonstrate variations greater than one standard deviation from mean age values will demonstrate even greater differences.

An advanced maturer reaches a particular maturation stage at an earlier chronologic age when compared with an average or delayed maturer. The delayed maturer reaches each SMI at a later chronologic age when compared with an average or advanced maturer. If maturation is proceeding at advanced or delayed levels, particularly if it occurs during the late childhood period and/or early adolescence, the child will usually have enough time to reach an average level of maturation during the later stages of maturation.[17] In this type of situation, mean chronologic age values of average maturity will most probably never be achieved but will be approached. It would be most unusual for an individual to alter more than one maturation level over the entire growth period. The delayed maturer demonstrates a strong tendency of catch-up growth, often delaying the ending of skeletal development until a significantly later chronologic age.

As seen in Fig 13-5, the length of periods between maturation stages varies relative to the maturation level (advanced vs average vs delayed), particularly during the later period of adolescence. During the low growth velocity period of late childhood and the accelerating and high velocity periods of adolescence, the lengths of time between maturation stages do not vary too much. During late adolescence (SMI 8 to 11) it becomes evident that delayed maturers attempt to catch up and take a significantly longer time between maturation stages and subsequently until growth is terminated. When the entire adolescent developmental period is considered, this trend for delayed maturers to take more time to complete full growth is evident. The overall length of adolescence for average and delayed maturing females is longer than for males.

Female and male individuals demonstrate the same percentages of total growth completed at the same maturation stage and level. In this regard, maturational age (stage plus level) can be considered a common denominator between individuals regardless of gender and serves as a useful yardstick to evaluate patient comparisons whether it be for clinical or research purposes. Since advanced maturers reach their respective maturation stages chronologically earlier than average or delayed maturers, variations in percentages of total growth completed exist. Figures 13-6 and 13-7 demonstrate female and male percentages of total growth completed relative to maturational stage and level. During adolescence, delayed maturers demonstrate less growth completed at every stage of maturation. This fact is of particular clinical significance because, even during the late stages of maturation, delayed maturers may continue to demonstrate an undesirable pattern of growth. For example, maxillary headgear treatment often needs to be continued well into the retention phase of therapy for delayed maturers, otherwise excessive downward and forward growth of the maxilla usually associated with skeletal Class II cases will result in a recurrence of skeletal and dental protrusion. For the same reasons, advanced maturers may often be considered as candidates for surgery before all facial growth is completed (SMI 11) because they have completed significantly more of their total growth.

As mentioned above, maturational timing of treatment will provide opportunities for taking advantage of more appropriate growth velocity periods relative to the nature of treatment.

Table 13-1 Childhood Chronologic Ages, SMIs, and Maturation Levels for Females

SMI	Age (y)							
		−1 SD		Mean		+1 SD		
G		6.69		7.84		8.99		
H	A	8.51	B	9.26	C	10.01	D	
I		8.68		9.50		10.32		
J		8.99		9.79		10.59		
K		9.14		10.11		11.08		

A = advanced growth; B = average to advanced growth; C = average to delayed growth; D = delayed growth.

Table 13-2 Childhood Chronologic Ages, SMIs, and Maturation Levels for Males

SMI	Age (y)							
		−1 SD		Mean		+1 SD		
F		7.61		8.82		10.03		
G	A	7.81	B	9.18	C	10.55	D	
H		9.18		10.18		11.18		
I		9.87		10.79		11.71		
J		9.95		11.07		12.09		
K		10.29		11.23		12.17		

A = advanced growth; B = average to advanced growth; C = average to delayed growth; D = delayed growth.

Table 13-3 Adolescent Chronologic Ages, SMIs, and Maturation Levels for Females

SMI	Age (y)							
		−1 SD		Mean		+1 SD		
1		9.357		10.230		11.302		
2	A	9.800	B	10.722	C	11.643	D	
3		9.914		10.872		11.831		
4		10.072		11.041		12.011		
5		10.549		11.708		12.867		
6		10.802		11.955		13.108		
7		11.369		12.512		13.655		
8		12.261		13.263		14.265		
9		12.636		13.967		15.298		
10		12.986		14.229		15.472		
11		14.291		16.008		17.725		

A = advanced growth; B = average to advanced growth; C = average to delayed growth; D = delayed growth.

Table 13-4 Adolescent Chronologic Ages, SMIs, and Maturation Levels for Males

SMI	Age (y)							
		−1 SD		Mean		+1 SD		
1		10.548		11.368		12.488		
2	A	10.955	B	11.951	C	12.887	D	
3		11.109		12.211		13.312		
4		11.351		12.574		13.797		
5		11.835		13.029		14.224		
6		12.571		13.779		14.987		
7		13.230		14.429		15.629		
8		14.185		15.194		16.203		
9		14.289		15.485		16.682		
10		14.815		16.079		17.343		
11		15.815		17.242		18.669		

A = advanced growth; B = average to advanced growth; C = average to delayed growth; D = delayed growth.

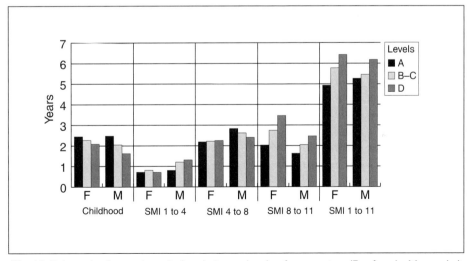

Fig 13-5 Length of growth periods relative to levels of maturation. (F = female; M = male.)

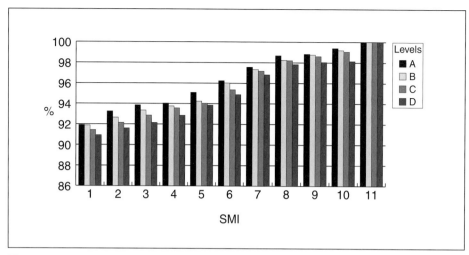

Fig 13-6 Percentage of total maxillary growth completed relative to maturation stage and level.

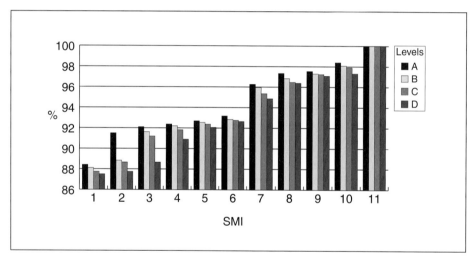

Fig 13-7 Percentage of total mandibular growth completed relative to maturation stage and level.

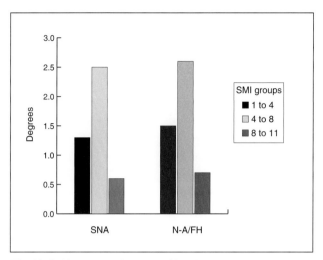

Fig 13-8 Maturational timing of headgear treatment.

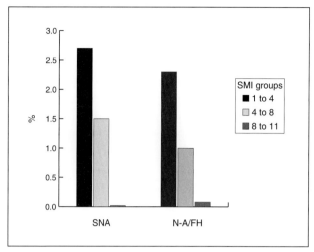

Fig 13-9 Maturational timing of face-mask treatment.

Figure 13-8 demonstrates the importance of properly timing headgear treatment.[18] Patients who were treated during the highest growth velocity period (SMI 4 to 8) underwent the most improvement. The next best time for headgear treatment was during the accelerating velocity period (SMI 1 to 4); the least desirable time was during a period of decelerating growth (SMI 8 to 11). This pattern was reflected in both SNA and Lande's angle (N-A/FH) measurements.

As a further example, Fig 13-9 demonstrates the importance of properly timing face-mask treatment.[19] The most desirable time to initiate face-mask treatment is during an early period of development. An insignificant amount of improvement took place during late adolescence. Only the early period of adolescence resulted in significant changes. These conclusions are also reflected in the SNA and N-A/FH measurements. This may imply that face-mask treatment during childhood may be even more desirable. Proper timing of this form of treatment is probably less associated with growth velocity variations than it is with less fusion of the midpalatal suture and a small maxilla.

Individualized evaluation of facial form

The fundamental objective of identifying the uniqueness of an individual may also be applied to the evaluation of facial form. Conventional numerically based cephalometric analyses do not address this objective rationally. So-called normative cephalometric populations are not similar enough skeletally to be designated as standards. Even when sample populations include individuals with good occlusion and satisfactory soft tissue profiles, their cephalometric measurements vary widely because their cranial base and other skeletal interrelationships are not significantly similar. It is common for interpretations of more than one measurement to disagree with each other because of this nonstandardization of the underlying sample. This nonconformity within the sample material is often reflected in wide numerical ranges of normalcy depicted by the mean and standard deviation values.

The challenge to the clinician is to be able to assess skeletal, dental, and soft tissue balance of the individual and then design a treatment plan that will provide a more harmonious morphologic environment for the individual to function within. If treatment is to be timed to achieve the best results, the maturational profile of the patient described previously must always be integrated into the planning process. If only chronologic age is considered, treatment may not be satisfactorily coordinated with the growth and development of the individual.

CentroGraphic Analysis (CGA)[20]

A nonnumerical *cephalomorphic* approach to the assessment of facial form allows for individualized evaluation of balance and harmony between skeletal, dental, and soft tissue structures. Facial morphology can be judged on an individualized patient basis without direct comparisons with other faces that do not reflect similar structural details. This is particularly beneficial when racial and ethnic variations in facial form are evident. The analysis allows for the pretreatment discovery of where satisfactory facial balance does not exist and also provides for the graphic visualization of the potential restoration of harmonious facial form. The term *cephalomorphic* is to be distinguished from the term *cephalometric*, as the former refers to evaluation of morphologic balance and harmony of anatomically derived spatial areas without relying on numbers. As mentioned previously, this cephalomorphic assessment has to be correlated with what can be expected relative to growth as revealed by the maturational analysis and what clinically exists relative to the dentition.

Some basic geometric characteristics relative to centroids and their relationships to the face are important to understand. The *centroid* of an area or mass represents its center of gravity. As seen in Fig 13-10, the centroid of a triangular area is constructed simply by drawing lines from the midpoints of each side to the opposing angle. The point of intersection of the three planes represents the centroid. It becomes evident that using only two of the three planes in this manner will accomplish the same result.

Interesting centroid relationships exist between two or more triangles. As also seen in Figs 13-10 and 13-11:

1. As triangles increase significantly in size and shape, their respective centroids move very little spatially from each other.
2. Centroids representing two adjacent equal triangles that share a common border and the centroid that represents the larger triangle composed of the two smaller triangles all fall within a straight line that is perpendicular to the shared side. Also, in this situation, the centroid that represents the two triangles is located on the shared side.
3. If the two triangles are not equal, then the centroids will deviate from the above description. If one triangle is smaller than the other, the centroid representing both triangles will be located vertically within the larger triangle. Horizontally, each centroid representing the two triangles will be located anterior or posterior to a vertical plane drawn perpendicular to the shared side through the centroid that represents both triangles.

Skeletal balance and harmony

Based on the triangular and associated centroid relationships illustrated above, Fig 13-12 illustrates the application of these same principles to a morphologic evaluation of facial form. The skeletally well-balanced face can be divided into two equal triangles representing the upper and lower faces. The upper facial triangle is constructed using the anatomical points nasion (Na), basion (Ba), and point A (A). The lower facial triangle is constructed using the anatomical points A, Ba, and gnathion (Gn). The total facial triangle is composed of the upper facial and lower facial triangles and is thereby formed by the anatomical points Na, Ba, and Gn. The centroids representing these three triangles are designated upper centroid (UC), lower centroid (LC), and facial centroid (FC), respectively. The common border shared by the upper and lower facial triangles is the Ba-A plane. A vertical line drawn perpendicular to the Ba-A plane through the facial centroid is designated the centroid plane. For the purposes of serial superimposition of cephalomorphic tracings, to be discussed later, a cranial centroid (CC) is constructed from the Na-Sella(S)-Ba landmarks. As illustrated in this tracing of a well-balanced face,

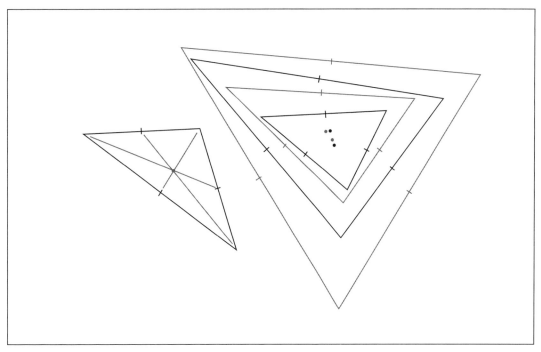

Fig 13-10 Construction of a centroid for a triangle and demonstration of centroid stability with change in size and shape.

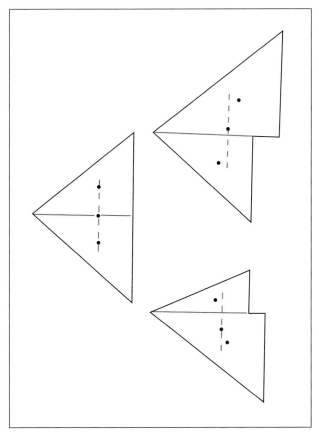

Fig 13-11 Centroid relationships between equal and un-equal triangles.

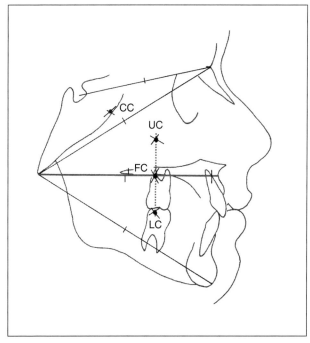

Fig 13-12 CentroGraphic Analysis. Skeletal relationships of a well-balanced face. (CC = cranial centroid; UC = upper centroid; FC = facial centroid; LC = lower centroid.)

all three facial centroids are located on the vertical centroid plane and the facial centroid is located on the Ba-A plane.

As described above, an important characteristic of centroids, as utilized in this analysis, is that they move positionally very little even if the areas they represent enlarge significantly and change shape. A face is in vertical skeletal balance if the facial centroid lies on the Ba-A plane. If the facial centroid is positioned above the Ba-A plane, a deficiency in lower facial height exists. This is characteristic of deep bite cases and suggests the need for vertical opening of the lower face through treatment with a resultant repositioning of the facial centroid closer to or on the Ba-A plane. Examples of treatment procedures that could accomplish this are a biteplate, utility arch, uprighting of molars utilizing a lip bumper, or a cervical headgear. If the facial centroid is positioned below the Ba-A plane, an excessive amount of lower facial vertical height exists. This is commonly associated with skeletal open bite cases and, to re-establish facial harmony with treatment, lower facial height needs to be decreased, thereby repositioning the facial centroid closer to or on the Ba-A plane. Treatment procedures that could accomplish this include depression of molars with a high-pull maxillary headgear and/or a posterior bite block.

Horizontal skeletal balance of the upper and lower facial areas is characterized by the upper and/or lower facial centroids being positioned anterior or posterior to the vertical centroid plane. The upper centroid, being positioned anterior to the centroid plane, is commonly associated with maxillary skeletal protrusion, as in Class II malocclusions. Successful maxillary headgear therapy results in a repositioning of the upper centroid closer to the centroid plane, thereby establishing an improvement in horizontal skeletal facial balance. Posterior positioning of the upper centroid reflects a midface maxillary skeletal retrusion. Face-mask therapy results in a repositioning of the upper centroid closer to the vertical centroid plane. Mandibular skeletal retrusion is depicted by the lower centroid being positioned posterior to the vertical centroid plane. Anterior positioning of the lower centroid is commonly associated with mandibular skeletal protrusion; posterior positioning of the lower centroid to the vertical centroid plane reflects mandibular skeletal retrusion. Surgical retropositioning of the mandible in severe cases results in a repositioning of the lower centroid relative to the centroid plane, thereby establishing better skeletal facial balance.

Longitudinal study of well-balanced faces reveals that the upper and lower facial triangles maintain a constant relationship within the total face from approximately the time of first permanent molar eruption until adulthood. The upper and lower facial triangles remain relatively equal in size (Fig 13-13). The Na-Ba-A angle and the A-Ba-Gn angle remain equal and relatively stable in dimension. Prior to eruption of the first permanent molars, the lower facial area is usually smaller than the upper facial area; it is thereby conjectured that vertical stability of the face is achieved after these permanent teeth assume their supportive positions within the lower face.

Dental balance and harmony

Analysis of dental balance and harmony is achieved by evaluating the positional and/or long axis relationships of the incisors and molars to both anatomically derived and construction planes. As seen in Fig 13-14, the mandibular incisor is positionally in facial balance if its labial surface is tangent to or slightly forward of the A-pogonion (Pog) plane and its incisal edge approximates the vertical level of a plane drawn horizontal to the Ba-A plane from the lower centroid. The angulation of the long axis of the mandibular incisor should approximate a point located one third the symphyseal distance along the Ba-Gn plane as measured from the posterior border of the symphysis. This will provide the mandibular incisor with a satisfactory amount of supporting alveolar bone regardless of the variation in mandibular morphology. The maxillary incisor is best positioned by relating it properly to the mandibular incisor with the long axis angularly positioned so its extension approximates orbitale. The maxillary molar is in the best positional balance if the vertical centroid plane passes approximately through the distal half of the root and crown. The mandibular molar should be positioned in a Class I relationship with the maxillary molar.

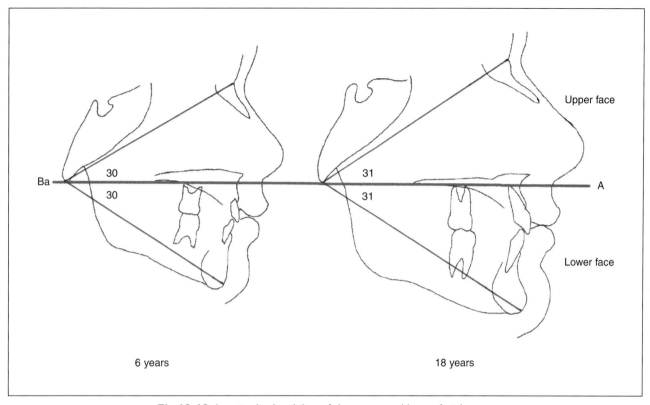

Fig 13-13 Longitudinal stability of the upper and lower facial areas.

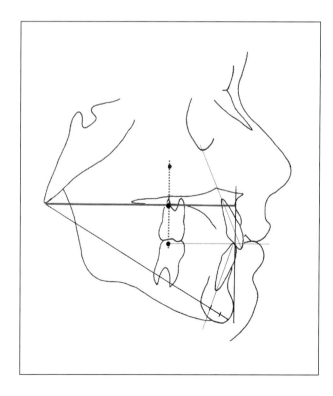

Fig 13-14 CentroGraphic Analysis. Dental relationships of a well-balanced face.

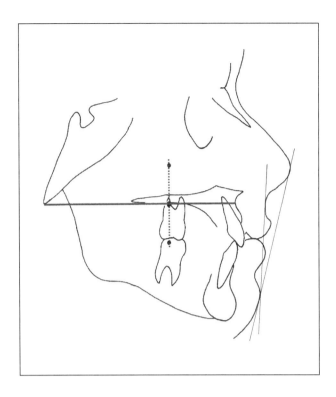

Fig 13-15 CentroGraphic Analysis. Soft tissue relationships of a well-balanced face.

Soft tissue balance and harmony

Soft tissue balance and harmony is best characterized by graphically utilizing inner and outer profile planes together. The inner profile plane is constructed between soft tissue pogonion and subnasale. The outer profile is constructed between soft tissue pogonion and the nasal tip. This provides a V-shaped triangular area to visualize the positional relationships of the upper and lower lips to the nose and chin. As seen in Fig 13-15, the lips are well positioned if they occupy approximately half the space within the two profile planes, the upper lip being more anteriorly positioned. Visualizing the profile in this manner enables us to evaluate the positional relationships of the nose and chin. For instance, if good skeletal and dental morphologic balance exists, yet the soft tissue relationships are not satisfactory, then the size and/or position of the nose and/or chin are considered to be the most likely problem.

An example of a Class II skeletal pattern and associated malocclusion is illustrated in Fig 13-16. The CentroGraphic Analysis (CGA) applied to this patient reveals the following:

Skeletal
- Vertical underdevelopment of lower face.
- Horizontal protrusion of upper face.
- Slight retrusion of lower face.

Dental
- Anteroposterior position of mandibular incisor is satisfactory.
- Vertical position of mandibular incisor is too high.
- Angulation of mandibular incisor is slightly procumbent.
- Maxillary incisor overjet is excessive.
- Maxillary incisor overbite is excessive.
- Angulation of maxillary incisor is very procumbent.
- Protrusive position of maxillary molars.

Soft tissue
- Upper lip is positioned too far anteriorly.
- Lower lip is positioned too far posteriorly.
- Sublabial furrow is excessive.

A second example of the utilization of the CentroGraphic Analysis is depicted in Fig 13-17:

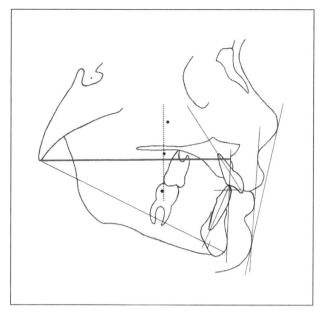

Fig 13-16 CentroGraphic Analysis. Class II skeletal pattern.

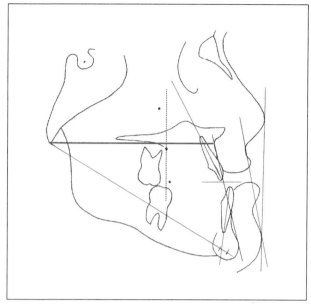

Fig 13-17 CentroGraphic Analysis. Class III skeletal pattern.

Skeletal
- Excessive vertical development of lower face.
- Skeletal open bite.
- Retrusive position of upper face.
- Protrusive position of lower face.

Dental
- Protrusive position of mandibular incisor.
- Vertical position of mandibular incisor is deficient.
- Angulation of mandibular incisor is slightly upright.
- Vertical position of maxillary incisor is deficient.
- Extremely retrusive position of maxillary incisor.
- Maxillary incisor angulation is satisfactory.
- Extremely retrusive position of maxillary molar.

Soft tissue
- Retrusive position of upper lip.
- Lack of lip seal.

CentroGraphic superimposition of serial tracings

The CentroGraphic Analysis graphically provides for an analysis of changes resulting from treatment. Even if the case is not growth-related, dental and soft tissue balance must be periodically assessed. Re-evaluation of a developing growth pattern is facilitated by relating serial cephalometric tracings, superimposing on their respective facial centroid axes (FCAs), and registering on the cranial centroid. As seen in Fig 13-18, the facial centroid axis is constructed by extending the plane drawn between the cranial centroid and facial centroid. This plane maintains a relatively stable angular relationship to the cranial base, deviating only one or two degrees throughout the entire growth period regardless of whether the patient is undergoing active treatment. This relative stability of the fa-

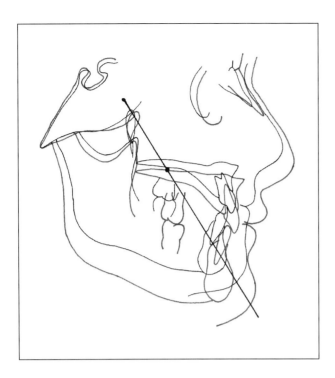

Fig 13-18 Superimposition of serial tracings using the facial centroid axis.

cial centroid axis occurs because the centroids move very little, even when they directly represent areas that change significantly in size and shape. This method of orientation provides a very rational depiction of downward and upward growth of the face. It demonstrates an upward and forward movement of nasion, thereby taking into account the continuing growth within the spheno-occipital suture. It properly depicts a rotation of the Ba-Na plane and upper and backward repositioning of sella.

Cephalomorphic CentroPrint

Another useful graphic technique of displaying the characterization of the developing growth pattern and/or treatment results is to employ

the construction of a serial CentroPrint. As seen in Fig 13-19, it is designed to illustrate the alterations in skeletal balance over a period of time. It usually provides a clearer depiction of facial changes than superimposing tracings of mid-sagittal-plane radiographs. The CentroPrint is constructed simply by overlaying the Ba-A plane with the vertical centroid planes, upper, lower and facial centroids of the serial records that were evaluated with the CentroGraphic Analysis. Figure 13-19 depicts the progress of a skeletal Class II patient who originally demonstrated a lack of vertical development of the lower face and upper face protrusion. As treatment progressed, the bite was opened, re-establishing more vertical balance to the face. This is illustrated by following the progressive relationship

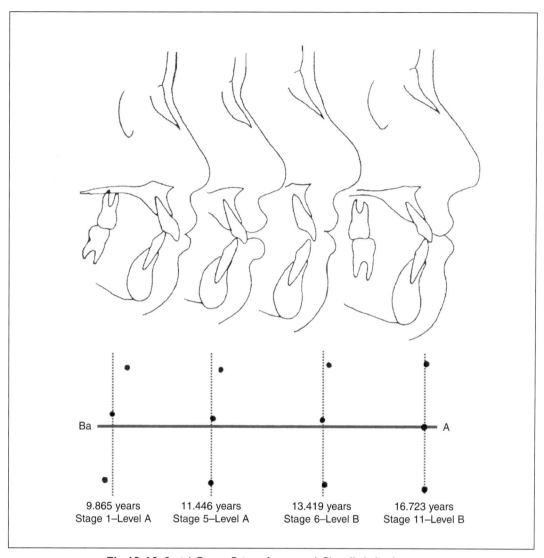

Fig 13-19 Serial CentroPrint of a treated Class II skeletal pattern.

of the facial centroid to the Ba-A plane. Maxillary headgear treatment reduced the relative protrusion of the upper face. This is illustrated by following the progressive relationship of the upper centroid to the vertical centroid plane. The CentroPrint provides an objective way for the clinician to periodically evaluate "how are we doing with treatment?"

Figure 13-20 illustrates a serial CentroPrint of a treated Class III skeletal pattern. The pretreatment CentroGraphic Analysis depicted excessive skeletal development of the lower face and a protrusive skeletal position of the lower

face. The final record demonstrates satisfactory improvement in reduction of lower facial protrusion and in decreasing the excessive development of the lower face.

The CentroPrint of an untreated patient who demonstrated a Class II skeletal pattern is depicted in Figure 13-21. The patient demonstrated excessive vertical development of the lower face and a protrusive relationship of the upper face. As expected, without treatment this patient maintained this skeletal pattern throughout the growth period.

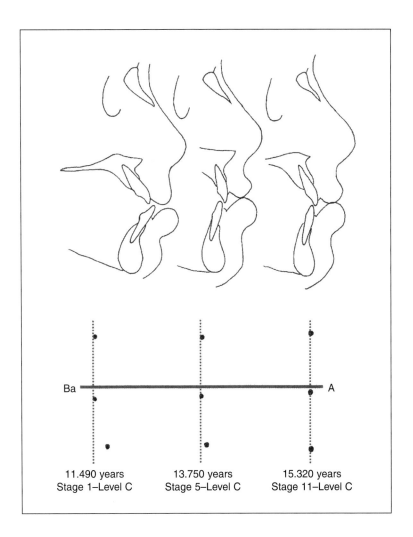

11.490 years
Stage 1–Level C

13.750 years
Stage 5–Level C

15.320 years
Stage 11–Level C

Fig 13-20 Serial CentroPrint of a treated Class III skeletal pattern.

When should maturational and cephalomorphic analyses be done?

It is important to assess the maturational age (stage plus level) of any young recall patient who visits the orthodontic office but may be considered too young to initiate active orthodontic treatment. In attempting to decide when to start treatment, the orthodontist is often exclusively focused on the stage of dental development, particularly if many primary teeth are present. Since no correlation exists between dental eruption time and skeletal development, this could easily be a mistake. Many children initiate their period of adolescent development at very young ages (SMI 1). Level A (advanced) and some level B maturers, especially, are starting to

demonstrate progressively increasing velocities of maxillary and mandibular growth at a very early period. One cannot reliably evaluate a child's maturational development by physical inspection alone. Significant skeletal height increases, pubertal development, as reflected by alterations in physical form, and onset of menstruation all occur well after the initiation of adolescent development.

Identification of a chronologically young patient who demonstrates more advanced skeletal age could certainly influence the clinician to initiate therapy, such as headgear wear, during the accelerating period of adolescent development (SMI 1 to 3) if a relatively severe skeletal discrepancy existed between the maxilla and mandible. If headgear therapy is indicated and the skeletal discrepancy is not overly

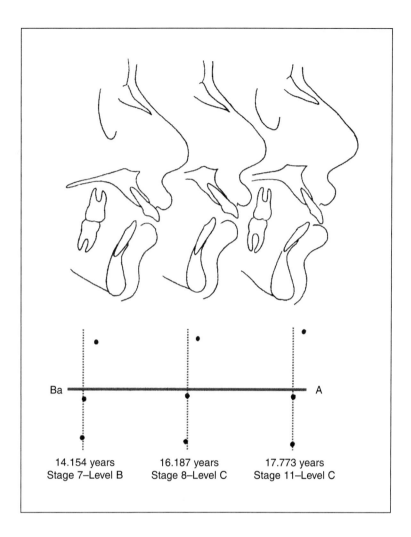

14.154 years
Stage 7–Level B

16.187 years
Stage 8–Level C

17.773 years
Stage 11–Level C

Fig 13-21 Serial CentroPrint of an untreated Class II skeletal pattern.

severe, it may be more appropriate to time its initiation at a later maturational age. As illustrated before, it has been clearly demonstrated that successful headgear treatment is dependent on proper timing of growth.[18] The rate of maxillary growth and the amount of favorable maxillary change that occurs are directly dependent on each other. Regardless of the patient's chronologic age, the decision when and if to initiate headgear therapy should depend almost exclusively on the maturational profile of the patient.

As described before, preadolescence and the very early stages of adolescence are the most appropriate times to initiate face-mask therapy in cases of maxillary retrusion. Face-mask therapy is progressively less successful as development toward the adult form proceeds.[19]

This may be due to the fact that the maxilla is much smaller at a younger age, but may also be due to the premaxillary and other maxillary sutures being significantly less fused during early development periods.[21] For example, only approximately 8% of the midpalatal suture is fused prior to SMI 4, thereby being the most ideal time for maxillary expansion. Prior to SMI 9, osseous interdigitation occurs with some fusion of the midpalatal suture, and at SMI 11 50% of the suture is fused. The posterior portion of the palatal suture fuses first.

Completing the cephalometric Centro-Graphic Analysis during this early developmental period is also of significant value. Usually the unique facial growth pattern of the young patient will reveal itself even during the childhood period of development. It is true that many patients demonstrate malocclusions that are associated with interarch space problems, whether it be an inadequacy or excessive amount of arch length to accommodate the dentition, but a definitive number of patients demonstrate significant skeletal growth problems and these are the ones that need identification and evaluation. The CentroGraphic Analysis provides for initial and subsequent follow-up analyses to confirm the diagnosis and to monitor treatment progress.

Maturational and cephalomorphic evaluations must be undertaken prior to retention. The cephalomorphic analysis will provide the clinician with information relative to the existing pattern of facial form and whether all treatment objectives were accomplished. For example, it is not uncommon at this late stage of active treatment to realize the need for continued lingual root torque of incisors. Before retention is initiated, it is of particular importance to evaluate the maturational profile of the patient at that time. It must be determined whether the patient will express significantly more maxillary and/or mandibular growth. Just as it is very difficult to assess maturity by physical inspection of the very young individual, it is equally difficult to utilize such an approach to determine whether growth has terminated. For example, if the facial growth pattern was originally characterized by upper face protrusion and a headgear was employed, it is very important to evaluate whether a similar pattern of growth will continue into the retention phase of treatment, if further growth will be occurring. In other words, the headgear may have to be continued into retention even when all other appliances have been removed.

Facial surgical cases certainly benefit from both cephalomorphic and maturational evaluations. Although the surgeon usually wants to wait for all jaw growth to have terminated, the maturational analysis can determine how much skeletal growth will be forthcoming, whether or not SMI 11 has been reached. Advanced maturers (Level A) demonstrate significantly more percentages of completed maxillary and mandibular growth at the same SMI as delayed maturers.[22] As a result, the advanced maturers can be seriously considered for surgery even at relatively young chronologic ages.

Conclusions

Skeletal facial growth disharmonies can often be modified or compensated for, but success of such is dependent on identifying patterns of growth and development that are unique to the patient. The timing of facial growth processes may be very pertinent to which orthodontic therapeutic procedures are instituted and when they are instituted. Indeed, this may be more relevant to the stage of development and maturation of the patient than the malocclusion itself. The system of skeletal maturation provides an objective methodology of assessing the maturational profile of a patient. The CentroGraphic Analysis provides the methodology to cephalomorphically evaluate facial balance. Correlation of these two basic factors, maturational age and facial balance, will allow the clinician to establish a treatment plan that is more rationally timed.

References

1. Grave KC, Brown T. Skeletal ossification and the adolescent growth spurt. Am J Orthod 1976;69:611–619.
2. Hunter C. The co-relation of facial growth with body height and skeletal maturation at adolescence. Angle Orthod 1966;36:44–53.
3. Fishman LS. Chronological versus skeletal age: An evaluation of cranio-facial growth. Angle Orthod 1979; 49:181,189.
4. Bambha JK. Longitudinal cephalometric roentgenographic study of the face and cranium in relation to body height. J Am Dent Assoc 1961;63:776–799.
5. Nanda RS. The rates of growth of several facial components measured from serial cephalometric roentgenograms. Am J Orthod 1975;41:658–673.
6. Krogman WM. Maturational age of the growing child in relation to the timing of statural and facial growth at puberty. Transactions and Studies of the College of Physicians of Philadelphia 1979;1:32–42.
7. Gray SW, Lamons FP. Skeletal development and tooth eruption in Atlanta children. Am J Orthod 1959;45: 272–277.
8. Gron AM. Prediction of tooth emergence. J Dent Res 1962;41:573–585.
9. Pyle SI, Waterhouse AM, Greulich WW. A Radiographic Standard of Reference for the Growing Hand and Wrist. Chicago: Press of Case Western Reserve Univ, 1971.
10. De Roo T, Schroder HJ. Pocket Atlas of Skeletal Age. Baltimore: Williams and Wilkins, 1977.

11. Tanner JM, Whitehouse RH, Marshall WA, Goldstein H. Assessment of Skeletal Maturity and Prediction of Adult Height: TW2 Method. London: Academic Press, 1975.

12. Roche AF, Chumlea WC, Thissen D. Assessing the Skeletal Maturity of the Hand-Wrist: Fels Method. Springfield, IL: Charles C Thomas, 1988.

13. Tofani MI. Mandibular growth at puberty. Am J Orthod 1972;62:176–195.

14. Bergersen EO. The male adolescent facial growth spurt: Its prediction and relation to skeletal maturation. Angle Orthod 1972;42:319–338.

15. Barakat R, Fishman LS. Indicators of Skeletal Maturational Development during Infancy and Childhood [senior research]. Rochester, NY: Eastman Dental Center, 1995.

16. Fishman LS. Radiographic evaluation of skeletal maturation: A clinically oriented study based on hand-wrist films. Angle Orthod 1982;52:88–112.

17. Fishman LS. Maturational patterns and prediction during adolescence. Angle Orthod 1987;57:178–193.

18. Kopecky GR, Fishman LS. Timing of cervical headgear treatment based on skeletal maturation. Am J Orthod Dentofac Orthop 1993;104:162–169.

19. Glauser J, Fishman LS. Timing of Face-Mask Treatment Based on Skeletal Maturation [senior research]. Rochester, NY: Eastman Dental Center, 1995.

20. Fishman LS. Individualized evaluation of facial form. Am J Orthod Dentofac Orthop 1997;111:510–517.

21. Revelo B, Fishman LS. Maturational evaluation of ossification of the midpalatal suture. Am J Orthod Dentofac Orthop 1994;105:288–292.

22. Silveira AM, Fishman LS, Subtelny JD, Kassebaum DK. Facial growth during adolescence in early, average, and late maturers. Angle Orthod 1992;62:185–189.

Chapter 14

Temporomandibular Joint Problems in Children

Scott Stein, DDS
Ross H. Tallents, DDS
Mark A. Moss, DDS, PhD

Orthodontic treatment and temporomandibular disorders (TMDs) have been the focus of much research and discussion in the past two decades. Signs and symptoms of temporomandibular joint disorders are common in the pediatric population. The occlusal, skeletal, and orthodontic implications will be evaluated in this chapter as they relate to the presence or absence of signs and symptoms of TMD. At times it will be necessary to draw information from adult samples because this information is not available in the pediatric literature. The etiology, diagnosis, and treatment of TMD is a controversial subject. Multifactorial etiology has been suggested, implying that the profession has no sound data implicating a single etiology. Clinical examination often reveals dental features (such as deep bite, skeletal abnormalities, dental occlusal observations, and plain film findings) that are thought to be the cause of the patient's pain. One must keep an open mind when making associations between clinical observations and the patient's TMD. The orthodontist planning early orthodontic treatment should be cognizant of the literature that examines the relationship between orthodontic treatment and TMD. These signs and symptoms, which may pose a risk for the development of TMD, are unknown at this time. The questions that one needs to answer are:

1. What is the prevalence of signs and symptoms of TMD in children?
2. Do these signs and symptoms change over time in growing children?
3. What percentage of children require treatment for TMD and which specific problems actually require active treatment?
4. What is the relationship, if any, between occlusion and signs and symptoms of TMD?
5. Is there a relationship between craniofacial morphology and signs and symptoms of TMD, including internal derangement?
6. What is the relationship, if any, between early orthodontic treatment and signs and symptoms of TMD?
7. Which are the most appropriate treatment modalities for children who develop signs and symptoms of TMD either before or during early orthodontic treatment?

Epidemiologic Studies of Signs and Symptoms of TMD in Children

The first two questions, which relate to the prevalence and temporal relationships of signs and symptoms, must be answered with the use of epidemiological data. One must remember that there is little agreement on which signs and symptoms should be included in a survey or clinical examination for signs and symptoms of TMD. There is controversy over which index surveys and tests should be used in the epidemiologic assessment of different populations.[1,2] Studies examining the prevalence of signs and symptoms of TMD have presented occurrence in children ranging from 3.5%[3] to over 90%.[4] Mintz[2] found a prevalence of signs or symptoms averaging over a range of 39.5% for the 22 articles he reviewed. Katzberg et al[5] found that 94% (29 of 31) of symptomatic pediatric patients studied by arthrography had internal derangement. Sanchez-Woodworth et al[6] found 85% of the 150 symptomatic pediatric patients studied with MRI had internal derangement. Ribeiro et al[7] found that 34% of the asymptomatic children and young adult volunteers (age 6 to 25) and 86% of the TMD patients studied with MRI had internal derangement. They concluded that disc displacement was relatively common and highly associated with symptomatic TMD patients. Several studies[8–10] suggest that signs and symptoms of TMD increase in frequency with age. McNamara's review[11] relating orthodontics and TMD found that studies of non-patient adult subjects showed a range of 33% to 75% of the adults reporting at least one TMJ symptom. He concluded that signs and symptoms of TMD increase with age. This conclusion was also drawn by Mintz[2] in his review.

The point to be stressed is that there is an increase in the prevalence of signs and symptoms of TMD in asymptomatic children over time,[11] whether they are undergoing orthodontic treatment or not. Therefore, one should expect to find an increase in signs and symptoms of TMD in their patients undergoing early orthodontic treatment due to the longitudinal aspects of orthodontic treatment. Volunteer studies suggest that there is over a 30% chance that pediatric and adult patients will have asymptomatic internal derangements undetected by clinical exam.[5,7,12–14]

Treatment Need for TMD: Which Problems Require Active Treatment?

This question, concerning increasing symptoms and the actual need for treatment, is difficult to ascertain due to the lack of longitudinal epidemiologic studies. The American Academy of Pediatric Dentistry published a consensus paper regarding treatment of TMJ disorders and concluded that 2% of children need treatment for TMJ symptoms.[15] Unfortunately, they did not make recommendations as to which symptoms require treatment. Ingerslev[16] studied 366 children, aged 6 to 16, referred for functional disturbances of the masticatory system. He suggested that approximately 83% needed treatment. No mention was made of the total number of children seen each year during this 4-year period. Rugh and Solberg estimated that 10% of the adult population may have some type of masticatory dysfunction and only 5% will seek treatment for it.[17] Schiffman et al[18] completed a cross-sectional study of prevalence of signs and symptoms of TMD in 269 female nursing students. Their findings showed that 6.7% had previously sought treatment for TMJ problems. After reviewing the pediatric literature, Okeson[19] believed that the percentages are even lower in children. Wanman and Agerberg[20] estimated that 5% of young adults in their study needed treatment; Ohno et al[21] estimated the number to be 11.5%. The most common symptoms reported by children and young adults include headache, pain on chewing or opening wide, facial pain, TMJ locking or clicking, jaw tiredness, and pain on palpation of the muscles of mastication.[16,22–25]

If the pediatric subjects experience subjective (eg, pain, clicking)[13,25–31] and/or objective (eg, degenerative joint disease [DJD], deviation on opening)[13,20,28,30–32] signs and symptoms, it must be surmised that a small segment of this population is at risk for further development of symptoms, regardless of the presence or absence of initiating factors. Longitudinal studies suggest, however, that not all individuals develop pain and dysfunction that require treatment. Although the relationship of both morphological and functional occlusion to signs and symptoms of TMD will be discussed later, perhaps Tallents et al[33] have summed it up best when they concluded that an asymptomatic population may not differ from a symptomatic population, with one exception: pain.

Occlusion and Signs and Symptoms of TMD

Many forms of malocclusion have been implicated as correlating factors in the development of signs and symptoms of TMD. These include deep bite (increase in vertical overlap), open bite, anterior maxillary crowding, anterior mandibular crowding, Class II division 1, Class II division 2, Class III, negative overjet, posterior crossbite, nonworking-side interferences, and retruded contact position–intercuspal position (RCP-ICP) slide.[10,26,28,34–45] Since there have been only a few longitudinal studies addressing this topic, many of the articles suggesting various malocclusions as causative factors in the development of signs and symptoms of TMD have been in the form of case reports, viewpoint articles, and sample studies.[11] Most lacked proper controls or were based on the author's opinion.[46] Furthermore, since most of these studies were not longitudinal in nature, one must bring up the question of the chronological relationship of malocclusion and signs and symptoms of TMD.

Mintz[2] points out that Williamson[34] and Gazit et al[35] found that deep bite contributed to muscle tenderness. Williamson evaluated 304 children, screened for orthodontic treatment, 6 to 16 years of age.[34] Palpation revealed that 35% complained of pain in the TMJ or muscles of mastication, and/or had discernible clicking. It is also suggested that there is a correlation with deep bite and predisposition for the development of TMD. In this adolescent group, observations concerning horizontal and vertical overlap of the anterior dentition should be viewed with caution, since the growth potential for a large segment of this age range may not have been attained. It should also be noted that Class II occurs to the same extent in both the asymptomatic and symptomatic groups. In the Williamson study, 54% of the symptomatic patients had 50% or greater vertical overlap.

Luther[46] points out that Williamson failed to report the prevalence of open bite, deep bite, and overjet in asymptomatic individuals, making cause and effect relationships "difficult to establish." Brandt[37] found in an evaluation of 1,337 children that 43.6% of the subjects had 4 to 5 mm of horizontal overlap and 24.5% had vertical overlap greater than 6 mm. Excessive vertical overlap reached a peak at ages 11 to 12 and decreased toward the end of the study. Additionally, TMJ dysfunction (sounds, luxation, locking and pain on movement) increased from 5.4% in the 6- to 8-year age group to 15.6% in the 15- to 17-year age group. This suggests that excessive vertical overlap, or deep bite, is normal in the growing pediatric population. Humerfelt[47] demonstrated a decrease in overlap (horizontal and vertical) that was greater in boys than in girls as growth potential was expressed. Björk[48] demonstrated similar findings in a longitudinal study of boys.

Brandt[37] found only weak correlations between TMD (TMJ sounds, TMJ tenderness, muscle tenderness, mandibular opening, pain on movement, patient-reported sounds, headache, tooth grinding) and horizontal overlap (overjet). He also found a weak correlation between TMD and vertical overlap (overbite), with the exception of mandibular opening and tooth grinding. Signs and symptoms of TMD increased with age and were more common in females. TMJ sounds were positively correlated with headache and pain during mandibular movement. Muscle tenderness and headache were positively correlated with pain during mandibular movement. It was also pointed out by Luther that Brandt failed to assess inter- or intra-examiner agreement.[46]

Egermark-Eriksson et al[49] carried out a 4-year longitudinal study on children and adolescents, examining the relationship between occlusal factors and mandibular dysfunction. No strong correlations were demonstrated. However, *weak* correlations were found in the 15-year-old group between Class II occlusion and a large RCP-ICP slide. Nonworking-side interferences were correlated with an anterior open bite as well as several other forms of malocclusion. Unilateral crossbite and horizontal overlap greater than 6 mm were weakly associated with signs and symptoms of TMD.

Nilner[26] found that functional disturbances were related to occlusal interferences and Class II occlusions; however, these relationships were not shown to be statistically significant. de Vis et al[3] studied children 3 to 6 years of age and found that crossbite, open bite, occlusal contacts on lateral excursion, and wear facets did not have a negative impact on function. Pullinger et al[50] found occlusal slides of less than 1 mm to be common in TMD patients and asymptomatic volunteers. The authors state that nonfunctional occlusal contacts were found by several investigators to be prevalent in both orthodontic and control groups 10 years after treatment. Grosfeld and Czarnecka[51] and Jamsa[52] carried out independent studies on children and adolescents and found no correlation between malocclusion and signs and symptoms of TMD in all but the oldest age groups. These results agree with the findings of Brandt,[37] suggesting that signs and symptoms increase with age.

Luther[46] states that "it is important not to equate (even when statistically significant) correlation with cause, even if the correlation coefficient is high." Correlation implies only an association, which is not the same as cause. In fact, in these studies, despite a "statistically significant" association, the correlation coefficients were generally low. In some cases, the malocclusion may be associated solely with nonworking-side interferences, rather than TMD signs/symptoms themselves. There is some evidence that specific types of craniofacial morphology and malocclusion may actually be an effect of TMD as opposed to a cause.

Relationship Between Craniofacial Morphology and Signs and Symptoms of TMD, Including Internal Derangement

The effect of internal derangement of the temporomandibular joint on craniofacial growth and morphology has come under increasing investigation in both the orthodontic and surgical literature. The one common thread running through any theory of growth is that of normality. Normal craniofacial growth and development assumes that there is normal growth potential, normal anatomic relationships, and normal physiologic systems. We have clear examples of what happens to craniofacial morphology when these entities are not present, as demonstrated by congenital craniofacial dysplasias. The normal relationship found in the temporomandibular joint finds the condyles in the glenoid fossa in the most superior position with the central area of the articular disc in contact with the articular surface of the condyles and with the articular eminences (Fig 14-1a). With jaw opening, the mandible rotates and translates anteriorly and inferiorly, with the central part of the disc remaining interposed between the condyle and articular eminence (Fig 14-1b). At maximal opening, the condyle may be positioned inferior and slightly anterior to the anterior band of the disc.[53]

An internal derangement of the TMJ has been defined as an abnormal relationship of the articular disc relative to the mandibular condyle, glenoid fossa, and articular eminence (Fig 14-2a). These may be categorized as disc displacement with and without reduction (Figs 14-2b and 14-3). Disc displacement with reduction is characterized by an anteriorly, medially, or laterally displaced disc that returns to a more normal position with jaw opening. Disc displacement without reduction may have the disc displaced in an anterior, anteromedial, lateral, or medial direction in the closed jaw position. Upon jaw opening, the disc does not return to the normal position on the mandibular condyle and remains displaced through the opening and closing cycles.[53]

From an epidemiologic standpoint, the prevalence of internal derangement in asymptomatic volunteers has been shown to be as high as 34%[7,12,13] and in TMD patients approximately 80% to 85%.[14,53] The prevalence of internal derangement in young adult autopsy specimens was 12%.[54] Kamelchuk et al[55] found that 45% of the 82 temporomandibular joints of asymptomatic adolescent subjects presenting for orthodontic treatment had an internal derangement when studied with MRI. As shown by Roberts et al,[14] the ability to predict the presence and stage of internal derangement by clinical examination has been demonstrated to be about 60%. It is

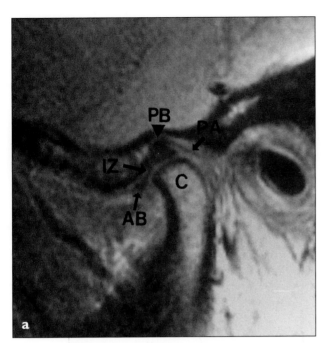 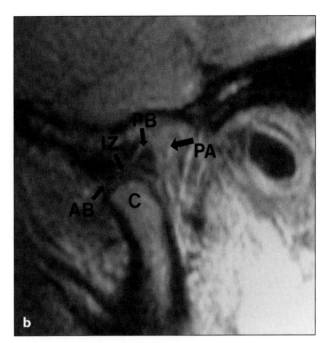

Fig 14-1 Closed and open sagittal magnetic resonance scan and cadaver sections of a temporomandibular joint with normal disc position. *(a)* Closed sagittal scan of a joint with normal disc position. (C = condyle; PA = posterior attachment; PB = posterior band; IZ = intermediate zone; AB = anterior band.) *(b)* Sagittal scan of the joint in Fig 14-1a in the open jaw position. The disc is located between the condyle and articular eminence and has a bow-tie configuration. Note the posterior attachment, posterior band, intermediate zone, and anterior band.

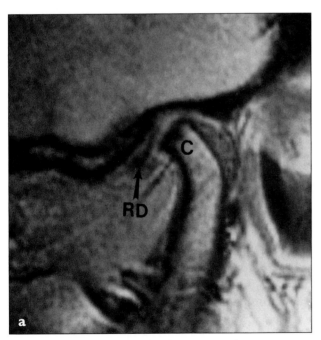 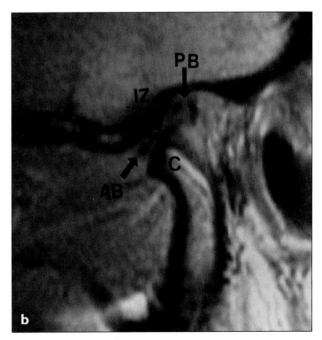

Fig 14-2 Closed and open sagittal magnetic resonance scan and cadaver sections of a temporomandibular joint with a displaced disc with reduction. *(a)* Closed sagittal scan of a joint with disc displacement. There is a remodeled disc (RD) anterior to the condyle. The bow-tie configuration seen in Figs 14-1a and 14-1b is not present. *(b)* Sagittal scan of the joint in Fig 14-2a in the open jaw position. Note that the disc is interposed between the condyle and articular eminence, similar to the scan in Fig 14-1b. This represents disc displacement with reduction. (PB = posterior band; IZ = intermediate zone; AB = anterior band.)

easy to surmise that many practitioners are treating patients with undiagnosed internal derangements of the TMJ.

There are opposing views as to the contribution of internal derangements to TMD. Hellsing and Holmlund[56] suggest that internal derangement is an anatomic variant. Mills et al[57] have studied partial displacements in rabbits. Morphological changes in the disc and posterior attachment were found to be similar to findings in humans. Dworkin and Massoth[58] suggest that patient complaints are not correlated with the degree of pathology. Disease is defined as an "objective biologic event" that involves disruption of specific body structures or organ systems caused by pathologic, anatomic, or physiologic changes. Internal derangement is often associated with anatomic changes in the articular disc, articular eminence, and mandibular condyle. Changes frequently occur in mandibular movement and function; when this represents a pathologic event or becomes painful is uncertain. Schiffman et al[59] have suggested that there is no correlation between the severity of derangement and pain in a sample of TMD patients. This would suggest that a joint with derangement need not be chronic (eg, DJD) to be painful and that the degree of pathology may not be as important as the presence of the derangement. The prevalence of internal derangement is greater in symptomatic patients when compared with asymptomatic volunteers[60,61]; this would suggest that internal derangement has some contribution to mandibular dysfunction, the severity of which does not correlate with pain. The prevalence of occult derangements may represent a risk factor and may be one explanation for why symptoms develop in a patient previously asymptomatic. If derangements are very common in symptomatic patients, it should be no surprise that occult derangements are present prior to treatment or trauma.

Hatala et al[62] evaluated the effect of surgically created unilateral disc displacement on growth changes in the New Zealand white rabbit. Fifteen female rabbits (age 10 weeks) were included in the study. Five experimental rabbits had surgically created anterior disc displacement, five had no surgery, and five controls had sham surgery. The five rabbits that had sham surgery showed no condylar deformity. Linear measurements were not done for these animals; only histologic sections were evaluated for this group. The rabbits were sacrificed at 22 weeks of age and the mandibles were hemisected and radiographed. Cephalograms were digitized and analyzed by conventional methods. The gross appearance showed shortening and flattening of the articulating surface in the experimental group (Fig 14-4). No significant shortening and flattening was found in the control group or on the contralateral side of the experimental animals. These observations suggest that surgically created internal derangement can produce altered growth in the mandible.

Quadan et al[63] used the same methodology to study changes in the cranial base and maxilla. Occlusal radiographs showed that the glenoid fossa on the experimental side was located more anteriorly (Fig 14-5). Oblique radiographs demonstrated that the root of the zygomatic arch on the experimental side was more inferior than the contralateral side. The anterior aspect of the fossa was more inferior on the experimental side as seen on the frontal radiograph. These two studies suggest a deficiency in ramal height and an alteration of the position of the articular fossa, leading to the supposition that disc displacement is capable of producing asymmetry in the developing mandible and cranial base.

In 1966 Boering[64] presented his thesis, *Temporomandibular Joint Arthrosis: A Clinical and Radiological Examination*. Patients were examined for objective symptoms, interviewed for reports of subjective symptoms, examined with lateral cephalometric and transpharyngeal contact radiographs. He concluded that: *(1)* TMJ dysfunction can lead to ramal shortening, and *(2)* it may originate at early ages, even before 17 years.

In 1983 Björk and Skieller[48] evaluated a 25-year longitudinal study on normal and abnormal growth of the mandible. Mandibles that had normal growth showed a forward rotation. Nearly every mandible showing a backward rotation featured some form of condylar problem. Unfortunately, none of these temporomandibular joints was studied with arthrography. It is interesting to note that Björk and Skieller allude to the fact that these mandibles may have an ef-

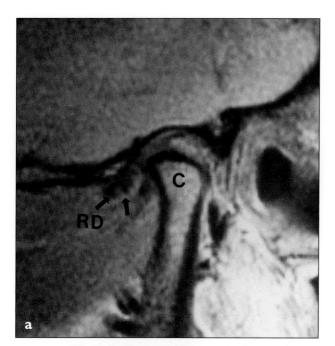
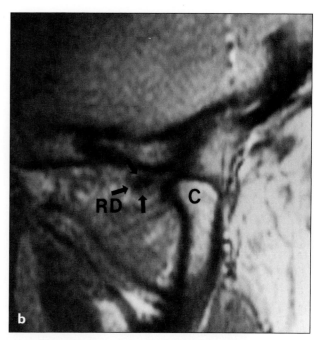

Fig 14-3 Closed and open sagittal magnetic resonance scan and cadaver sections of a temporomandibular joint with a displaced disc without reduction. *(a)* Closed sagittal scan of a joint with disc displacement. There is a remodeled disc (RD) anterior to the condyle. *(b)* Sagittal scan of the joint in open jaw position. Note that the disc is not interposed between the condyle and articular eminence. The disc is deformed and does not have any similarities to the disc in Figs 14-1b or 14-2b in the open jaw position. The remodeled disc (RD) remains anterior to the condyle in the open jaw position.

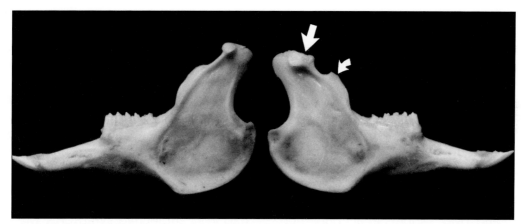

Fig 14-4 Lateral profile of the right and left mandible of an experimental animal. The condyle on the experimental side demonstrates shortening and flattening of the condylar head *(arrow)* and changes in shape of the coronoid process *(arrow)*. Also note the erosion of the articular surface on the anterior aspect of the condylar head.

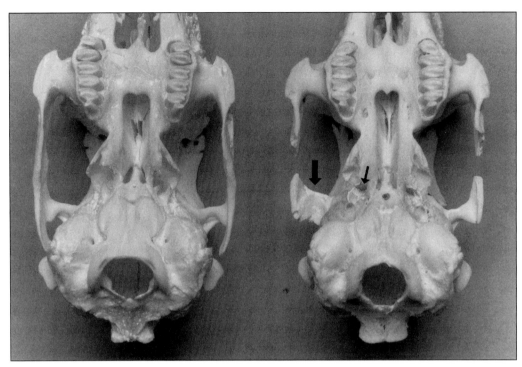

Fig 14-5 Occlusal view of a control *(left)* and experimental animal *(right)*. There has been remodeling of the right temporomandibular joint fossa. Note the anterior position of the anterior limit of the fossa *(large arrow)* compared with the contralateral side and control animal. Also note the anterior position of the right alar foramina on the experimental side compared with the contralateral side *(small arrow)*.

fect on the morphology of other parts of the developing face when they state, "It is not known to what extent maxillary growth is primarily affected ... It is obvious however from the maxillary implants and from the inclination of the anterior surface of the zygomatic process that there was increasing backward rotation of the maxillary corpus, probably secondary to the rotation of the mandibular corpus."

In 1985 two papers[29,65] evaluated craniofacial morphology and TMD. Dibbets et al[65] published a longitudinal study, started in 1969, that included 165 children exhibiting Class I or Class II division 1 or 2 occlusion requiring orthodontic treatment. Lateral and frontal cephalometric radiographs, as well as transpharyngeal radiographs, were taken on all patients. He evaluated the craniofacial morphology of two groups, those who had subjective and/or objective signs and symptoms or radiographic signs of condylar deformity and those who did not. The comparison showed that the group with dysfunction had

an approximately 2.5 mm shorter corpus, 1.3 mm shorter ramus, and a gonial angle that was 2.7 degrees larger. The larger gonial angle did not help offset the diagonal measurement of the mandible, which was still 2.3 mm shorter than the non-dysfunctional group. The posterior face height was 1.9 mm less and the mandibular plane angle was shown to be 2.1 degrees steeper relative to sella-nasion.

Dibbets et al[65] also compared those who had only subjective symptoms with asymptomatic subjects, evaluating deformities as visualized on radiographs. In the children solely with subjective reports of symptoms, the ramus appeared to "lean backward" along with gonial angles that were larger than those seen in normals, which seemed to compensate somewhat for reduced corpus length. Articulare was also seen to occupy a more inferior position. The group exhibiting deformities on radiographs had distinct morphologies, featuring a shorter mandibular corpus, smaller posterior facial height, and a profile that appeared to be more Class II. When these mandibles were studied to assess their growth pattern, it was shown that they were backward-rotating and had formed antegonial notches.

An interesting case study in the form of a pair of female monozygotic twins that presented for orthodontic treatment was reported. Although their faces appeared quite similar in the frontal examination, it was clear that in profile they were dissimilar. Superimposition demonstrated that the upper faces of these girls were quite similar, while the lower faces differed considerably. The twin with the more retrognathic profile had symptoms of TMD combined with radiographic evidence of right condylar deformation.

Dibbets et al[65] showed three distinct morphologic patterns in (1) those with objective symptoms, (2) those with subjective symptoms, and (3) those with radiographic evidence of joint degeneration. He stated that the potential of condylar cartilage to contribute to considerable growth fails in children with arthrosis deformans juvenilis (ADJ), which was the term given to temporomandibular joints that appeared deformed radiographically. The backward-rotating mandible, in an effort to express whatever it can to growth and enlargement of the mandible, starts to grow in a straight line.

Schellhas and Keck[66] presented case reports on 10 patients who had originally presented for consultation for abnormal occlusion and/or cosmetic facial deformity. There was one male and nine females. All patients were studied by clinical exam, TMJ radiography, and either arthrography or MRI. Progressive occlusal deficits, such as asymmetric anterior open bite, bilateral posterior open bite, and developing retrognathia correlated with the radiological observations of condylar destruction, articular surface degeneration, and/or loss of vertical dimension. It should be noted that the MRI findings were not longitudinal in nature and therefore do not correlate with changes over time.

Link and Nickerson[67] examined 39 patients referred for orthognathic surgery. Patients had either Class I open bite or unilateral or bilateral Class II with or without open bite. Patients included were evaluated by arthrography (n = 35)

or presented with clearly deformed condyles (n = 4) with transpharyngeal evaluation. The mean age was 29 years. Condylar morphology was defined by transpharyngeal radiography and labeled as being normal, small, or deformed. All 24 deformed joints evaluated by arthrography had disc displacement without reduction. All condyles with small morphology and 80% of the condyles with normal morphology also had internal derangement. The six patients with mandibular deviation had either small or deformed condyles with internal derangement on the side to which they deviated. The six contralateral joints had normal bony morphology. In the patients with deviation, those who had normal morphology and a normal disc were Class I on the ipsilateral side and Class II on the contralateral side with internal derangement. The three other patients with deviation had bilateral derangement. The more advanced derangement was on the side that demonstrated the greater degree of Class II molar relationship and small or deformed condyle. Of the 30 symmetrical Class II patients (with or without open bite), 43% had bilateral deformed condyles or a combination of deformed and small condyles. All open bite patients and 88% of the patients with Class II malocclusion had bilateral derangements.

The patients with facial deviation offered the greatest support for the hypothesis that disc displacement has a significant influence on the position of the jaws. The mandibular deviation was toward the side with the disc displacement in three patients when the contralateral disc was in a normal position and, in the three patients with bilateral disc displacement, toward the side with the more advanced displacement.

Schellhas et al[68] retrospectively evaluated 100 orthognathic surgery patients with retrognathic facial skeletal morphology, with or without lateral chin displacement and/or open bite. There were 85 females and 15 males aged 11 to 65. All subjects had bilateral TMJ MRI. The author stressed that the skeletal deformities were of primary concern. The imaging studies were performed because of a suspected role of internal derangement in cases of unstable occlusion and facial asymmetry. Patients were divided into stable and unstable groups, based on the presence or absence of changes in their facial contour and/or occlusion in the 24-month period prior to the investigation. However, it should be noted that the groups were based on patient responses to a questionnaire and not on clinical observations over the previous 24-month period. Sixty-one patients denied pain and 45 denied any mechanical TMJ symptoms such as clicking, locking, and masticatory dysfunction in a routine questionnaire. Fifty-eight patients in the study with unstable facial deformity and/or occlusal disturbances exhibited internal derangement of at least one joint were included in the study. The degree of joint degeneration and remodeling directly paralleled the deviation of facial deformity in most cases. Thirty of 42 patients with stable deformities (stability of a deformity was based on patients' self-reports during the prestudy interviews) were found to have internal derangements of at least one temporomandibular joint. When lateral displacement of the chin was evident clinically, this displacement was noted to be uniformly toward the smaller or more degenerated TMJ. Two patients showed an enlarged condyle. In those patients diagnosed with condylar hyperplasia, the chin was deviated away from the enlarged condyle, toward the smaller condyle, which had internal derangement. The authors suggest that skeletal abnormalities such as retrognathia and facial asymmetry, with or without malocclusion, may be the only presenting symptoms of underlying TMJ disease in orthognathic surgery candidates. They cite Nickerson and Moystad[69] in stating that pain-free, non-clicking temporomandibular joints have internal derangement and may contribute to skeletal remodeling.

Schellhas et al[70] studied 128 consecutive children suspected of having intracapsular TMJ disease because of inflammatory, mechanical, or structural symptoms such as retrognathia and mandibular asymmetry. They were retrospectively examined with radiographic and MR imaging. Results showed that the lateral deviation of the chin was always toward the smaller and more degenerated TMJ. MRI findings showed that 112 children exhibited at least one internally deranged joint, and 85 had bilateral derangements. Fifty-six of 60 retrognathic patients were found to have at least one internally de-

ranged TMJ. Advanced stages of TMJ derangement were almost invariably noted in cases of severe retrognathia or lateral asymmetry.

Brand et al[71] compared 23 female volunteers and bilateral normal temporomandibular joints with 24 female TMD patients with various internal derangements, diagnosed with MRI. All patients were adults; no attempt was made to group patients with internal derangements by specific diagnosis, and no patients with degenerative joint disease were included in the study. Each female in the study had lateral cephalometric radiographs taken. There were 24 landmarks used to make 23 angular and 26 linear measurements. The experimental group had significantly shorter linear measurements in the maxilla and mandible. Even through there were some statistically significant differences between the experimental and control groups, the authors concluded that the two groups could not be differentiated using cephalometric analysis.

Stein et al[72] studied 198 consecutive patients from the Temporomandibular Disorders Clinic at the Eastman Dental Center and 80 asymptomatic volunteers. Each subject had had a standard lateral cephalometric radiograph taken and had been studied with bilateral TMJ MRIs. Right and left full profile TMJ laminagraphic radiographs were taken on 128 of the patients and each of the volunteers. After examination, the asymptomatic volunteers were determined to have no subjective or objective symptoms of temporomandibular joint dysfunction. Groups were divided according to MRI diagnosis of their TMJs (normal, internal derangement, degenerative joint disease). Eighty volunteers had bilateral MRI; 33% (n = 26) were found to have internal derangement of the TMJ. Seventy-eight percent (n = 153) of the symptomatic patients were diagnosed as having internal derangement. Groups were also divided by sex due to significant gender differences that became apparent during statistical analysis (Table 14-1, Fig 14-6). Females with bilateral DDN/DJD (disc displacement without reduction and degenerative joint disease) had a shorter S-N (69.5 mm vs 73.4 mm), a shorter Ba-N (106 mm vs 110.4 mm), a more retrusive maxillary (SNA 78.9 degrees vs 83.1 degrees) and mandibular (SNB 75.2 degrees vs 79.6 degrees)

Table 14-1 Female Cephalometric Analysis, Values for Selected Measurements for Bilateral Normal Volunteers, and Patients with Bilateral Degenerative Joint Disease

	Bilateral normal	Bilateral DDN/DJD
Cranial base		
S-N-Ba	131.4	133.3
S-N (mm)	73.4*	69.5*
S-Ba (mm)	47.2	45.6
Ba-N (mm)	110.4*	106.0*
Skeletal pattern		
Maxillary		
Lande's (FH-NA)	91.6	88.4
S-N-A	83.1*	78.9*
ANS-PNS (mm)	54.9	55.1
Mandibular		
FAC-ANG	88.9	86.0
S-N-B	79.6*	75.2*
Mandibular plane	24.5*	30.5*
Y-axis	58.1*	63.1*
Intermaxillary		
NA-APo (convexity)	5.0	5.1
A-B to N-Po (facial plane)	−5.9	−6.6
A-N-B	3.1	3.6
FH-OP (occlusal cant)	5.5*	10.8*
PP-OP	6.3*	11.3*
PP-MP	25.2*	31.0*
PP-FH	−0.8	−0.5
Denture pattern		
Intermaxillary		
Horizontal overlap	3.1*	5.2*
Vertical overlap	2.9	2.1
Vertical relations		
Ar-Go (lower posterior facial height)	47.1*	45.6*

*P < 0.05.

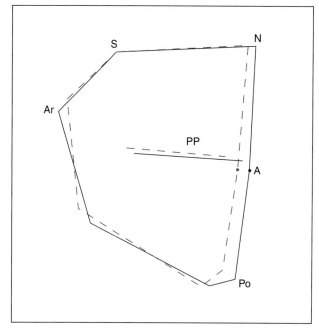

Fig 14-6 Cephalometric polygons constructed for the female control subjects with bilateral normal joints (solid line) and symptomatic patients with disc displacement without reduction and degenerative joint disease (dotted line). The cephalometric polygons were superimposed on the sella-nasion line registered at sella.

denture base, a steeper mandibular plane (30.5 degrees vs 24.5 degrees), a larger Y-axis (63.1 degrees vs 58.1 degrees) and a greater overjet (5.2 mm vs 3.1 mm) when compared to controls. There was a more divergent relationship of palatal plane (PP) to the occlusal plane (OP) (11.3 degrees vs 6.3 degrees), Frankfort horizontal plane (FH) to occlusal plane (10.8 degrees vs 5.5 degrees), and palatal plane to mandibular plane (MP) (31 degrees vs 25.2 degrees). There was also a smaller posterior face height (45.6 mm vs 47.1 mm), giving a retrognathic appearance. Dentally, a second group of

female patients emerged with respect to incisor position. Female patients with bilateral disc displacement with reduction (DDR) had maxillary and mandibular incisors that were less proclined to several reference planes as compared with those found in female volunteers without internal derangement (Table 14-2).

The laminagraphic data showed that there was more mandibular asymmetry in female patients with unilateral internal derangement and DJD than in female volunteers with bilateral normal joints. Furthermore, the data generated from the group with unilateral DJD showed that

Table 14-2 Female Cephalometric Analysis, Values for Selected Measurements for Bilateral Normal Volunteers, and Patients with Bilateral Disc Displacement with Reduction

	Bilateral normal	Bilateral DDR
Denture pattern		
Maxillary		
UI-SN	102.0*	94.8*
UI-FH	110.7*	105.3*
UI-PP	109.9*	104.2*
UI-APo (deg)	24.7*	19.7*
UI-APo (mm)	7.5	6.5
Mandibular		
LI-MP	6.6*	2.1*
LI-OP	25.5	22.1
LI-APo (deg)	27.0*	22.1*
LI-APo (mm)	4.2*	2.8*
Intermaxillary		
Interincisal angle	128.0*	137.3*

*$P < 0.05$.

Table 14-3 Laminagraphic Measurements for Mean Side-to-Side Differences for Female Bilateral Normal Volunteers and Bilateral DDN/DJD Patients

	Bilateral normal	Unilateral DDN/DJD
Ramus	1.5*	4.6*
Effective length	2.1*	5.2*
Body	2.5	1.9

*$P < 0.05$.

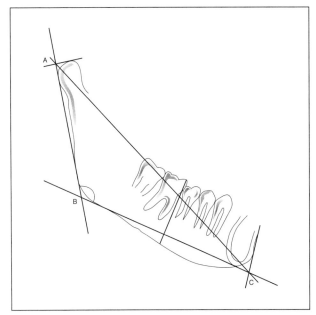

Fig 14-7 Laminagraphic measurements: mandibular ramus length (A-B), body length (B-C), and effective length (A-C).

the side with joint degeneration was asymmetric (shorter ramus) when compared with the side without DJD and that the differences can be traced to the mandibular ramus, body, effective length, and gonial angle. Much of the significant deviation in skeletal form was limited to the mandible and its relation to other craniofacial structures. There was also some suggestion that patients affected by more severe forms of unilateral internal derangement show greater side-to-side differences (4.6 mm vs 1.5 mm for ramus height and 5.2 mm vs 2.1 mm for effective length) for mandibular measurements than other groups of subjects (Table 14-3, Fig 14-7).

Nebbe et al[73] conducted a pilot study comparing the craniofacial morphology of 25 preorthodontic patients with age- and sex-matched normals from the Craniofacial Growth Series. The preorthodontic patients were studied with MRI to assess disc position. Results showed that internal derangement in adolescents may be associated with reduced ramal and posterior face height, reduced maxillary molar dentoalveolar height, clockwise rotation of the palatal and mandibular planes, and a more anterior direction of maxillary development.

These previously presented studies suggest a link between TMJ internal derangement and craniofacial dysmorphology. Longitudinal prospective studies are needed to elucidate the relationship of internal derangement and its effect, if any, on craniofacial growth.

Early Orthodontic Treatment and TMD: Appropriate Treatment Modalities

Of necessity, the relationship between early orthodontic treatment and signs and symptoms of TMD at this time is extrapolated from studies in older populations. Early orthodontics is often undertaken to correct skeletal and asymmetry problems, provide room for permanent teeth, and correct destructive functional habits. The necessity of early treatment to prevent future TMJ problems, however, is more difficult to prove because no particular occlusal scheme has been shown to prophylactically prevent signs and symptoms of TMD. Posterior unilateral crossbite is the one problem that seems to merit special consideration. One reviewer points to the findings of Pullinger et al,[50] which showed a potential link between unilateral crossbite and TMJ internal derangement.[11] This study suggested that some children's temporomandibular joints may not be able to adapt to the functional shift that often goes along with unilateral crossbite. This may result in internal derangement; it is the authors' opinion that the correction of this particular problem early in life may be the one case type that could benefit from orthodontic correction to help prevent TMJ internal derangement. A longitudinal, well-controlled study is needed to confirm this hypothesis.

A retrospective study by Sadowsky and Polson[74] compared patients treated orthodontically at least 10 years previously at the University of Illinois and at the Eastman Dental Center, with a nontreated sample. There were no statistically significant differences between the treatment and control groups for signs and symptoms of TMD. Three exhaustive reviews of the literature examining orthodontics and signs and symptoms of TMD have concluded that orthodontic treatment (including fixed, functional, orthopedic, extraction, and nonextraction treatment) does not cause or prevent the development of TMJ signs or symptoms.[1,2,11] These reviews concluded that orthodontic treatment does not lead to posterior condylar positioning incident to retraction of anterior teeth or to an increase in centric discrepancies between intercuspal and retruded contact position, when compared with control groups.[74–88] More conclusive data may be generated by ongoing prospective studies comparing two-phase orthodontic treatment with one-phase treatment. The generation of data on TMJ signs, symptoms, and function may help to analyze any effect early orthodontic treatment may have on the temporomandibular joints of growing patients.

Treatment of child and adolescent patients presenting with complaints of TMJ pain either before or during early orthodontic treatment is complicated by the fact that they are growing during treatment. There are no studies that have analyzed how different TMD treatment modalities affect pain, dysfunction, or early orthodontic treatment in children. Most authors have stressed conservative, reversible methods to help alleviate pain. It is difficult to find studies examining specific TMJ signs or symptoms to determine which, if any, need to be treated. Even though most epidemiologic studies survey many different signs and symptoms of TMD, the one that seems to get the vast majority of attention is pain. The American Academy of Pediatric Dentistry recommended simple, conservative, and reversible treatment in its 1990 position paper.[15] This opinion is in agreement with Ingerslev[16] and Skeppar et al,[22] who used various hard and soft flat plane splints in their studies to bring relief to children and young adults complaining of TMD.

Summary

Signs and symptoms of TMD are common in adolescent subjects. Symptoms seem to increase with age; however, by and large the majority do not require active treatment. Dental occlusal factors seem to have some correlation with signs and symptoms, but may be a result of joint remodeling rather than a single etiologic factor. No particular occlusal scheme has been demonstrated to prevent or cause TMD. There seems to be a relationship between craniofacial dysmorphology and the presence of temporomandibular joint internal derangement (DJD, arthrosis, regressive remodeling, arthrosis juvenilis deformans). The literature suggests that orthodontic treatment neither causes nor cures TMD. The adolescent symptomatic patient is best treated with simple, conservative, and reversible treatment in agreement with the American Academy of Pediatric Dentistry.

References

1. Luther F. Orthodontics and the temporomandibular joint: Where are we now? I: Orthodontic treatment and temporomandibular disorders. Angle Orthod 1998;68:295–304.
2. Mintz S. Craniomandibular dysfunction in children and adolescents: A review. J Craniomandibular Pract 1993;11:224–231.
3. de Vis H, De Boever JA, van Cauwenberghe P. Epidemiologic survey of functional conditions of the masticatory system in Belgian children aged 3-6 years. Community Dent Oral Epidemiol 1984;12:203–207.
4. Magnusson T, Egermark-Eriksson I, Carlsson GE. Four year longitudinal study of mandibular dysfunction in children. Community Dent Oral Epidemiol 1984;13:117–120.
5. Katzberg RW, Tallents RH, Hayakawa K, Miller, Goske MJ, Wood BP. Internal derangements of the temporomandibular joint: Findings in a pediatric age group. Radiol 1985;154:125–127.
6. Sanchez-Woodworth R, Katzberg RW, Tallents RH, Guay JA. Radiographic assessment of temporomandibular joint pain and dysfunction in the pediatric age group. J Dent Child 1988;55:278–281.
7. Ribeiro RF, Tallents RH, Katzberg RW, Murphy WC, Moss ME, Magalhaes AC, Tavano O. The prevalence of disc displacement in symptomatic and asymptomatic volunteers aged 6 to 25 years. J Orofac Pain 1997;11:37–47.
8. Agerberg G, Bergenholtz A. Craniomandibular disorders in adult population of West Bothnia, Sweden. Acta Odontol Scand 1989;47:129–140.
9. Salonen L, Hellden L, Carlsson GE. Prevalence of signs and symptoms of dysfunction in the masticatory system: An epidemiologic study in an adult Swedish population. J Craniomandib Disord Facial Oral Pain 1990;4:241–250.
10. Egermark-Eriksson I, Carlsson GE, Magnusson T. A long-term epidemiologic study of the relationship between occlusal factors and mandibular dysfunction in children and adolescents. J Dent Res 1987;67:67–71.
11. McNamara JA Jr. Orthodontic treatment and temporomandibular disorders. Oral Surg Oral Med Oral Pathol Oral Radiol Endod 1997;83:107–117.
12. Westesson PL, Eriksson L, Kurita K. Prevalence of disc displacement in symptom-free normal volunteers. Abstract, presented at the Farrar-Norgaard Society meeting, Rochester, NY, August 1989.
13. Kirkos LT, Ortendahl DA, Mark AS, Arakawa M. Magnetic resonance imaging of the TMJ disc in asymptomatic volunteers. J Oral Maxillofac Surg 1987;45:852–854.
14. Roberts CA, Katzberg RW, Tallents RH, Espeland MA, Handelman SL. Correlation of clinical parameters to the arthrographic depiction of TMJ internal derangement. Oral Surg Oral Med Oral Pathol 1988;66:32–36.
15. American Academy of Pediatric Dentistry. Treatment of temporomandibular disorders in children: Summary statements and recommendations. J Am Dent Assoc 1990;120:265–269.
16. Ingerslev H. Functional disturbances of the masticatory system in school children. J Dent Child 1983;50:445–450.
17. Rugh JD, Solberg WK. Oral health status in the United States, temporomandibular disorders. J Dent Educ 1985;49:398–404.
18. Schiffman EL, Fricton JR, Haley D, Shapiro BL. The prevalence and treatment needs of subjects with temporomandibular disorders. J Am Dent Assoc 1990;120:295–303.
19. Okeson JP. Temporomandibular disorders in children. Pediatr Dent 1989;11:326.
20. Wanman A, Agerberg G. Etiology of craniomandibular disorders: Evaluation of some occlusal and psychosocial factors in 19-year-olds. J Craniomandib Disord Facial Oral Pain 1991;5:35–44.
21. Ohno H, Morinush T, Ohno K, Ogur A. Comparative subjective evaluation and prevalence study of TMJ dysfunction in Japanese adolescents based on clinical examination. Community Dent Oral Epidemiol 1988;16:122–126.
22. Skeppar J, Nilner M. Treatment of craniomandibular disorders in children and young adults. J Orofac Pain 1993;7:362–369.
23. Kononen M, Nystrom M, Kleemola-Kujala E, Evalaht M, Laine P, Peck L. Signs and symptoms of craniomandibular disorders in a series of Finnish children. Acta Odontol Scand 1987;2:109–114.
24. Deng Y, Fu M, Hagg U. Prevalence of temporomandibular joint dysfunction (TMJD) in Chinese children and adolescents: A cross-sectional epidemiological study. Eur J Orthod 1995;17:305–309.
25. Gordfeld O, Jackowska M, Czarnecka B. Results of epidemiological examinations of the temporomandibular joint in adolescents and young adults. J Oral Rehabil 1985;12:95–105.

26. Nilner M. Prevalence of functional disturbances and diseases of stomatognathic system in 15-18 year olds. Swed Dent J 1981;5:189–197.

27. Magnusson T, Egermark-Eriksson I, Carlsson GE. Four year longitudinal study of mandibular dysfunction in children. Community Dent Oral Epidemiol 1985;13: 117–120.

28. Egermark-Eriksson I, Carlsson GE, Ingervall B. Prevalence of mandibular dysfunction and oralfacial parafunction in 7, 11, and 15 year old Swedish children. Eur J Orthod 1981;3:163–172.

29. Dibbets JMH, van der Weele LT. Prevalence of TMJ symptoms and X-ray findings. Eur J Orthod 1989;11: 31–36.

30. Stewart CL, Standish SM. Osteoarthritis of the TMJ in teenage females: Report of cases. J Am Dent Assoc 1983;106:638–640.

31. Tallents RH, Hatala MA, Katzberg RW, Westesson PL, Murphy W, Proskin H. Temporomandibular joint sounds in asymptomatic volunteers. J Prosthet Dent 1993;69: 298–304.

32. Wanaman A, Agerberg G. Mandibular dysfunction in adolescents, I: Prevalence of symptoms. Acta Odontol Scand 1986;44:47–54.

33. Tallents RH, Catania J, Sommers E. Temporomandibular joint findings in pediatric populations and young adults: A critical review. Angle Orthod 1991;61:7–16.

34. Williamson E. Temporomandibular dysfunction in pretreatment adolescent patients. Am J Orthod 1977;72: 429–433.

35. Gazit E, Lieberman M, Eini R, Hirsh N, Serfaty V, Fuchs C, Lilos P. Prevalence of mandibular dysfunction in 10–18 year old Israeli school children. J Oral Rehabil 1984;11:307–317.

36. Solberg WK, Woo MW, Houston JB. Prevalence of mandibular dysfunction in young adults. J Am Dent Assoc 1979;98:25–34.

37. Brandt D. Temporomandibular disorders and their association with morphologic malocclusion in children. In: Carlson DS, McNamara JA Jr, Ribbens KA (eds). Development Aspects of Temporomandibular Joint Disorders, monograph 16, Craniofacial Growth Series. Ann Arbor: Univ of Michigan, 1985.

38. Mohlin B, Kopp S. A clinical study on the relationship between malocclusions, occlusal interferences and mandibular pain and dysfunction. Swed Dent J 1978;2: 105–112.

39. Mohlin B, Ingervall B, Thilander B. Relation between malocclusion and mandibular dysfunction in Swedish men. Eur J Orthod 1980;2:229–238.

40. Mohlin B, Thilander B. The importance of the relationship between malocclusion and mandibular dysfunction and some clinical applications in adults. Eur J Orthod 1984;6:192–204.

41. Jamsa T, Kirveskari P, Alanen P. Malocclusion and its association with clinical signs of craniomandibular disorder in 5, 10, and 15 year old children in Finland. Proc Finn Dent Soc 1988;84:235–240.

42. Motegi E, Miyazaki H, Ogura I, Konishi H, Sebata M. An orthodontic study of temporomandibular joint disorders, Part 1: Epidemiological research in Japanese 6–18 year olds. Angle Orthod 1992;62:249–255.

43. Keeling SD, McGorray S, Wheeler TT, King GJ. Risk factors associated with temporomandibular joint sounds in children 6 to 12 years of age. Am J Orthod Dentofac Orthop 1994;105:279–287.

44. Riolo ML, Brandt D, TenHave MPH. Associations between occlusal characteristics and signs and symptoms of TMJ dysfunction in children and young adults. Am J Orthod Dentofac Orthop 1987;92:467–477.

45. de Boever JA, van den Berghe L. Longitudinal study of functional conditions in the masticatory system in Flemish children. Community Dent Oral Epidemiol 1987;15: 100–103.

46. Luther F. Orthodontics and the temporomandibular joint: Where are we now? Part 2. Functional occlusion, malocclusion, and TMD. Angle Orthod 1998;68: 305–318.

47. Humerfelt A, Slagsvold O. Changes in occlusion and craniofacial pattern between 11 and 25 years of age. Trans Eur Soc Orthod 1972;2:113–122.

48. Björk A, Skieller V. Normal and abnormal growth of the mandible. A synthesis of longitudinal cephalometric implant studies over a period of 25 years. Eur J Orthod 1983;5:1–46.

49. Egermark-Eriksson I, Carlsson GE, Magnusson T, Thilander B. A longitudinal study on malocclusion in relation to signs and symptoms of cranio-mandibular disorders in children and adolescents. Eur J Orthod 1990;12: 399–407.

50. Pullinger AG, Solberg WK, Hollender L, Petersson A. Relationship of mandibular condylar position to dental occlusion factors in an asymptomatic population. Am J Orthod Dentofac Orthop 1987;91:201–206.

51. Grosfeld O, Czarnecka B. Musculo-articular disorders of the stomatognathic system in school children examined according to clinical criteria. J Oral Rehabil 1977;4: 193–200.

52. Jamsa T. Malocclusion and its association with clinical signs of craniomandibular disorders in 5-10-15 year old children in Finland. Proc Finn Dent Soc 1988;4: 235–240.

53. Paesani D, Westesson PL, Hatala M, Tallents RH, Kurita K. Prevalence of temporomandibular joint internal derangement in patients with craniomandibular disorders. Am J Orthod Dentofac Orthop 1992;101:41–47.

54. Solberg WK, Hansson TL, Nordstrom B. The temporomandibular joint in young adults at autopsy: A morphologic classification and evaluation. J Oral Rehabil 1985; 12:303–321.

55. Kamelchuk L, Nebbe B, Major P. Adolescent TMJ tomography and magnetic imaging: A comparative analysis. J Orofac Pain 1997;11:321–327.

56. Hellsing G, Holmlund A. Development of anterior disc displacement in the temporomandibular joint: An autopsy study. J Prosthet Dent 1985;53:397–401.

57. Mills DK, Daniel JC, Herzog S, Scapino RP. An animal model for studying mechanisms in human temporomandibular joint disc displacement. J Oral Maxillofac Surg 1994;52:1279–1292.

58. Dworkin SF, Massoth DL. Temporomandibular joint disorders and chronic pain. Disease or illness. J Prosthet Dent 1994;72:29–38.

59. Schiffman EL, Anderson GC, Fricton JR, Lindgren BR. The relationship between level of mandibular pain and dysfunction and stage of temporomandibular joint internal derangement. J Dent Res 1992;71:1812–1815.

60. Tallents RH, Katzberg RW, Murphy WC, Proskin H. Magnetic resonance imaging findings in asymptomatic volunteers and symptomatic TMD patients. J Prosthet Dent 1996;75:529–533.

61. Katzberg RW, Westesson PL, Tallents RH, Drake CM. Orthodontics and temporomandibular joint disorders. Am J Orthod Dentofac Orthod 1996;109:515–520.

62. Hatala MP, Macher DJ, Tallents RH, Spoon M, Subtelny JD, Kyrkanides S. Effect of a surgically created disk displacement on mandibular symmetry in the growing rabbit. Oral Surg Oral Med Oral Pathol Oral Radiol Endod 1996;82:625–633.

63. Qadan S, Macher DJ, Tallents RH, Kyrkanides S, Moss ME. The Effect of Surgically Induced Anterior Disc Displacement of the Temporomandibular Joint on the Midface and Cranial Base [senior research]. Rochester, NY: Eastman Dental Center, 1998.

64. Boering G. Arthrosis Deforman van Het Kaakgewrict. Leiden, The Netherlands: Stafleu en Tholen, 1966.

65. Dibbets JMH, Van Der Weele, Uildriks AKJ. Symptoms of TMJ dysfunction: Indicators of growth patterns? J Pedod 1985;7:265–284.

66. Schellhas KP, Keck RJ. Disorders of skeletal occlusion and temporomandibular joint disease. Northwest Dent 1989;68:35–39.

67. Link JJ, Nickerson JW. Temporomandibular joint internal derangements in an orthognathic surgery population. Int J Adult Orthodon Orthognath Surg 1992;7:161–169.

68. Schellhas KP, Piper MA, Bessette RW, Wilkes CH. Mandibular retrusion, temporomandibular joint derangement, and orthognathic surgery planning. Plast Reconstr Surg 1992;90:218–232.

69. Nickerson JW, Moystad A. Observations on individuals with radiographic bilateral condylar remodeling. J Cranio Mand Pract 1982;1:20–37.

70. Schellhas KP, Pollei SR, Wilkes CH. Pediatric internal derangements of the temporomandibular joint: Effect on facial development. Am J Orthod Dentofac Orthop 1993;104:51–59.

71. Brand JW, Nielson KJ, Tallents RH, Nanda RS, Currier GF, Owen WL. Lateral cephalometric analysis of skeletal patterns in patients with and without internal derangement of the temporomandibular joint. Am J Orthod Dentofac Orthop 1995;107:121–128.

72. Stein S, et al. A Comparison of the Craniofacial Morphology of Asymptomatic Volunteers and TMD Patients [senior research]. Rochester, NY: Eastman Dental Center, 1995.

73. Nebbe B, Major PW, Prasad NG, Grace M, Kamelchuk LS. TMJ internal derangement and adolescent craniofacial morphology: A pilot study. Angle Orthod 1997;67:407–414.

74. Sadowsky C, Polson AM. Temporomandibular disorders and functional occlusion after orthodontic treatment: results of two long-term studies. Am J Orthod 1984;86:386–390.

75. Larrson E, Ronnerman A. Mandibular dysfunction symptoms in orthodontically treated patients ten years after completion of treatment. Eur J Orthod 1981;3:89–94.

76. Janson M, Hasund A. Functional problems in orthodontic patients out of retention. Eur J Orthod 1981;3:173–178.

77. Dibbets J, van der Weele L. Orthodontic treatment in relation to symptoms attributed to dysfunction of the temporomandibular joint. Am J Orthod Dentofac Orthop 1987;81:193–199.

78. Sadowsky C, BeGole E. Long term status of temporomandibular joint function and functional occlusion after orthodontic treatment. Am J Orthod 1980;78:201–212.

79. Dahl BL, Krogstad BS, Ogaard B, Eckersberg T. Signs and symptoms of craniomandibular disorders in two groups of 19 year-olds, one treated orthodontically and the other not. Acta Odontol Scand 1988;46:89–93.

80. Dibbets JMH, van der Wheele LTh. Prevalence of TMJ symptoms and X-ray findings. Eur J Orthod 1989;11:31–36.

81. Dibbets JMH, van der Wheele LTh. Extraction, orthodontic treatment, and craniomandibular dysfunction. Am J Orthod Dentofac Orthop 1991;99:210–219.

82. Dibbets JMH, van der Wheele LTh. Long-term effects of orthodontic treatment, including extraction, on findings and symptoms attributed to CMD. Eur J Orthod 1992;14:16–20.

83. Kess K, Bakopoulos K, Witt E. TMJ function with and without orthodontic treatment. Eur J Orthod 1991;13:192–196.

84. Hirata RH, Heft MW, Hernandez B, King GJ. Longitudinal study of findings of temporomandibular disorders (TMD) in orthodontically treated and nontreated groups. Am J Orthod Dentofac Orthop 1992;101:35–40.

85. Egermark I, Thilander B. Craniomandibular disorders with special reference to orthodontic treatment: An evaluation from childhood to adulthood. Am J Orthod Dentofac Orthop 1992;101:28–34.

86. Kremenak CR, Kinser DD, Harman HA, Menard CC, Jakobsen JR. Orthodontic risk factors for temporomandibular disorders (TMD). I: Premolar extractions. Am J Orthod Dentofac Orthop 1992;101:13–20.

87. Rendell JK, Norton LA, Gay T. Orthodontic treatment and temporomandibular joint disorders. Am J Orthod Dentofac Orthop 1992;101:84–87.

88. Dibbets JMH. Juvenile Temporomandibular Joint Dysfunction and Craniofacial Growth: A Statistical Analysis. Leiden, The Netherlands: Stafleu and Tholen, 1977:1–112.

Chapter 15

Other Considerations Relative to Early Orthodontic Treatment: Concluding Observations

Facial Appearance and Self-Image

Physical appearance is generally recognized to be an important parameter in individuals' self-esteem, in their behavioral patterns, and in their success in personal interactions. It is generally acknowledged that personal interactions with others, as well as self-image, can be influenced by facial esthetics. When we meet someone, it is usual to first glance at the face, then generally to the rest of the person, and subsequently to return to the face—a face that is clearly visible as well as a center of speech communication.[1] Both children and adults have been shown to gaze longer at a face they consider attractive than at an unattractive face.[2] This bias seems apparent even in preschool children where the most popular children among their peers seem to be the more attractive ones in the group,[3] although facial body image may not emerge until a child is 4 or 5 years of age.[4] In the earlier developing years, much vacillation seems to occur, as youngsters test the environment, seeking reaffirmation and approval. Preadolescence and adolescence are fragile transitional stages in emotional development—stages that are very difficult to deal with, and yet ones that are extremely important to deal with effectively. These young ages seem to be ones of rebellion, and yet a period of time when a need to conform and to be just like all other youngsters is evi-

dent; self-image and self-evaluation are very important. With this as the focus of attention, some highlights from a study could be briefly, but perhaps profitably, reviewed. It was a study[5] designed to evaluate the impact of a handicap on the personality of near-adolescent individuals. Two groups of children, 10 and 11 years of age, were studied; one group was handicapped and the other was not. They were children from different states and of differing social and cultural backgrounds. They were studied over a 2-year period while attending summer camps or public schools. They were shown series of drawings of children, some with visible handicaps and some with no visible physical handicap. The drawings were randomized according to all the precepts necessary for a controlled study. The drawings were placed in front of the children, who were asked to pick out the picture in order of their personal preference. Based on six drawings, there were six preference levels, basically from most preferred to least preferred.

Some very significant as well as revealing findings emerged from this study. From the ranked choices and verbal expressions of these children, a very definite pattern of feelings seemed to evolve. First, the nonhandicapped child was clearly preferred to a handicapped child. Second, a marked uniformity became apparent in the preference order for the different handicapping disabilities as expressed by both the handicapped and the nonhandicapped children. Of course, the nonhandicapped child was ranked highest; the child with a leg brace and crutches was ranked second in order of preference, the child in a wheelchair with a blanket covering both legs was ranked third, the child with a missing left hand was ranked fourth, and the child with a "facial disfigurement on the left side of the mouth" was ranked fifth, or next to last, in preference, followed only by an obese child. In the author's interpretation, the orthopedically handicapped child in a wheelchair had a great functional disability, yet all the children preferred a severe functional handicap to a difference in facial appearance. The impact of facial disfigurement was just as difficult to accept for the child who had the disfigurement as it was for the child who had none. The implication to be derived from this is one that does not allow us to depreciate the value of acceptable facial appearance and cosmetic revision for young children. In fact, procedures for improvement in appearance might well be encouraged for many preadolescents and adolescents; the potential impact on psychosocial health should be thoughtfully considered.

What is being suggested is that a strong focus be aimed at consideration of treatment at young age levels in the correction of visible facial discrepancies to provide the psychosocial and emotional support that may be needed at these ages. The conclusion is also drawn that the face is very important in forming an opinion of another person. Studies seem to indicate that the eye has a tendency to focus and periodically refocus on another's face. Craniofacial malformations, inclusive of more than moderate jaw malocclusions, can affect attractiveness as perceived by others. As a consequence, physical attractiveness or lack of it can affect self-image and the development of adequate interpersonal relationships. Any facial deformity appears to have a direct bearing upon personality structure and attitudes toward one's self, one's appearance, and one's behavior. A poor self-image may not result from malocclusion or craniofacial malformation alone, but also may be a function of our society, which sometimes attaches a stigma to those who are different. Individuals with facial dysconfiguration may receive a nega-

tive social message, and the result may be self-devaluation.

One can postulate that an individual's facial appearance is an important factor in his or her interactions with society. It can affect how society reacts to that person, as well as how the individual perceives his or her acceptance within the social structure. Being born with a serious craniofacial anomaly may make it more difficult for a child to adapt to his or her environment. A common example of an individual with such a developmental anomaly is the child born with extensive facial clefts or severe hemifacial microsomia. The psychosocial impact on the child may produce negative sequelae that may affect him or her to as great an extent as those produced by the physical deformation itself. For example, in a revealing study,[6] investigators presented colored slides of three noncleft children and six children with clefts to a large group of second, third, and fourth grade students. The students were asked to rate each slide on 15 semantic differential variables such as boring, stupid, sad, dirty, mean, and bad. The children with clefts were rated more negatively on all the objective scales employed. In addition, the children with bilateral clefts received greater negative ratings associated with physical or psychosocial attributes than did the unilateral cleft lip group. These data suggest that children may hold a "what is facially disfigured or deformed is bad" stereotype. In another study,[7] photographic slides of children with cleft lip and palate were presented to four different age groups (8 to 16 years). Individuals with unilateral or bilateral cleft lip and palate were depicted as they actually appeared, and the photos were also retouched to remove scarring and nasal deformity. The raters responded to questions about friendliness, popularity, intelligence, attractiveness, and how likely they would be to choose this person as a friend. The results indicated that the deformed faces were rated more negatively than the retouched faces. Ratings of facial deformity were not significantly related to either age or gender of the raters; however, female faces were rated more negatively than male faces. Similar findings were noted in a study where a facial birth defect was solely evident, but variance in dentofacial configurations were presented. In this study,[8] portrait photographs of an attractive boy and girl and an unattractive boy and girl were modified so that, for each face, five different photographic versions were available. In each version, the child's face was standardized, except that a different dentofacial arrangement was demonstrated. These were: normal incisors, prominent incisors, missing maxillary lateral incisors, severely crowded incisors, and unilateral cleft lip. Each photograph was viewed by a different group of 42 children and 42 adults. Their impressions of each depicted child's social attractiveness were recorded. The central hypothesis that photographs of children with normal dental appearance will be judged to be better looking, more desirable as friends, more intelligent, and less likely to behave aggressively was clearly upheld.

Several significant considerations could be gleaned from the aforementioned investigations. Concern for physical attractiveness (specifically, facial attractiveness) seems to begin relatively early in childhood; the finding of low self-esteem could be manifested as early as 7 years of age. There may be a relationship between the degree of facial disfiguration, or deviation from accepted norms, and the child's adjustment level. From this, an implication can be drawn for the need—or at least the desirability—of early treatment. This, of course, may be more true for the congenital facial defect.

Our levels of clinical success have improved tremendously over the years and our focus of attention is clearly shifting toward further refinement in clinical correction. Clinicians need no longer be concerned with the *how* and *whether;* facial disfigurement should be treated orthodontically. Within the precepts of this book, it seems that a focus of attention should progress rapidly toward how ideal a result can be achieved at as early an age as possible. Unquestionably, the more ideal the improvement, the more the potentially adverse problems stemming from any facial disfiguration might be avoided at any age.

Finally, over the past years many changes have taken place in the focus of attention as well as in the corrective procedures for unharmonious jaw malocclusions. However, the primary objectives in the treatment of individuals with these jaw disharmonies have not changed. Every change and procedure is still being directed toward attaining an adequate and desirable result: that of providing for the many needs of young individuals so that they may mature into well-adjusted, contributing members of society. To accomplish this objective, it is necessary for all procedures to be directed toward making an individual look as normal as possible, toward permitting that individual to function as normally as possible, and toward helping that young individual to feel as normal as possible. This focus of attention must not ever change.

References

1. McGregor FC. Social and psychological implications of dentofacial disfigurement. Angle Orthod 1970;40:231–233.
2. Dion KK. The incentive value of physical attractiveness for young children. J Pers Soc Psychol Bull 1977;3:67–70.
3. Dion KK. What is beautiful is good. J Pers Soc Psychol Bull 1972;24:285–290.
4. Knorr NJ, Hoopes JE, Edgerton MT. Psychiatric-surgical approach to adolescent disturbance in self image. Plast Reconstr Surg 1968;41:248–253.
5. Richardson SA, Goodman N, Hastorf AH, Dornbusch SM. Cultural uniformity in reaction to physical disabilities. Am Sociologic Rev 1961;26:241–247.
6. Schneiderman CR, Harding JB. Social ratings of children with cleft lip by school peers. Cleft Palate J 1985;21:219–223.
7. Tobiasen JM. Social judgments of facial deformity. Cleft Palate J 1987;24:323–327.
8. Shaw WC. The influence of children's dentofacial appearance on their social attractiveness as judged by peers and lay adults. Am J Orthod 1981;79:399–415.

Index